Michael Dooley is a leading consultant gynaecologist and Fellow of the Royal College of Obstetricians and Gynaecologists, with practices in London and Dorset. He has established a pioneering women's health clinic that provides an integrated approach to care.

Sarah Stacey is an award-winning journalist and best-selling author of *Feel Fabulous Forever: The Anti-ageing Health & Beauty Bible*. She is currently Health Editor of the *Mail on Sunday's You* Magazine and a Vice President of the Guild of Health Writers UK.

D0732289

Michael Dooley FRCOG & Sarah Stacey

YOUR CHANGE
YOUR CHOICE

The Integrated Guide to Looking
and Feeling Good Through the
Menopause – and Beyond

HODDER
MOBIUS

Hodder & Stoughton

Copyright © 2004 by Michael Dooley, FRCOG and Sarah Stacey

First published in Great Britain in 2004 by Hodder and Stoughton
A division of Hodder Headline

The right of Michael Dooley and Sarah Stacey to be identified as the Authors of the Work has been asserted by them in accordance with the Copyright, Designs and Patents Act 1988

A Mobius Book

1 3 5 7 9 10 8 6 4 2

A CIP catalogue record for this title is available from the British Library

ISBN 0340828854

Typeset in Sabon by
Palimpsest Book Production Limited,
Polmont, Stirlingshire

Printed and bound by
Clays Ltd, St Ives plc

Hodder Headline's policy is to use papers that are natural, renewable and recyclable products and made from wood grown in sustainable forests. The logging and manufacturing processes are expected to conform to the environmental regulations of the country of origin

Hodder and Stoughton Ltd
A division of Hodder Headline
338 Euston Road
London NW1 3BH

Dedication

To Michael's wife Barbara for her patience and guidance

To Sarah's horse Keats and cats William and Fred
for keeping her more or less sane when there were
just too many hormones

Acknowledgements

We're hugely grateful to everyone who has helped with this book. To Michael's patients and Sarah's friends for sharing their experiences and tips. To many scientists and other experts worldwide for their generous help and advice, particularly: consultant rheumatologist Dr Tom Palferman, GP and flower remedies practitioner Dr Andrew Tresidder, GP Dr Karen Kirkham, integrated medicine practitioner Dr Mosaraf Ali, nutritionists Gillian Hamer and Kathryn Marsden, naturopath Roderick Lane, medical herbalist Andrew Chevallier, bio-energetic medicine practitioner Thomas Marshall-Manifold, women's health expert Marilyn Glenville, yoga teacher Hannah Lovegrove, exercise physiologist David Macutkiewicz, make up artists Jenny Jordan and Barbara Daly, Aveda hair colour guru Ian Black, Geraldine Howard of Aromatherapy Associates, tantric sex expert Val Sampson and alchemical aromatherapist Ixchel Susan Leigh for her menopause cocktail recipe.

To Hilary Boyd, Fiona North, Kate Saunders, Daisy Warner, Felicity Warner and Anne Woodham for their help.

To Michael's assistants, Paula Eastwell and Pat Mcauley, and menopause nurse Lesley Woodward.

To our agent Kay McCauley.

To fashion artist David Downton for his wonderful cover illustration.

To Rowena Webb, Kerry Hood, Jacqui Lewis, Emma Heyworth-Dunn and Helen Coyle at Hodder Mobius, and copy editor Morag Lyall.

Contents

GLOSSARY

A lot of medical words and phrases you'll come across on the menopause journey are quite complex. You'll find a glossary of terms on page 415.

INTRODUCING IMT

**– Integrated Menopausal Therapy –
A new way of thinking about your healthcare**

This chapter covers:
* what makes up IMT
* choosing a practitioner
* integrated healthcare consent form and co-operation card

Since you've picked up this book, it's a good bet that you are approaching or going through the menopause – the change of life. And you're looking for some help: maybe a little, maybe a lot.

You may have irregular periods, hot flushes during the day and sweats at night. You may feel sad for no particular reason, forget where you put things, fret about extra bulges, miss your growing-up children (or be anguished because you never had them), wonder why you ever enjoyed sex (and how long you need contraception) – and where your life is going ... (And that's just for starters.)

Or you may feel absolutely fine and have picked up this book because you want information – about the menopause and about all your options.

This book doesn't only tell you about Hormone Replacement Therapy (HRT) or other drugs (though they're in here, with *all* the latest research), or about natural therapies (though they're in here too). What we're suggesting is a new way of thinking about yourself and your body. We set out a new way of looking at how you organise your healthcare that embraces your mind and spirit as well as your body. It's a new way of being prepared and travelling well through this stage of life – and the rest.

We'd like to start off by asking you to do something that might sound a bit dotty but bear with us!

- take a moment to think about yourself.
- what are you?
- a physical body?
- yes, of course. You feel hungry, thirsty, hot, cold; you sleep, wake, move, talk and so on.
- but you also have thoughts, feelings, desires, instincts ... millions and millions of them every day of your life.
- you are an amazingly wonderful and complex mixture of mind, body and spirit.
- what's more, everything is interconnected and interdependent.
- what happens in your mind and your spirit profoundly affects your body and vice versa.
- feel happy, you'll feel well. Feel healthy, you'll likely feel happy.
- it works the other way too: if you're physically low or in pain, your mood tends to be low – and if you're stressed or depressed, you're much more likely to have health problems.
- so you need to care for yourself on every level. That's the basis of this book.

"The truthful message is that the body changes gear, and so does life. Discomfort can be ameliorated but, for many, navigating the menopause is the grit in the oyster.

*It brings reappraisal of ambition, goals, personal rela-
tionships. Many women testify that, post-Change, life
can and does get better. Those on HRT, of course, will
never know."*

Yvonne Roberts,
The Observer, August, 2003

In the past, doctors approached women going through
the menopause in a 'one size fits all' way – invariably from
a physical perspective. That is wrong. If you think about
your situation, you'll see that your problems fall into several
categories: physical, mental and emotional/psychological.
There is another category, which even comes into scientific
research papers now, and that is the spiritual side of life.
That's why we talk about mind, body and spirit.

By 'spiritual' we don't mean religious – as in Christian,
Muslim, Buddhist and other formal belief systems, although
that may come into it – we mean the side of your life that
inspires you, which gives you those moments of sheer joy and
which makes you think there is a purpose in living, even on
charcoal-grey days and even if you don't know what it is.

Common sense alone says that one magic bullet pill can't
sort every problem. You can think of your life as a big jigsaw
with lots of little scenes going on – all of them interconnecting. You need to get the right bits in the right places
to make the whole. In the same way, you need different and
interconnecting forms of help for the different pieces of your
life – physical, mental, emotional and spiritual. Then you
can see the lovely big picture.

We wrote this book to help the whole of you. It's based
on what's now called 'integrated medicine' or 'integrated
health care'. We call our approach Integrated Menopausal
Therapy – IMT for short.

WHAT IMT MEANS

Integrated Menopausal Therapy offers you a range of choices, both self-help and professional, conventional and traditional, to help you manage your menopause in the way that is best for you and your lifestyle.

To explain a little more. There are two recent buzz words in healthcare. One is 'integrate', the other is 'holistic'. According to the *Oxford English Dictionary*, 'integrate' means 'combine or be combined to form a whole'. 'Holistic' means 'the treating of the whole person rather than just the symptoms of the disease'. In practice, this means using conventional Western (allopathic) medicine and traditional medical systems, plus complementary therapies, to treat the whole person.

> *"Integrated health is the gathering together of all the factors that contribute to your continued wellbeing and balancing them so that you can attain your full potential all of the time."*
>
> Dr Mosaraf Ali, founder of the
> Integrated Medical Centre, London

IMT is built on the following approach:

- **day-to-day wellbeing:** you should aim to be as healthy and feel as happy as you possibly can on a daily basis. You do this by 'controlling the controllables'. That means taking excellent care of the basics of your daily life – the ones you can do something about: eating well and regularly, drinking lots of water, exercising, keeping mentally stimulated, doing things you enjoy, laughing and spending time with people you love. Living like this minimises stress of all kinds and helps you not to worry about the things you can't control. As well as keeping you healthy and happy, it gives you a much better chance of avoiding menopausal symptoms including hot flushes, insomnia and depression, or only having minimal ones.

- **treats and rewards – doing nice things for yourself**: we urge you to add TLC for you to your daily basics; for example, have an aromatherapy bath, give yourself a facial, massage your feet and legs, buy yourself a bunch of flowers, listen to your favourite music. Michael sometimes advises his patients to buy themselves a reward when they've achieved something or when things go well. It doesn't have to be expensive: a trinket from the market is as meaningful as something costly. The important thing is that you see it daily and remember the positive things about your life. Sarah's favourite tip is to keep a Happy Box with lovely letters, inspiring quotes and pictures, and mementoes of happy days: you can keep a rolling pinboard too, reminding yourself of all the good things that are going on.

- **preventing problems**: as well as controlling the controllables, we suggest you take sensible precautions such as regular health checkups and screens, including cervical smears, mammograms and blood pressure checks.

- **treating problems if and when they occur, and preventing more serious ones**: take notice of any symptoms or disease immediately, take self-help measures if appropriate, and/or consult appropriate practitioners.

It is vital that you recognise you are not just a physical machine. Get used to thinking of yourself and your wellbeing in this holistic way and you will understand IMT and how to apply it to your life. Look after your mind, your body and your spirit. Be your own best friend.

SELF-HELP AND PROFESSIONAL HELP

If you look at the IMT approach above, you will see that the goals divide into two categories: what you can do for yourself and treatment from healthcare professionals. Day-to-day wellbeing and treats are largely DIY, whereas you would invariably go to a health professional to prevent and treat problems. There are overlaps of course: you might choose, say, to do yoga with a teacher as well as on your own or go to an aromatherapist for a treat. Equally, looking after your day-to-day wellbeing helps prevent health problems and aids healing if you do get ill. It's a virtuous circle!

YOUR CHOICE

We want you to know that you have choices. It is your life. Think about what you want. This book lays them out so that you can put together your own menu to manage your menopause – and the rest of your life. The combination is flexible. You can pick and mix, add in and take out, at different times as you want or need. You'll see that we have grouped the professional therapies under different headings, including mind, touch, movement and so on. Once you get the idea of looking at the different aspects of yourself and your situation in an integrated way, you will see how you can pick from the menu and mix it to create balance and harmony. You will find that you feel better and better – possibly better than you ever have in your life.

HOW TO CHOOSE

Throughout the book you will find guidelines to help you choose. In some cases, it's very clear: for instance with contraception you're going to go to a conventional doctor not an aromatherapist or psychotherapist. And if you have a bad back, you'll choose from a medical doctor, physiotherapist, osteopath or chiropractor. In others, such as depression, you will need to look at what is really affecting you and build up your own holistic treatment programme, based on our information and suggestions – and of course input from your own health professionals.

You may be surprised by how many options we have listed. Michael's philosophy is that he never wants a patient to come in and say, 'Why didn't you tell me about X?' Of course, there are bound to be ones we don't know about – so do write in or e-mail us (gynaecology@mdooley.co.uk) and tell us what has helped you so we can think about it for the next edition.

BOOST YOUR WELLBEING: MIND, BODY, SPIRIT

Control the controllables:

10 daily basics

- eat fresh wholesome food, three meals a day with snacks between
- never miss breakfast
- have five portions of fruit and veg minimum a day
- drink lots of still pure water, at least eight big glasses daily
- take exercise you enjoy, aim for half an hour or more daily
- get out in the fresh air
- live in the present but plan the days ahead: organise work and play
- take relaxing time for you, 45 minutes or more a day
- be loving and have fun
- don't worry about the things you can't control

Remember: HALT, the tried and tested axiom of many self-help programmes: don't get Hungry, Angry, Lonely or Tired.

Mind, body, spirit connections:

Live your life like this

Mind
- have fun – laugh!
- give yourself treats
- set attainable goals
- be positive
- share meals with friends
- be assertive: think of what you want and ask for it
- learn to say no (nicely) to things you can't really do without getting stressed
- learn something new and interesting
- be creative
- dejunk! Clean a cupboard
- listen to your favourite music, watch your favourite film

Body
- eat well and regularly
- don't miss meals
- choose food you like
- buy fresh, organic, locally grown food wherever possible
- take supplements if necessary

BOOST YOUR WELLBEING: MIND, BODY, SPIRIT

* drink lots of water
* do exercise you enjoy and vary it
* practise breathing exercises and yoga
* have regular medical check-ups and screens
* give yourself some beauty therapy
* massage yourself
* stop smoking
* drink less alcohol
* avoid toxic environments

Spirit
* be loving
* accept love
* hug someone – and yourself
* listen to other people without interrupting
* say what you want to say, straight from your heart
* do something – anything – you really enjoy
* express yourself: dance, sing, paint
* practise meditation and/ or creative visualisation

* light a candle and make a wish
* pray if you choose

DIY therapies for mind, body, spirit wellbeing

(You can do these with professionals, too)

* aromatherapy (see page 200)
* art therapy (paint, draw, splodge!) (see page 214)
* creative visualisation (see page 218)
* dance therapy (turn on the music and move!) (see page 214)
* flower remedies (see page 220)
* hydrotherapy (bath/ shower/swim) (see page 210)
* light therapy (buy a light box) (see page 212)
* massage (see page 207)
* meditation (see page 230)
* music therapy (play your favourite music/sing) (see page 232)

HELP FROM PROFESSIONALS: YOUR CHOICES

You go to a professional because you have a problem that you want help with. Having the problem investigated by your health professional (often your conventional Western doctor) is the first step. Then you can consider your choice of therapy/therapies from an integrated perspective, looking at the range below. You should always choose an appropriately trained and qualified professional in all branches of healthcare who has the expertise to help with your problem. There is a natural overlap with conventional and so-called alternative and complementary therapies in some cases. For instance, some Western doctors integrate some of these therapies into their practice.

Conventional Western (allopathic) medicine
- investigation/diagnosis
- screening
- medical including HRT and other drugs; contraception
- surgery
- physiotherapy
- counselling

Traditional medical therapies
- acupuncture
- ayurveda
- chinese herbal medicine
- homeopathy
- naturopathy
- nutritional therapy
- western herbalism

Manipulative therapies
- chiropractic and McTimoney chiropractic
- osteopathy and cranial osteopathy (the manipulation is almost undetectable)
- physiotherapy

Touch therapies
- acupressure
- aromatherapy
- cranio-sacral therapy
- massage
- reflexology
- reiki

Nature therapies
- hydrotherapy
- light therapy

Movement therapies
- alexander technique
- dance therapy

Psychological/emotional 'mind and spirit' therapies
- art therapy
- bereavement counselling
- biofeedback
- counselling
- creative visualisation
- flower remedies
- healing
- hypnotherapy
- laughter therapy
- life/work coaching
- meditation
- music therapy
- psychotherapy
- radionics

DON'T DO IT ON YOUR OWN

Although we're encouraging you to take charge of your health and your life, you must remember that you're not in it alone. You can and should ask for advice and help and support. This isn't a solo voyage round the globe in a rowing boat (though it might feel like that sometimes). Pick your team carefully from family, friends and healthcare professionals. But remember, they must be people you like and trust. Doesn't matter if it's your oldest friend, most gorgeous George Clooney look-alike beau, or eminent doctor: if they don't make you feel good, move on! Trust your gut feeling.

REMEMBER – YOU'RE A WINNER
(AND A GODDESS. . .)

Winning the game of life is a lot simpler than most of us think it is. And it needn't bust your budget. Control the controllables. Love life and be kind. And if you have a problem, don't get stuck in it – live in the solution. That's how to start. It all flows from there.

Something a tad trivial perhaps: we've noticed an undesirable tendency for books about the menopause to talk about women becoming crones. That word is banned here. In our book, you're all goddesses.

INTEGRATED MEDICINE: THE WAY AHEAD FOR HEALTHCARE

Many people believe that integrated medicine – centred round the individual patient – is the way ahead for healthcare. This isn't new of course: it was the way medicine was practised for centuries and still is in so-called Third World countries. Increasingly, Western doctors are recognising that treating

the physical body alone is not enough and are acknowledging that the mind and spirit need healing too. Indeed
many doctors now practise some form of complementary
therapy and/or refer patients to other practitioners.

The key initiative in the United Kingdom is the Prince of
Wales' Foundation for Integrated Health (FIH). Its principles,
which we've adapted below, are a guide for all integrated
healthcare approaches including IMT.

• healthcare should look after all aspects of a patient's being
  including mind, body and spirit, and take into considera-
  tion their lifestyle, including nutrition, relationships and
  environment.
• it's vital that individuals take more responsibility for their
  own healthcare; this requires teamwork among patients
  and healthcare practitioners.
• integrated healthcare acknowledges the intrinsic healing
  capacity of every person.
• different approaches and interventions may need to be
  combined to restore health and wellbeing.
• healthcare services should be provided by appropriately
  educated, safe, competent and regulated practitioners.
• all therapies should be investigated for safety and effectiveness and their practice regulated.
• everyone should have access to the treatment approach of
  their choice, after investigation and regulation as above.

HOW DO YOU KNOW A TREATMENT IS SAFE AND EFFECTIVE?

As with a lot of things in life, the more you know about
treatments of all kinds, the more questions arise. The whole
question of proving that a drug, herbal medicine, operation
or technique is safe and effective is a minefield. This applies

to both conventional and complementary therapies. In the 1980s, for instance, many doctors felt that every menopausal woman should be given HRT. Now that has changed because of evidence that's emerged since, which we explain in Chapter Five. Equally, many doctors have said loudly in the past that complementary and alternative medicine (CAM) is worthless: that too has changed because the value is, in many cases, evident – although not always proven by scientific evidence.

The common complaint about CAM is there is often little rigorous scientific evidence to support its safety and effectiveness. The key questions about any health procedure are: Does it work? Is it safe? Is there proof? In fact these questions often can't be satisfactorily answered when it comes to conventional medicine, right across the board. Recognising this, a new discipline has emerged called Evidence Based Medicine or EBM, which is now the gold standard for treatment.

EBM is trying to produce as much evidence as possible of what any sort of treatment will do. However, this is far from complete and until then the most important thing you can do is to apply common sense. One of the major difficulties is that the biggest source of funding for scientific trials comes from drug companies and they are, on the whole, unlikely to fund research into complementary therapies. They may not always be the most reliable collaborators, in any case. In September 2001, 13 leading international medical journals, including the *Lancet* in the UK, warned that the promise of big financial rewards was corrupting human clinical drug trials. Since then, there have been further similar attacks. What is urgently needed in the interests of consumers worldwide is an independent source of funding to evaluate health treatments of all kinds.

For now, your best guides to making a decision are up to date information, good practitioners and common sense.

Be a critical consumer as well as a patient

- find out as much as you can about your problem and the possible solutions: read books, talk to support groups and get their information leaflets, trawl the Net.
- with all therapies, weigh up benefit and risk for you individually.
- distinguish between invasive and non-invasive treatments: invasive treatments for body and mind – including surgery, drugs, herbal medicines, physical manipulation and mind-altering therapies – have the greatest risk potential.
- if you are prescribed drugs, always read the patient literature that comes with them.
- choose your practitioners carefully (see below) and don't hesitate to question them: don't buy into the notion that the doctor or any other health professional is God and automatically knows best.
- use the same common sense when it comes to looking after your health as you would for looking after your car.

CHOOSING A PRACTITIONER

The relationship you have with your health professional is unique. You are putting yourself in their hands. That makes you vulnerable. You must have someone you can trust both as a practitioner and a person.

Here are some suggestions for choosing a practitioner:

- ask for recommendations from other health professionals and friends.
- ensure practitioners belong to a professional organisation and are fully qualified and insured. (It's usually easiest to do this on the phone before you make the first appointment; you can also ask for any written material.) Alternatively,

contact the relevant professional organisation (see Directory) for a list of local practitioners; those organisations require that members are fully insured and qualified and that they abide by a code of conduct, practice or ethics.

- consider the location: is it easy to get to?
- look for a practitioner with knowledge of, and interest in, your particular problem: you don't want to be the first person they treat.
- establish costs, if any, and waiting times; make sure they are willing to communicate with other practitioners.
- make sure you will be able to see the same health professional at each appointment.
- assess how easy they are to communicate with; if you feel you're not being listened to, point it out and move on.

The Patients Association suggests that healthcare professionals should:

- listen to you and respect your views.
- treat you politely and considerately.
- respect your privacy.
- treat information about you as confidential.
- give information to you in a way you can understand.
- ensure, wherever possible, you have understood what is proposed and have consented to it before investigations are carried out or treatment provided.
- respect your right to be fully involved in decisions about your care.
- respect your right to decline treatment or to take part in teaching or research.
- respect your right to a second opinion.
- a good rule of thumb with a CAM practitioner is that if they try to persuade you to abandon your conventional treatment it's wise to move on. Equally, with a conventional doctor, you should expect them to be interested in and respect your wishes to try out CAM.

COMMUNICATION: KEEPING EVERYONE IN THE PICTURE

Adverse interactions between different drugs are well known. For example, you must avoid aspirin if you're on warfarin. That's sometimes true of food too: eating grapefruit affects the action of several blood pressure-lowering drugs. Also herbs: St John's wort may affect the way the Pill and other drugs work. There's a similar potential for problems if you are consulting different types of practitioner. So to avoid any risk, we encourage you to get all your practitioners to communicate with each other. Since practitioners are ethically bound to keep your details confidential, we have devised two forms (pages 18 and 19) which we suggest you photocopy. The first is a Consent Form for you to sign and give to each practitioner, giving them permission to discuss your treatment. The second is a Co-operation Card, which is simple to use but allows you to notify each practitioner about what you are doing. This way you help your practitioners and yourself and get a total integrated package.

CONSENT FORM

Consent to disclosure of identifying information about treatment

I ....

Address: ....

e-mail: ....

consent to information about my treatment with ....
being sent to:

GP:
Of: ....
e-mail: ....

Other practitioners:

1 Name: ....
Address: ....
     ....
e-mail: ....

2 Name: ....
Address: ....
     ....
e-mail: ....

3 Name: ....
Address: ....
     ....
e-mail: ....

I do not want information disclosed to:
Name: ....
Address: ....

I would like copies of all correspondence sent to me: YES/NO

By mail:
By e-mail:

Signed .... Date ....

INTEGRATED HEALTHCARE CO-OPERATION CARD

Name:

Date:

Address:

Card No.:

Contacts:

The aim of this card is to improve communication between different health practitioners. Please carry it with you so that it can be filled in at every visit.

MAIN CONCERNS

	Date first noticed	Date improved
1	. . . .	. . . .
2	. . . .	. . . .
3	. . . .	. . . .
4	. . . .	. . . .
5	. . . .	. . . .

Practitioner	Date	Problem/s reported	Advice/Drugs/Supplements	Follow up
. . . . .	. . . . .	. . . . .	. . . . .	. . . . .
. . . . .	. . . . .	. . . . .	. . . . .	. . . . .
. . . . .	. . . . .	. . . . .	. . . . .	. . . . .
. . . . .	. . . . .	. . . . .	. . . . .	. . . . .
. . . . .	. . . . .	. . . . .	. . . . .	. . . . .

2

THE MENOPAUSE:

What's It All About?

This chapter covers:
- good things about the menopause
- very short guide to the menopause
- longer Q&A
- a bit more biology, including what happens at menstruation
- a simple drawing of the reproductive cycle

There's a strange thing about the menopause. It seems to take many women by surprise, however well-informed they are otherwise. There's a taboo about discussing it, even acknowledging it. While many women openly discuss periods, pregnancy, even their sex lives, the menopause tends to get pushed under the carpet.

Some admit it's because the thought of hot flushes and all the connotations of becoming a wrinkly 'crone' are too much to cope with. 'We just don't want to know,' one recently married 47-year-old professional told us. 'We're sorry for women drenched in sweat but we can't bear the thought of it all happening to us. And we know it will. So we're in denial.'

The taboo may also be because going through the menopause is a comparatively recent phenomenon for most women.

The average age of the menopause – 51 years – has not changed since medieval times but until the twentieth century, fewer than 30 per cent of women reached it. Surprisingly perhaps, the Bible (both the Old and New Testaments) does mention periods stopping. 'It ceased with Sarah after the manner of women,' records the book of Genesis, 'and her womb was dead.' No details about whether she had hot flushes or anything like that (well, presumably the writer was a chap). When it comes to medical literature, however, menopausal symptoms didn't really feature until the end of the nineteenth century.

For most menopausal women today, there were only two generations who went through it before and they tended to be pretty buttoned-up. In spite of being a health journalist, Sarah was baffled when, aged 47, she started getting hot and bothered at 2 a.m. When she went to the doctor, the word 'menopause' came through clearly but the rest – like 'peri-menopause' and 'FSH tests' – was a fog of medical jargon. Talking to women friends the same age was comforting in one way because almost no one (not even the nurses) seemed to know much more than the usual old myths. *But* ... there's a big downside to not knowing because it means you can't make informed decisions about how to cope with any troublesome symptoms and the choice of possible treatments.

Here's a very simple guide so that you can decode 'doctor-speak' and put yourself in control. Incidentally, quite a few men we know have found this section helpful too.

Before you go on: remember, you may not get symptoms like hot flushes – some women don't feel a thing or only experience very mild symptoms. If you do have problems, there are simple, effective ways of coping with them. If you haven't got there yet, a few simple lifestyle shifts can help keep you symptom-free and feeling (and looking) great. It's all in this book.

GOOD THINGS ABOUT THE MENOPAUSE

Periods tail off so no PMS and no tampons
'I was thrilled when I went through the menopause – at last I could travel round India without having to worry about tampons.'

No need to worry about contraception
'Not having to worry about getting pregnant is the best aphrodisiac ever.'

More free time for yourself
'I'm doing all the things I wanted to do when I was 20, 30 and 40 but never had the time – seeing films and plays, visiting gardens and redoing mine, helping an interesting charity, learning to paint and having holidays!'

Often fewer responsibilities
'The children have flown the nest so my husband and I have got a new lease of life.'

More fun, adventure, romance!
'I'm having the best time ever; just let yourself go and you'll enjoy every moment – and don't ever believe that falling in love stops at 35 ...'

THE MENOPAUSE

In brief

If you're in a tearing hurry, here's the short version! When you have a bit more time, you can read the rest.

* menopause literally means your last natural period; this

happens because your ovaries have run out of eggs, medically called ovarian failure.

- symptoms occur because of falling levels of the reproductive hormones oestrogen and progesterone.
- symptoms like hot flushes may start several years before your last period, or afterwards; they are likely to stop between one and five years after menopause.
- there are other reasons for not having periods such as pregnancy, weight loss and other hormonal imbalances – if in doubt, consult your doctor.
- the average age of menopause in the UK is 51; premature menopause is usually taken as when your last period is before 45 in the developed world and 40 in developing countries.
- surgical menopause occurs when your ovaries have been removed (oophorectomy): this often takes place when your womb is removed (hysterectomy). If you've had a hysterectomy and your ovaries have *not* been removed, it's important to consult your doctor and to have an annual check-up and blood test. This is because the ovaries may stop working early and that brings an increased risk of osteoporosis and possibly heart disease.

The longer version

Q What is the menopause exactly?
A Menopause comes from the Greek *menos* meaning 'monthly', and *pausis* meaning 'ending'. It is a shortened form of the term 'La Menespausie' which was first used in medical writings published in France in the early 19th century. The term is confusing to non-medics because, strictly speaking, menopause means the point at which a woman has her final period (whereas laymen tend to use it to refer to the years leading up to and after the final period; see

next paragraph). The snag is, you can only date the actual menopause with hindsight – when you haven't had a period for 12 months. Sometimes, women think they've been through it and then one sneaks up and gets them unprepared (literally ... so take precautions).

Doctors may also use the word 'climacteric', referring to the whole transitional time (or 'change of life'). This can be as long as 15 to 20 years, lasting from the stage when periods stop being regular and normal up to the time after menopause when symptoms like hot flushes are over.

Q What age does natural menopause happen?
A The average age for a final period is 51 in the UK and most Western countries, although some women carry on having periods into their early and even mid 50s. The latest recorded age for menopause is 58.

Some traditional communities worldwide start their periods later and have their last one earlier – for more on this, see pages 42 to 48. Interestingly, around 50 years has been the average age of menopause for centuries although the onset of puberty, now 13 in the West, has got earlier.

Smoking is known to hasten the onset of menopause by about 18 months. Your genes may also play a part: if your mother had an early menopause, you may too.

Q What is premature menopause?
A Premature menopause is when your periods stop before the age of 45 in the developed world or 40 in the developing world. This happens to about 2 in 100 women in the West. Often the cause is unknown but it may be due to disease or to surgery, as we explain below.

Disease and its treatment can cause premature menopause. Cancer treatments (radiotherapy and chemotherapy) can provoke the ovaries to shut down early. Some auto-immune disorders may be linked to early menopause. The thinking is that the body starts to attack its own ovaries and the eggs inside them, resulting in ovarian failure. Women with Down's Syndrome tend to have early menopause. Because premature menopause may run in families, if it happened to your mother it is important to discuss this with your doctor.

In a tiny number of cases, the last period can happen as early as 16 due to very rare genetic problems. In Turner's syndrome, the woman never gets a period at all so menopause happens by default.

Premature surgical menopause happens when periods stop because the womb and ovaries are removed by surgery; in medical terms that's a hysterectomy and bilateral oophorectomy (taking both ovaries away).

If you have a hysterectomy and your ovaries are removed, you will obviously not get the hormones from your ovaries and you will go into menopause immediately.

If the ovaries are *not* removed with the hysterectomy, there are two scenarios. Firstly, they may continue working as usual, the woman will continue to produce oestrogen and can even get PMS. So – although she doesn't have a womb or periods and has technically been through menopause – she will experience the same passage through the change of life as women with wombs.

Secondly, even if your ovaries are not removed, you may still go through the menopause early. This is because the ovaries' blood supply may be disrupted by the hysterectomy and there's a significant chance that they will then stop working. If they have stopped working early, you have a higher risk of osteoporosis (see pages 241 to 243). That's why women who go into premature menopause are invariably prescribed HRT; see page 244. So if you have had a hysterectomy before the age of 50 and kept your ovaries, you should have a yearly blood test for FSH (follicle stimulating hormone; see Tests, page 27) levels to check what's happening with your ovaries. You should discuss this with your doctor and have an annual check-up.

Q What's perimenopause?
A Perimenopause refers to the time before the menopause when you experience physical changes (and possibly symptoms like hot flushes) and the first year after your last period.

You may also hear the term 'premenopause'. The meaning of this is a bit fuzzy: it's used to refer to both the time when periods are normal and also to the early years when the menstrual cycle changes and periods may get irregular and/or heavy and/or very frequent.

'Postmenopause' is a word you probably won't ever hear but in case you do it's the time from your last period to when you kick up the daisies. However, the term 'post-menopausal bleeding' is sometimes used. If you do bleed after the menopause, you should see your doctor.

Q Why does the menopause happen?
A People often think the menopause occurs because oestrogen levels drop and that's partly true. Falling oestrogen causes the symptoms. But the actual ending of periods – the menopause – happens when the ovaries run out of eggs so the woman stops ovulating (releasing eggs). This is medically called ovarian failure. That leads to decreasing oestrogen levels and, in turn, to periods stopping. One estimate is that women experience an 85 per cent drop in oestrogen between the ages of 35 and 55.

Q How do I know when I'm coming up to menopause?
A Around 45, sometimes earlier, women start noticing changes – often small – in their periods, due to erratic production of oestrogen and progesterone. Periods may get

heavier or lighter. The cycle length may be shorter or you may skip a period. If you're a PMS sufferer, you may notice variations in your premenstrual symptoms. Additionally, because the ovaries need more stimulation from the age of 35, the levels of FSH increase, which is why these are tested to establish what stage women are at.

Q If I notice changes do I need to do anything? Should I tell the doctor?
A The best thing is to start keeping a diary of your periods and bleeding patterns (including irregular cycles, bleeding between periods, bleeding after intercourse, heavy bleeding and any changes in your normal pattern) and your most distressing symptoms (see Chapter Four).

If you're at all concerned about anything, consult your doctor or health professional. ('If in doubt, give a shout!' is Michael's mantra for patients.)

Q Are there tests to see if I'm coming up to my last natural period?
A Your doctor may do a blood test to measure levels of follicle stimulating hormone (FSH); this can give a crude assessment of the stage of menopause and any significant hormonal deficiency but it's a signpost rather than a firm measurement. Hormone levels go up and down like yo-yos so the blood tests may need to be repeated. (One-off blood tests are generally considered unreliable.) It is important that tests are done at the correct time of the month (i.e. the early part of your cycle), and they will almost certainly need to be repeated several times to get a true picture. If you're not having periods, then they should be done on two or three occasions across a calendar month. If you are already on HRT or some form of hormonal contraceptive, turn to page 138.

There are two new blood tests under investigation, which may prove useful. One test is inhibin B, the other anti-Mullerian hormone.

Q What does oestrogen do?
A Oestrogen is in fact a group of female reproductive hormones: oestriol, oestradiol and oestrone. These rise and fall at different stages of a woman's life:

- oestriol increases during pregnancy.
- oestradiol is higher during the reproductive years.
- oestrone remains more constant because the adrenal glands can, if they're working well, produce androgens (male hormones) which are then converted to oestrone in the fat tissue (see below).

For simplicity's sake, we'll call them all oestrogen (or estrogen if you're American).

Oestrogen and progesterone, both of which are produced by the ovaries, where the eggs, or 'ova', are stored, are the main hormones that control women's sexuality and reproduction. Oestrogen stimulates the womb lining to grow and progesterone makes it more nourishing for a fertilised egg. Women also have a bit of the male hormone testosterone, which zips up the libido; again the ratio is greater after menopause because of lower oestrogen levels.

Oestrogen plays a key part in many non-reproductive organs. Cells in the vagina, breasts, skin, bones, heart and brain all contain receptors for this hormone to carry out their normal cell functions. It makes you feminine, keeping hair lustrous, skin moist and smooth and voice soft. Oestrogen also keeps your internal thermostat operating optimally: when oestrogen levels fall around menopause, this may get disrupted and that's why so many women get hot flushes (for more on this, including how to prevent them, see page 71).

Progesterone, on the other hand, usually has a calming effect on the brain but is sometimes linked to PMS.

Q Is there a point at which women stop producing oestrogen altogether?
A Overall oestrogen levels drop gradually as the ovaries stop releasing eggs. After menopause, oestradiol levels will have fallen significantly, up to a factor of ten. But there is still some circulating oestrogen, in the form of oestrone produced by your fat tissue. The adrenal glands also produce androgens, which are then converted to oestrogen (oestrone). This is an important source around menopause but the adrenals are also responsible for our stress hormones (adrenalin, noradrenalin and cortisol) and these may take priority. So it's very important to keep stress levels down so that the adrenals can help keep your oestrogen levels from plunging too far and too fast. This is one of the reasons why stressed-out women are more likely to have symptoms such as hot flushes and night sweats.

Q What about progesterone?
A Progesterone is only made in effective quantities during the time that the ovaries are producing oestrogen. Women also produce a small amount of testosterone from the adrenal glands and ovaries. As oestrogen levels tail off, the ratio of testosterone to oestrogen becomes higher and the more active testosterone is available.

Q What's a hormone exactly?
A Hormones are body chemicals produced by different glands and organs, which carry messages from one part of the body to another via the bloodstream. Different hormones control all the many different functions of our body and brain.

Individual hormone molecules are so small you can't even see them under a microscope. But they're so powerful that, in some cases, less than a millionth of an ounce of a hormone can have an effect.

Q So what's Hormone Replacement Therapy?
A Hormone Replacement Therapy, or HRT, aims to replace the falling levels of oestrogen and progesterone, also in some cases testosterone. Once hailed as the fountain of youth and the panacea for all menopausal women, international research over the last decade has thrown up many negatives about taking HRT. However, it may still be useful for some women if it's carefully prescribed and monitored. Because there is so much to say, we have devoted a whole chapter to HRT starting on page 129. With big question marks over the safety and effectiveness of HRT, scientists are increasingly interested in phyto (plant) oestrogens like soya and herbs such as black cohosh. (You could call them nature's HRT.)

Q When is it safe to have unprotected sex without the risk of pregnancy?
A Pregnancy can occur around the menopause although it's rare. The oldest natural birth recorded was in a woman of 56. The standard guideline is that if your last period occurs before the age of 50, you need to use contraception for two years; if it's after 50, take precautions for one year. There's a lot more information about this, including different choices for contraception, on pages 349 to 386.

Q Will HRT stop me getting pregnant?
A No.

Q Falling oestrogen levels are always said to be risky for people with a risk of osteoporosis. What's the link?
A There are various causes of bone density loss but the most common is post-menopausal osteoporosis. How bad it gets

depends on the peak bone mass the woman has achieved as an adult (remember that happens at about age 30 to 35, so it's vital to eat and exercise well from childhood on, particularly if there's osteoporosis in your family) and how fast the bone mass deteriorates after that. Women have 30 to 50 per cent lower bone density than men. Bone loss starts after 35 and continues gradually until the menopause when the fall-off of oestrogen, which protects the skeleton, stimulates rapid loss that goes on for about five years. Just how oestrogen helps bones is unclear, although oestradiol receptors have now been found on the bone-making cells (osteoblasts) showing that there is a direct connection. For more on osteoporosis, turn to page 237.

A BIT MORE BIOLOGY

If you're interested, this section gives you more details about how our reproductive hormones work.

The Reproductive Hormone Cycle

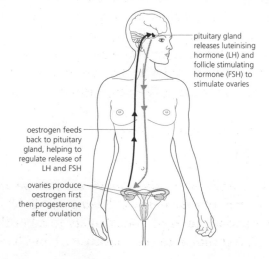

pituitary gland releases luteinising hormone (LH) and follicle stimulating hormone (FSH) to stimulate ovaries

oestrogen feeds back to pituitary gland, helping to regulate release of LH and FSH

ovaries produce oestrogen first then progesterone after ovulation

Everything to do with reproduction is gradual. In fact you could say that the menopause – the process of the ovaries running out of eggs – starts before birth. At about 20 weeks old in the womb, a girl baby has some five million eggs. At birth there's around one million, and by puberty that's halved. Ovarian activity starts long before puberty however; if you scan a girl toddler's ovaries, even at two years old, you can see something going on. It may seem as if we've got so many eggs that we would never run out but in order to produce one egg for release each cycle (ovulation), about 1,000 eggs are recruited and literally the fittest goes to the top.

What Happens Where in Reproduction

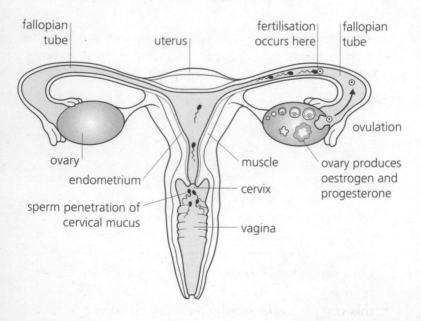

fallopian tube | uterus | fertilisation occurs here | fallopian tube | ovulation | ovary | endometrium | muscle | ovary produces oestrogen and progesterone | cervix | sperm penetration of cervical mucus | vagina

Over a year a 25-year-old woman will probably have 13 menstrual cycles, release one egg in 11 of those, produce two eggs in one and no egg in one (called 'anovulatory'). At 45, women with regular cycles will follow the same pattern but if you have irregular periods as you get older you're much less likely to ovulate – an egg won't be released in up to 30 per cent of cycles.

Puberty is kicked off by a chain reaction of several different hormones but in fact the ovaries often don't release eggs straight away; it can take up to a couple of years. That's why teenage girls often have irregular heavy periods. One big thing that's changed over the last century is the number of menstrual cycles women have. Today, an average woman has about 400 periods in her lifetime. In Victorian times, women had more like ten to 20, due to more or less continual pregnancies and breast-feeding. Also, girls nowadays start menstruating about 13, on average. Until about a century ago, the average age was 15 or 16.

The peak reproductive time is before the age of 30. By the age of 35 in most women, the ovaries need more stimulation (from follicle stimulating hormone; see below) to release an egg.

WHAT HAPPENS AT MENSTRUATION

* around the age of 11 or 12 in most girls, an increase in growth hormone triggers the growth spurt that makes them shoot up before starting periods.
* next, the hypothalamus (the hormone headquarters in the brain) starts producing another hormone called gonadotrophin releasing hormone (GnRH) more regularly.
* this stimulates the nearby pituitary gland to produce follicle stimulating hormone (FSH) and luteinising hormone (LH).

- every month, FSH gets to work on the follicles, or cells, surrounding the eggs (ova) in the girl's ovaries. (A follicle is like a balloon starting off at 2 mm in diameter and growing up to 20mm, and the egg is the smallest thing you can see with the naked eye – you can't see a sperm without a microscope.) FSH triggers one or more eggs to ripen, ready for release into the Fallopian tubes and fertilisation by any passing sperm. FSH also tells the ovaries to produce the female sex hormone, oestrogen.
- the role of oestrogen is to stimulate growth of the womb lining, ready for a fertilised egg to settle down there, so oestrogen levels rise over the first half of the menstrual cycle as the womb lining thickens until it looks like raspberry jam. Then, in the middle of the cycle, Abracadabra! LH triggers the release of an egg (ovulation) from one ovary.
- after a temporary dip of oestrogen, there is a gradual increase of both oestrogen and progesterone. Progesterone stimulates the glands in the womb to produce a nourishing fluid that generally makes the womb receptive to implantation.
- if the egg is not fertilised, the progesterone and oestrogen levels fall, causing a period as the womb lining is expelled from the body.
- if the egg is fertilised, the developing baby (embryo) produces its own hormone (HCG) and oestrogen / progesterone production goes on.

The Normal Menstrual Cycle

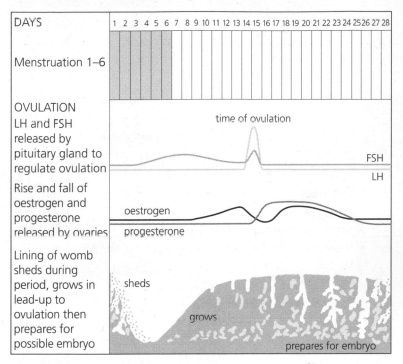

3

THE MENOPAUSE JOURNEY:

What's Going On in Your Life

This chapter covers:
- the menopause journey: what's it like living through this time?
- symptoms: what are the most common, how many women suffer what, and for how long?
- how women experience the menopause in different cultures world wide
- your symptoms questionnaire
- your wellbeing assessment
- general health guidelines

THE MENOPAUSE JOURNEY

Rush, rush, rush. Dash, dash, dash. If you're like most of the women we know, you're reading this feeling tired and a bit (or very) stressed out. You might have elderly parents leaning on you. Your partner – if you have one – may be driving you up the wall (and sex is a non-starter). Teenagers are multiplying round the house, needing feeding, ferrying and understanding – or they're leaving the nest (wonderful and awful). The dog/cat/hamster seems to have been sick on the carpet and your Little Black Dress, which you thought you could wear tonight, is – well – just too little.

You might be wondering what's in store for the rest of your life.

Not for nothing is menopause called the change of life. For most women, the decade from your mid 40s to mid 50s is a non-stop soap opera. As well as the physical changes that we've talked about in the first chapter, there are invariably all sorts of shifts happening in your family as well as in the way you think about yourself and your life. If you go out to work, there may be changes there too.

If you're feeling under pressure, that affects how you go through the physical side of the menopause, and crucially what symptoms you get. How severe, how many, how long.

What happens in our minds has a profound effect on our bodies. It's not just falling levels of oestrogen that are behind the potential cascade of symptoms. It's the whole shooting match of physical, mental and emotional bullets bombarding you.

Interestingly, researchers worldwide are now adding a spiritual category when they assess how women cope with menopausal symptoms. There are stacks of research showing that people who have faith in something greater than themselves – who believe in some guiding principle – are generally happier and in turn healthier than those who don't. This can be any form of religious or spiritual belief. What it gives people is a sense of security and self-worth, of being connected with others and often that there is a purpose in life (although you may not know what that is).

It's well-known that being under stress makes all physical conditions worse – and sure enough women who lead pressured lives are more likely to have severe hot flushes and other symptoms. Since stress is part of everyday life in the twenty-first century, it's not surprising that up to 80 per cent of women suffer hot flushes.

What we're getting at is that symptoms that are put under the heading of menopause are likely to be caused not just by falling oestrogen levels but by a combination of factors. Anxiety and depression – which many women put down to the menopause – is a good example. Careering hormones may affect your mood but it would be strange if you were not also affected by, say, an ill or dying parent, missing your children, or a partner being made redundant. Again, poor sleep – waking up at 2 a.m. in a battlefield of a bed – is more likely due to anxiety combined with night sweats due to falling oestrogen. Falling levels of serotonin may also play a part, (see page 97.) And almost everyone feels edgy and low if they don't get enough sleep because of night sweats. Equally, poor memory and lack of concentration are more likely to be due to anxiety, tiredness and general stress than to oestrogen deficiency.

Sexual changes can obviously be a huge issue for women at this time. Vaginal dryness and thus pain with making love are fairly common, which can put a big strain on relationships. It's not helped by the fact that the man in your life may also be feeling stressed – and left out. Men go through the events that are affecting you – children leaving, sick parents, job insecurity – and often a male change of life. Many men are interested in what happens at menopause but don't like to ask. One husband whose first marriage split up in synch with his wife's menopause (possibly the only thing that was in synch) said our second chapter should be required reading for all men.

So you see the thinking. Unless you're superlucky or superwoman, you're probably stressed in all sorts of ways. One magic bullet – be it HRT, vitamins, herbs, massage, a daily run, or whatever! – can't possibly deal with all those different sorts of problem. You need an all-round solution that covers physical, mental, emotional and perhaps spiritual issues.

That's why we have developed the concept of Integrated Menopausal Therapy, as we explained in Chapter One.

You can think of the menopause as part of your journey through life. There is a beginning and end to the specific physical symptoms but the other parts – the way you feel about yourself and what's going on in your life – are much less clearly defined. We've outlined the picture below in our list of landmarks. You may have different things to add in but it gives you a general picture.

After that there is a symptoms questionnaire to fill in every three months plus guidelines for your general health. It's really important to keep as well as you possibly can. Remember: you control the controllables, and the treats and rewards you give yourself.

Everyone's experience is different. You don't have the same life situation as your friends and colleagues and you may not have the same symptoms. Just because they have hot flushes and put on weight doesn't mean you will too. Equally, the same solution may not work for everyone: that's why we give you the choices laid out in Chapter One.

THE MENOPAUSE JOURNEY: LANDMARKS

When you look at these, remember that this is a two-way street so look both ways: the stressful situations (right-hand column) can make your symptoms (left-hand column) worse and vice versa.

Common physical/mental symptoms	*Psychological/emotional upheavals*
Period changes	Relationship shifts: old ones ending and/or new ones starting (or not)
Hot flushes/night sweats	
Insomnia	

Less energy/fatigue

Aches and pains

Weight changes

Bowel changes

Skin/hair changes

Decreased libido

Vaginal dryness

Pain with intercourse

Bladder problems

Possible long-term health problems: osteoporosis, heart disease, general health problems

Loneliness

Children moving on/empty nest syndrome

Realisation of end of fertility

Self-image changes, both physically and emotionally

'Peter Pan' worries: difficulty with accepting that you're getting older

Sexual changes

Family problems with sick or dying parents and/or friends

Work changes

Financial problems

Work/career problems and/or changes

Facing retirement

Surveys

There is surprisingly little research on how many women suffer what menopausal symptoms. One of the most comprehensive recent surveys was carried out in July 2003 by the National Consumers League in Washington, USA (www.nclnet.org/menopause). This involved 851 women aged from 45 to 59. Their responses were divided into three categories of severity: mild, moderate and severe. The survey showed that:

- 49 per cent had mild symptoms, which had little impact on their everyday lives.
- 34 per cent had moderate symptoms, which had a greater impact on their everyday lives.
- 17 per cent had severe symptoms, which had a major impact on their everyday lives.

This survey confirmed that menopausal symptoms add to your general stress levels. In the group with severe symptoms, 49 per cent felt they were 'not as nice to be around since menopause', 39 per cent lost 'a lot of self-confidence' and 43 per cent had 'less confidence in sexual intimacy' and the same number said their symptoms 'put a strain on their relationships with family and friends'. 60 per cent felt moody and irritable, and cried at times.

In Great Britain, the Menopause Awareness Alliance (which includes two women's charities and the manufacturers of a nutritional supplement) surveyed 362 women over 45 who were going through, or had been through, the menopause. These are the results of the survey.

Menopause Awareness Alliance survey

Most common symptoms	%		%
Hot flushes	68	Depression	16
Night sweats	49	Anxiety	19
Poorer skin and hair	41	Lack of energy	31
Day sweats	26	Palpitations	16
Water retention	21	Vaginal dryness	13
Poor concentration	21	Sexual problems	5

How long did the symptoms last?	%
Under 1 year	21
2–3 years	36
4–6 years	17
Longer	26

How the menopause affects women worldwide

Here's a strange thing. Although women's bodies all work in the same way, their experience of menopause varies dramatically. Research comparing different cultures shows that symptoms from hot flushes and insomnia to low mood and loss of libido vary significantly from one country to the next and from one ethnic group to another. The cross-cultural experiences of menopause are particularly relevant because they give clear signposts about what natural approaches can help women cope well with the menopause.

The biggest factors are these:

- the influence of mind and brain over body: what we believe about menopause has a direct bearing on what happens to us (remember, Western science has shown that what we feel affects our physical state profoundly).
- there is a clear link between lifestyle – including diet, physical activity and wellbeing – and the frequency and severity of symptoms, both physical and psychological.

Social scientists believe that your attitude towards the menopause can directly influence the sort of experience you have – troublesome and negative or liberating and positive.

Low mood and depression around the menopause may well be due as much to your expectation of suffering – seeing it as a disease with physical symptoms that need treating, the end of femininity, a fast track to old age – as to plummeting oestrogen and/or tough life events.

The biggest divide, unsurprisingly, is West versus East, or so-called 'civilised' societies compared with so-called 'primitive' ones. Western doctors, in tandem with the pharmaceutical industry, tend to medicalise the change of life. The menopause is described as an 'oestrogen deficiency disease' and the whole gamut of symptoms – physical, mental and emotional – put down simply to that lack. Small wonder that Western women see it as the start of old age and degeneration. In contrast, traditional cultures see the menopause as a natural transition that often brings lots of benefits, including worry-free sex, less work and more respect. Typically, women in such cultures are less likely to have distressing symptoms and if they do, they'll probably take it in their stride rather than looking for medical help (where that's available).

In less developed countries where the standard of education is extremely poor compared to the West, rural women living simple lives show few or no signs of distress at menopause, according to research. Among the Hmong hill tribes of Laos, women become 'clean like a man' when they have stopped menstruating and can relax more. Mayan women in an ancient farming culture in south-eastern Yucatan, Mexico, generally said they looked forward to menopause, comparing it to being young and free again. None reported hot flushes (or cold), and they reported better sexual relations with their husbands because they weren't worried about getting pregnant. (Interestingly, the Hmong women usually go through menopause in their early to mid 40s, compared to a Western average of 51.)

In a recent American study, black women of African origin, who reached menopause significantly earlier than white Americans, said their mothers told them how to cope with menopausal problems. They felt they could mostly manage on their own and were generally unwilling to follow their doctors' advice and take HRT. Whereas women of European descent didn't have the same connection with their mothers and felt more dependent on a medical solution to menopausal problems.

The West/East divide is becoming blurred, however, as Western culture crashes into urban populations the world over, eroding traditional beliefs. It seems that women are having more problems with menopause as a result. In Thailand, for instance, the menopause has historically been accepted as a normal life stage. However, in a recent study, Thai women in the capital Bangkok reported hot flushes as well as dizziness, headache, joint pain and backache. Medical bills are soaring there as increasing numbers demand HRT to treat their symptoms. In Beirut, Lebanon, where many women are highly educated, 45 per cent reported hot flushes (nearer to the average of women in America, Canada and Sweden), 39 per cent sought medical help and 15 per cent used HRT (compared with about one-third in the UK).

There is conspicuous reluctance on the part of many Western doctors and their women patients about acknowledging the risks of HRT. The reason may be, in part at least, that they don't recognise any form of alternative treatment. A headline in the *Sunday Telegraph* in Britain, for 6 April 2003, above a feature written by a doctor about the American Women's Health Initiative (WHI) study (which was stopped because of the risks) screams: 'I was wrong. You can't escape the hot flushes'. The clear message was that nothing else will help, whereas many women and health practitioners in traditional cultures know there is a whole range of herbs and other natural substances plus therapies including acupuncture and yoga, that can alleviate symptoms.

Interestingly, when researchers in Taiwan reviewed all the research on HRT in June 2003, they concluded that there was no benefit for their countrywomen and emphatically praised the writers of the WHI study for their 'conscientiousness and integrity' in cautioning doctors not to prescribe combined HRT.

Goddess or crone?

Although a growing number of Western baby-boomer celebrities such as Joanna Lumley, Goldie Hawn and Susan Sarandon are emphatically flaunting their 50- and 60-plus birthdays, many women in the 'younger-is-much-much-better' West still feel insecure about their age. How women view growing old seems to contribute greatly to how they see the menopause. How you look, how you'll be treated, what life holds in store is a big concern.

There is a wide variation in the way older people are treated around the world, ranging from extreme reverence and respect to abandonment and deprivation. The more 'civilised' the society, the more value is placed on being, or at least looking, young – and conversely the less on maturity – and the more likely it is to fear growing old. Sadly, the facts are clear: women in these societies have more difficulties coping with the menopause than women in more simple communities.

When 70 perimenopausal Australian women were compared over three years with the same number of Filipinos, some fascinating differences emerged. The Australian women had fewer children and tended to live alone or with a partner, whereas the Filipinos lived with an average of four others.

While the Filipino women were almost all practising Catholics, the Australians were much less committed. When it came to symptoms, the surprise was that although the physical experiences were reported to be quite similar, emotionally they had a very different time. Almost all the Filipinos were positive in outlook and said they felt only minor, if any, psychological irritations during this time, whereas one in four of their Australian counterparts were definitely not having a good time. They found it difficult to come to terms with the whole ageing process, saying they experienced depression, irritability, fear of ageing, loneliness, mood swings and unhappiness plus loss of self-esteem, respect and admiration.

Having religious or spiritual faith of some kind is well recognised as making people happier. From ancient times, native Aboriginal people have seen the menopause as a time of spiritual renewal, a time when their duties of birthing and mothering could be exchanged for a clearer focus on more intense spiritual work.

Late Fragment by Raymond Carver

And did you get what
you wanted from this life, even so?
I did.
And what did you want?
To call myself beloved, to feel myself
beloved on the earth.

What we believe about death is also a key point of difference between East and West. In Western society, death is still a taboo subject. Doctors do everything they can to preserve life of any kind, whether there is quality or not. We don't see dying as a natural and inevitable part of the life cycle. So hitting menopause at 50-something may set off a slide into grief as women mourn their lost youth and see only grey nothingness ahead. Whereas women in cultures where they are valued as much or more as they become ripe, mature and wise – and where death is not something to be feared – have little to worry about and lots to look forward to.

Food and fitness

Chinese women report far fewer difficulties during menopause than Western women. Japanese women too have a much lower incidence of hot flushes (in fact, they don't have a word for it) and depression: one big study suggested that 85 per cent of Japanese women have no symptoms at all, although that is likely, at least in part, because it's not done to admit problems.

Dr T. Colin Campbell, Professor Emeritus of Nutritional Biochemistry at Cornell University who led the research in China, believes that diet may be a potent factor. In much of Asia (as in other Third World cultures), food is low fat, low sugar and rich in phyto (plant) oestrogens, including soy and whole grains such as brown rice and legumes. Several studies have found a decrease in the frequency of hot flushes in women consuming soy, either as food or supplements. Traditional Chinese Medicine practitioners (as with many ancient medical systems) advise that women going through the change of life should keep blood sugar levels stable, eat lots of vegetables and fruit (we say both these too! See page 259) and avoid red meat, spicy foods, sugar, caffeine and alcohol, which are thought to promote hot flushes and aggravate mood swings. They also recommend not smoking or being near smokers – because it dries up body fluid (think of vaginal dryness here ...) and avoiding stress, tension and anxiety as much as possible.

Generally, the research studies suggested that women who had fewer menopausal symptoms were leading more active lives. In primitive cultures, physical activity is a necessary part of daily survival – not an add-in as it tends to be in the West. Other forms of exercise have ancient roots and are well-respected for helping mind and body. A form of gentle meditative stretching exercise called qigung is widely practised in China, as yoga is in India, and dancing of one kind or another is also commonplace.

What's the message?

The experience of women worldwide shows that simple natural measures can help minimise problems of the menopause. The main ones, which you will find reflected throughout this book, are:

- positive attitude towards this stage of your life
- feeling good about yourself
- hopefulness about the rest of your life
- good support network with family and/or friends
- faith
- diet based on fresh organic food with plenty of phyto-estrogens
- physical activity
- minimal stress and anxiety
- relaxation

YOUR THREE-MONTHLY SYMPTOMS QUESTIONNAIRE

We've developed this questionnaire to help you know where you are. Predicting what will happen is almost impossible but by doing this questionnaire every three months you can check your position – like looking out of a train window. But remember – just to push the rail journey idea a bit further – some people will take a slow train which stops at every station (and sometimes in between) and others will leap on a high-speed through train which gets there in no time, almost without them noticing. In other words, you may get through the change of life with virtually no symptoms – it has been known! Or you may take a bit longer and have more to cope with.

Sometimes you may find that everything has been going great and then you suddenly seem to be caught in a web of problems. Using our questionnaire regularly will allow you to chart what's happening and if necessary make some of the small adjustments we suggest to get you back on track. You might find you simply haven't been eating well enough or drinking enough water – or that taking a daily walk or doing yoga makes all the difference. Or it could be that you need to deal with a long-term physical problem like a frozen shoulder, or an emotional one such as divorce or bereavement.

Remember, this is only for you. So you can be completely honest. That puts you in control. It may help to photocopy the questionnaire and pop a copy in a file so you can refer back easily.

A tip: we've said it before but it bears repeating! One of the most useful things you can do at this time is to keep a – very basic – daily diary of your symptoms. Then when you come to fill in the questionnaire at the end of three months, you won't have forgotten anything.

Finally: if you have any concerns do go and discuss them with your GP or health professional. (Remember: 'If in doubt, shout!') Take your filled-in questionnaire/s with you so that you have a ready reference.

Date:

Your Age:

Your Symptoms:

You'll see the numbers 0 1 2 3 after each symptom. These are to indicate your experience of the symptom.

0=none   1=mild   2=moderate   3=severe

VERY IMPORTANT: if there's an asterisk like this * by a symptom and you experience it at all, you should discuss it with your doctor or health professional as soon as possible.

Vasomotor and associated symptoms	None	Mild	Moderate	Severe
Hot flushes	0	1	2	3
Night sweats	0	1	2	3
Blip-outs (nanosecond losses of consciousness)	0	1	2	3
Sleeping problems	0	1	2	3
Giddy spells*	0	1	2	3
Palpitations*	0	1	2	3
Restless legs	0	1	2	3

Period problems				
Irregular cycles: long	0	1	2	3
shorter	0	1	2	3
varied	0	1	2	3
Bleeding between periods*	0	1	2	3
Bleeding after intercourse*	0	1	2	3
Bloody vaginal discharge*	0	1	2	3
Lighter periods	0	1	2	3
Increased pain with periods*	0	1	2	3
No periods	0	1	2	3

Weight gain/loss

Weight now in kg:

Height in m:

Waist circumference (see below):

BMI (see below):

Body fat (see below):

Bowel/gut changes

Constipation	0	1	2	3
Diarrhoea	0	1	2	3
Bloating	0	1	2	3

NB Any change in bowel habit that lasts longer than 14 days should be discussed with your GP.

Sexual problems

Vaginal dryness	0	1	2	3
Increase/change in vaginal discharge*	0	1	2	3
Smelly vaginal discharge*	0	1	2	3
Vaginal itching*	0	1	2	3
Vaginal burning	0	1	2	3
Painful sex (on entrance or on deep penetration)*	0	1	2	3
Feeling of something coming down/lump in your vagina (prolapse)*	0	1	2	3
Decreased libido (sexual desire)	0	1	2	3
Bleeding after intercourse*	0	1	2	3

Urinary symptoms

Frequency of passing urine (peeing often)*	0	1	2	3
Urgency (sudden urge to pee)*	0	1	2	3
Urge incontinence (sudden urge to pee, and wetting yourself)*	0	1	2	3
Stress incontinence (wetting yourself when you cough, laugh, exercise, make love etc.)*	0	1	2	3
Discomfort or pain peeing*	0	1	2	3
Recurrent urinary infections, e.g. cystitis*	0	1	2	3
Blood in urine*	0	1	2	3

Skin/hair/mouth/eye problems

Dry, flaky, thinning skin with less elasticity and more wrinkles	0	1	2	3
Crawling feeling over skin (formication)	0	1	2	3
Tendency to bruise easily	0	1	2	3
Dry, breaking, flaking nails	0	1	2	3
Dry hair	0	1	2	3
Hair loss (temples or general thinning)	0	1	2	3
Increase in facial hair*	0	1	2	3
Bleeding gums	0	1	2	3
Dry mouth	0	1	2	3
Dry eyes	0	1	2	3

Aches and pains

General aches and pains	0	1	2	3
Backache	0	1	2	3
Headache/migraine*	0	1	2	3

Psychological symptoms

Anxiety	0	1	2	3
Depressed mood/depression*	0	1	2	3
Irritability	0	1	2	3

Anger	0	1	2	3
Mood swings	0	1	2	3
Lethargy	0	1	2	3
Lack of energy	0	1	2	3
Poor memory	0	1	2	3
Lack of concentration	0	1	2	3
Loss of self-confidence/self-esteem	0	1	2	3

YOUR WELLBEING SELF-ASSESSMENT

Experts in the UK Wellbeing 2002 study agreed that people with wellbeing have a sense of being broadly in control of their lives and feel that in general they can shape the direction it takes. They can manage the increasing range of choices in modern life and benefit from them. They can also accept that there are parts of everyone's life that can't be controlled. They mostly feel balanced and secure, whatever life throws at them.

The questions below are entirely for you. They are based on the key 'drivers' of wellbeing identified in the Wellbeing 2002 study (also look at the report on menopause worldwide on page 42, which brings up these issues). Few people will feel positive about them all but you may compensate for a low rating in one by high ones in others. Even if, say, you had an unhappy childhood and don't feel financially comfortable, you may make up the difference in other categories such as having a strong network of friends and a positive working environment.

We suggest that you do this self-audit every six months, just to see what's going on. Then fill in the section below, called Living in the Solution. Put a note in your diary to remind yourself to do it again.

Assess Your Wellbeing

	Yes	Mostly	Sometimes	Seldom	No
Do you feel generally in control of your life?					
Are you generally optimistic?					
Are you comfortable with the way you look?					
Do you believe that most people think well of you?					
Are you confident about managing as you get older?					
Do you have a partner you feel content with?					
Do you have a good sex life – if you want one?					
Do you feel well and healthy, with sufficient energy to do what you want?					
Do you have religious or spiritual beliefs that guide the way you live?					
Are you interested and enthusiastic – not bored – most of the time?					
Do you have positive people around you and an environment you like?					
Do you have sufficient financial resources, with no particular worries?					
Did you have a good childhood, which made you feel loved and supported?					
Do you have good family relationships?					
Do you have a strong network of friends?					
Do you feel that you can deal well with the stress in your life?					
Do you have personal goals and are you working towards them?					

Living in the solution

One of our favourite sayings is 'Don't live in the problem, live in the solution.' Bearing in mind the results of your self-audit, try the following exercise:

List five positive things you do for your health and happiness that you could do more of (these can be physical, mental, emotional or spiritual):

_____

_____

_____

_____

_____

List five negative things associated with menopause/your stage of life that you would like to change and how you are going to do that (these can be physical, mental, emotional or spiritual):

_____

_____

_____

_____

_____

YOUR GENERAL HEALTH

It's vital to look after your whole health, not just concentrate on the menopause. So here goes. Is there any health matter you need to see your doctor/health professional about now? Should you be having a routine check-up? If yes, book that appointment today.

Things to discuss with your doctor

Have you had or do you have a family history of:

- heart disease
- stroke
- blood clots in your leg or lungs
- breast cancer
- ovarian cancer
- colon cancer

Have you had or do you have any of these conditions?

- endometriosis
- fibroids
- diabetes
- hysterectomy
- ovaries removed
- an abnormal smear

Assessing your risk of a heart attack or stroke

Heart disease is a hugely neglected ladykiller. It's often seen as a male disease but in fact more women are likely to die of it than men – more on this on page 255. Please take the time to discuss this with your health professional.

The risks of heart disease or stroke involve your lifestyle, family history and medical condition, including:

- smoking cigarettes.
- lack of exercise.
- overweight/obesity.
- poor diet, i.e. too many saturated fats, white sugar, white flour, salt, alcohol and too little fresh fruit and vegetables, plant oils and whole grains.

- drinking over four alcoholic drinks daily (*But* drinking one or two glasses of good red wine daily lowers the risk).
- taking certain drugs including some types of HRT.
- diabetes.
- family history.
- high blood pressure: you should have your blood pressure (BP) checked every year.
- high levels of blood lipids (types of fat): if you're suspected to be at high risk, i.e. with family history of premature heart disease or risk factors, your doctor should make sure that your blood lipid levels are checked regularly. For women with no obvious risk factors, the expert advice is that they should have their lipids checked at least once, preferably after the menopause, which can be regarded as a risk factor in itself, especially if it occurs prematurely.

You may also want to discuss

- contraception (see page 349).
- IMPORTANT: have you had any unexpected vaginal bleeding? If yes, you must go and see your doctor.
- bone density: fill in the osteoporosis risk test on page 241; if you are concerned and especially if you have osteoporosis in the family, talk to your doctor about a bone density scan.

Reminders

We suggest you have breast and cervical cancer checks regularly. Ovarian cancer screening is not currently available, because its benefit is unproven (see below for more details).

Cancer screening

In general, screening is not the same as diagnosing illness. The purpose of screening is to spot risky situations in apparently healthy people and encourage them to have diagnostic tests. It's also important that you realise that no test is 100 per cent accurate: so please don't get too worried if a screen throws up something, always wait for a firm diagnosis.

In the UK, you are offered free screening for cervical and breast cancer by the National Health Service (NHS). There is clear evidence that screening for these two diseases saves lives. For more information, talk to your doctor who should have leaflets at the surgery, call NHS Direct on 0854 54647, or log on to www.cancerscreening.nhs.uk Be aware that the results, which are sent by letter to your GP, may take up to 12 weeks.

Cervical screening: every three to five years

The cervical screening programme aims to help detect early, pre-malignant abnormalities of the cervix, which may progress to cancer of the cervix (cervical cancer). In the UK this programme starts at the age of 25. The disease is very rare in women under that age. Your doctor should take a sample of cervical cells, brushed from the neck of the womb, every three years up to the age of 49 years, and five-yearly from 50 to 64 (unless of course an abnormality occurs). After 65, only those women who have not been screened since the age of 50 or who have had recent abnormal tests will be screened.

Two methods are used to prepare samples: with the Pap smear, the sample is smeared on a microscope slide and assessed by a cytologist (an expert in the study and structure of cells). With Liquid Based Cytology, a new and more accurate method of testing which is used in America and now being introduced in Britain, the cells are treated in a laboratory before being assessed under the microscope by a cytologist.

There is no evidence that you need to increase the frequency of smears if you are on HRT.

Breast screening: every three years

In the UK, the NHS routinely offers women aged between 50 and 64 years (from 2004, this will be 70 years) breast screening in the form of a mammogram every three years. Older women may request the screens on the NHS. A mammogram is an X-ray, which is done on an outpatient basis. The gold standard is two views per breast, which is now being done routinely. As with cervical smears, there is no reason why women taking HRT should have a mammogram more frequently.

There is some controversy in the medical establishment about whether younger women (i.e. under 50) should be screened routinely. Although this is not available on the NHS, it can, if you wish it, be done privately. The argument is whether it's possible to detect changes in premenopausal breasts, because the greater density of breast tissue means that changes may not show up on the X-ray.

If, however, you have a family history of breast cancer (see table below), you should talk to your doctor about having a mammogram yearly from the age of 35 or, if younger, at five years before the age at which the youngest relative developed cancer. Additionally, if you are worried about any breast problem, you can ask your doctor to refer you to a hospital breast clinic.

FAMILY RISK FACTORS FOR BREAST CANCER

Although heredity does play a part in breast cancer, only five to ten per cent of cases are linked to genes.

- mother, sister, aunt or grandmother had breast cancer when over 60 (low risk).
- four close relatives on the same side of the family have had breast or ovarian cancer at any age (moderate risk).
- close relative has had both breast and ovarian cancer (moderate risk).
- three close relatives on the same side of the family have had breast cancer when they were under 70 (moderate risk).
- mother, sister or daughter had breast cancer when they were under 40 (moderate risk).
- mother, sister or daughter has had cancer in both breasts (high risk).
- father or brother with breast cancer (high risk).

If you develop any of the following breast symptoms, or any other abnormalities, it is important to discuss them with your GP:

- pain
- nipple discharge/bleeding
- a lump
- itching

Ovarian cancer screening

If ovarian cancer – sometimes called the silent killer – is detected early, the outlook is good. Sadly, at the moment it is often not detected until the disease has progressed when the changes of survival are greatly reduced.

As with breast cancer, between 5 and 10 per cent of ovarian cancers have a genetic basis. If you have two or more close relatives on one side of your family with ovarian cancer, or one with ovarian and another with early breast cancer (under 50), you should discuss this with your doctor.

Currently, there is no routine screening anywhere in the world for women who are not at increased risk. This is because there is as yet no evidence that screening will save lives. Trials are under way in the USA and UK to answer this question. The current tests available are ultrasound scanning of the ovaries and a blood test for CA125. These will probably pick up 80 per cent of the ovarian cancers but what is not known is whether the disease will be picked up early enough to cure the disease. In addition, like all other screening tests, there are false positive results, which can lead to unnecessary surgery with its risk of complications and anxiety. New and more reliable tests are likely to become available in the next few years.

There are two UK studies going on nationwide:

The UK Collaborative Trial of Ovarian Cancer Screening (UKCTOCS) will finally report in 2011. This trial is for women who do *not* have a strong family history of ovarian cancer (that is, no first-degree relative with ovarian cancer or only one) and aims to answer the crucial question of whether early detection saves lives. The study will recruit 200,000 women between 50 and 74, who will be randomised to receive screening or no screening. Screening will either use ultrasound or measure a tumour market in the blood called CA125.

The UK Familial Ovarian Cancer Screening Study looks at women who have a strong family history, with two or more cases of ovarian cancer or ovarian cancer and breast cancer at an early age (under 50) on the same side of the family. The criteria for being included in the trial are rigorous but candidates should have access to expert advice about prevention as well as screening through referral to a specialist centre.

If you are worried about your family history, discuss it with your doctor who may refer you to a local genetics clinic for risk assessment. Advice is also available through the charity OVACOME or by referral to the Ovarian Cancer Family History Clinic at St Bartholomew's Hospital in London, which specialises in managing women at increased risk of developing the disease.

DIY body weight checks

You can calculate the following simply. If you fall outside the normal range, it's wise to discuss this with your doctor or health professional.

Body mass index (BMI)

This gives you a good picture of whether you are under- or overweight, healthy or obese. Remember however that BMI does not differentiate between fat and muscle, so if you exercise vigorously you may seem overweight but in fact be very fit. You may want to check your BMI figure against a Body Fat (BIA) Monitor; see below.

To calculate your BMI, divide your weight in kilograms by your height in metres squared, as below. (You'll need a calculator.) Or use the table on page 63.

$$\frac{\text{Weight (kg)}}{\text{Height (m}^2)} = \text{BMI}$$

	Height (in metres)											
	1,50	1,55	1,60	1,65	1,70	1,75	1,80	1,85	1,90	1,95	2,00	BMI
kg	32	34	36	38	40	43	45	48	51	53	56	14
kg	36	38	41	44	46	49	52	55	58	61	64	16
kg	41	43	46	49	52	55	58	62	65	68	72	18
kg	45	48	51	54	58	61	65	68	72	76	80	20
kg	50	53	56	60	64	67	71	75	79	84	88	22
Weight (in kilograms)	54	58	61	65	69	74	78	82	87	91	96	24
	59	62	67	71	75	80	84	89	94	99	104	26
	63	67	72	76	81	86	91	96	101	106	102	28
	68	72	77	82	87	92	97	103	108	114	120	30
kg	72	77	82	87	92	98	104	110	116	122	128	32
kg	77	82	87	93	98	104	110	116	123	129	136	34
kg	81	86	92	98	104	110	117	123	130	137	144	36
kg	86	91	97	103	110	116	123	130	137	144	152	38
kg	90	96	102	109	116	123	130	137	144	152	160	40

BMI scores

Under 20: you are underweight

20–24: normal healthy range

25–26: overweight

27–29: veering towards obese; consult your GP or health professional

Over 30: this is medically termed obese; consult your GP or health professional

Waist circumference

If your BMI is 25 or more, calculate your waist circumference. A high waist measurement is associated with an increased risk for type two diabetes, abnormal lipids, hypertension and heart disease in patients with a BMI in a range between 25 and 34.9. Monitoring changes in waist circumference over time may be helpful (in addition to measuring BMI) since it can provide an estimate of increased abdominal fat even in the absence of a change in BMI. Furthermore, in obese patients with metabolic complications, changes in waist circumference are useful predictors of changes in risk factors for heart disease.

Measure your waist without holding the tape too tightly (or too loosely). As a rough guide, your waist is the narrowest part of your trunk, or approximately one inch above your belly button.

- waist circumference of over 31 inches (about 80 cm) indicates slight health risk.
- waist of over 35 inches (about 90 cm) indicates substantially increased health risk.

Body fat

You can also calculate any excess weight with a Fat Monitor. This is a simple electrical device that assesses the amount of body fat. It works by measuring the rate at which a minute electrical pulse flows through the body. The technology is called bio-electrical impedance analysis or BIA. Most BIA monitors have a memory so you can record and store readings, then compare them. Costing from about £50 ($75), these gizmos aren't cheap but they have the advantage of being able to differentiate between fat and muscle, unlike the Body Mass Index, so that you have a more accurate measurement of the fat you need to lose.

Waist/hip ratio

The ratio of your waist to your hip is a simple indicator of whether you are overweight or not, even if your BMI is not in the obese range.

* measure waist midway between the bottom of the ribs and the top of the hip bone.
* measure hips at the widest point between the hips and buttocks.
* divide your waist size at its smallest by your hip size at its largest and you get a waist-to-hip ratio.

Ideally, women should have a waist-to-hip ratio of 0.8 or less. Over 0.85 is seen as an increased risk for health and you should try to reduce your body weight by sensible dieting and exercise (see chapters on Food, Exercise and Yoga).

4

SOLVING YOUR
SYMPTOMS

This chapter covers:
- quick guide to feeling better all round
- how to deal with:
  - hot flushes and night sweats, including recipes for menopause cocktail and menopause smoothie
  - period changes
  - weight gain
  - gut and bowel problems
  - sexual problems including vaginal dryness
  - urinary incontinence
  - restless legs syndrome
  - aches and pains

In this chapter we take a trip through the possible symptoms of the menopause – the ones you'd prefer not to encounter but might. We explain what they are and, crucially, the simple measures you can take to deal with them and feel great.

Remember too that if you are under 45 and/or have no symptoms, a few simple lifestyle changes really can help prevent problems and keep you as fit as a fiddle. We want to emphasise that our general lifestyle recommendations apply whatever age you are: it's really important that you understand it's never too late – or too early – to think, be, do healthy.

Some of the most interesting research we looked at for this book shows that the simple things are the most important. You need to realise that nothing in your body and mind works in isolation: everything is interconnected and interdependent and that includes all your hormones. Think of how you feel when you've had a really good laugh: body tension melts away and so does anxiety. That's because smiling and laughing – even if you act it – releases a cascade of feel-good hormones. Your body lightens up and so does your mind.

So the message is this: think IMT – Integrated Menopausal Therapy – before you consider HRT. That means establishing a foundation of good mind and body health so that when – if – blips happen to you, they won't be too severe and you won't get too shaken. (But if you try it all and nothing stops the hot flushes, then read our chapter on HRT and consider whether it might suit you to try it out for a short time.)

Here's the short version: you will find all the research and relevant books listed at the back.

• many hormonal conditions are known to be linked to upsets in blood sugar levels, including Polycystic Ovary Syndrome (PCOS), which causes irregular periods. Eating good food every three hours keeps blood sugar levels steady and helps period problems and hot flushes; it also helps you not to get stressy. Blood sugar starts to drop two to three hours after you have eaten. A small study in Texas suggests that falling oestrogen may impair the body's ability to send glucose (its essential fuel) to the brain – the situation is made worse if your blood sugar level drops. The researchers hypothesise that hot flushes are the body's way of trying to increase blood flow – and thus glucose supplies – to the brain. Many practitioners of traditional medicine, including naturopathy and Traditional Chinese Medicine, say that maintaining constant blood sugar levels is vital in helping menopausal symptoms, period problems and hormonal imbalances in general.

- don't eat a high-fat, processed food diet: research worldwide points to a correlation between Western diet and menopausal symptoms: the hypothesis is that a high animal fat, high sugar Western diet pushes oestrogen levels unnaturally high so that menopause brings not a gentle decline, as nature probably intended, but a series of crashes that unbalance the body and brain; problems may start in puberty so you need to clean up your diet as early as possible.

- eat good fats, especially fish and plant oils: it's now recognised that good fats from fish and plant oils are essential (they're called Essential Fatty Acids or EFAs), not only for the smooth working of our bodies, including our hormonal system, but also for our brains; lack of EFAs, particularly the omega 3 fats found in fish and flax seed (linseed), is now linked to depression and anxiety of all kinds. EFAs are also essential for good skin, hair and nails.

- drinking lots of still water between meals helps everything in your body and brain function so you feel well; stops headaches and constipation; makes your skin clear and glowing. Michael was a team doctor at the last Olympics: the atheletes were told that if they were two per cent dehydrated, their overall performance would go down 20 per cent.

- regular daily exercise helps your body and mind function well; it also seems to trigger the release of hormones (androgens) from the adrenal glands that convert to a form of oestrogen and thus reduce hot flushes and other menopausal symptoms. Physical activity in daylight also helps boost serotonin levels, as we explain below.

- get out in the light: as oestrogen falls so do levels of the hormone serotonin, often called the feel-good hormone. Lack of serotonin can make you feel mildly anxious or depressed, lead to poor sleep and low energy; you may want to eat more (which tends to happen anyway with falling oestrogen), have difficulty concentrating, be drowsy in the daytime and feel unusually vulnerable and sensitive to criticism. American researchers who devised the LEVITY (Light, Exercise and Vitamin Interventional Therapy) programme established that simply getting out in the light for an extra hour a day can help redress the balance, supported by a good balanced diet and daily moderate exercise.
- keep stress levels under control, relax and laugh! Just as unwelcome stress makes everything worse so being relaxed improves your whole life; some research suggests that feeling too stressed may impair the release of the oestrogen-forming hormones above. Stress also depletes serotonin levels. Have fun, laugh – get those feel-good hormones whizzing round your body.
- deep slow breathing can calm you down, help you sleep and stop a hot flush in its tracks, according to research. Practise daily, as often as possible.
- ask for help: research suggests that the placebo effect of getting attention and TLC helps as many as half of women with hot flushes and other problems.

Remember: Positive thinking and positive actions lead to positive results – it's as simple as that.

SYMPTOMS AND SOLUTIONS

Joanne: *"I suffered mental problems that always occurred immediately before or during menstruation and some doctors advised a hysterectomy and HRT to counter my 'unbalanced' nature. Contrary to what I was told, menopause has been a very easy transition. I only noticed occasional night sweats over about six months. My diet was almost vegetarian, with a little chicken and fish. With osteoporosis in mind my daily diet included tofu, miso, kelp, sesame seeds, hummus, soya milk powder, fresh vegetables and fruit, plus pulses. I excluded red meat, caffeine and sugar and consumed few dairy products. I experienced no mood swings at all; I felt and still feel more grounded than ever before."*

Here are your choices for dealing with the more bothersome symptoms of the menopause. Many things are DIY and can be combined safely but of course you need to be cautious so here are a few guidelines. Remember what we've said above though: the foundation is good health – this is Integrated Menopausal Therapy! Don't forget to do our Symptom Questionnaire on page 51 before you start and consult your health professional if you have any concerns at all. You may want to discuss priorities and/or have a health check as we suggest on page 56.

Always start by following the simple suggestions above. If you currently have a generally unhealthy lifestyle, please try these for at least one to two months before adding in other helpers, such as herbs. However, the relaxation therapies such as massage and aromatherapy, and perhaps a general 'tonic' therapy such as acupuncture, could well help you establish a healthy balanced lifestyle. When you are back on a relatively even keel, reassess your symptoms, talk to your health professional and decide where to go from there.

A few words of warning:

- don't mix herbs (other than the ones we've listed below) without professional advice. Remember that herbs are powerful drugs: always read the label, respect any con-traindications or warnings and take the correct dose. Ideally consult an appropriately trained practitioner, if your budget and other constraints allow. Spending money on consulting an expert at an early stage could save you a fortune later.
- if you're taking medication, check with your doctor before starting anything, particularly herbs or nutritional supplements.
- when you're Pick 'n' Mixing, be sensible: try one approach first for at least four weeks to see if it works before adding in more. Otherwise you won't know what works and you could spend a lot of money on things that you don't need.
- ideally, consult an appropriately trained practitioner who can direct your treatment programme and help you choose combinations of therapy. If you go to more than one practitioner, including your doctor, let everyone know what you're doing. See our Co-op Card (page 19).

SYMPTOM: *hot flushes and night sweats*
(medically called vasomotor symptoms)

Hot flushes and night sweats are often the first complaint women encounter with perimenopause, though they may not occur until the menopause, or even after. They are very common, with about 70 per cent of women suffering them to some degree (though some surveys show lower incidences, of about 65 per cent). Generally, thin women are more likely to get them because their background oestrogen levels are lower. That's not an excuse for getting fat, but you certainly don't want to go on crash diets now (or ever).

Hot flushes, which are also known as hot flashes or midlife glows (even, perhaps optimistically, as power surges ...), have been recognised for thousands of years. They're mentioned in the Ebers Papyrii, an ancient Egyptian text from about 1500 BC. Some women suffer them so mildly that they hardly notice. Others are badly affected. One woman, a senior executive in London, describes 'personal tidal waves abruptly surging through my body, each one stopping me from thinking'.

These symptoms can occur any time of the day or night and although harmless in themselves, they can severely disrupt your life and, if they happen at night, your sleep. In fact, the psychological problems that demonise some menopausal women may be due more to sleep deprivation than to hormonal chaos. Think of the results of insomnia: irritability, anxiety, mood changes, tearfulness, giddiness, inability to cope, loss of self-confidence and sex drive, and, not least, difficulties with memory and concentration.

The vicious cycle can continue because there is also an increased risk of falls and injuries due to the lack of concentration: this is a big risk factor if you have osteoporosis (fragile bones).

The big question is how long will you have them for? The simple answer is that it's as long as a piece of string. Women often get them first some time before the menopause, as the menstrual cycles become more irregular. The hormones that the ovaries produce become erratic and hot flushes begin. Sometimes they stop for a while and then return. Up to 25 per cent of women suffer them for more than five years, before and after menopause.

Often, women experience headaches and poor sleep alongside hot flushes and night sweats. When you get on top of the hot flushes, the headaches should ease. Similarly, poor sleep patterns invariably improve when night sweats stop. (But remember other hormones such as serotonin are involved in sleep, as well as stress, so you must adopt a whole body/whole mind integrated approach.)

Why do hot flushes happen?

Hot flushes appear to be related to an upset in your ability to control the temperature in your skin. (Interestingly, however, other mammals don't seem to have the same problem.) They're categorised medically as a 'vasomotor disturbance': 'vaso' means 'blood vessel' and 'motor' means 'muscle', so it refers to an upset, or abnormal response, in the message from the brain to the blood vessels. What seems to happen is that the falling levels of oestrogen and other reproductive hormones cause an imbalance of hormones in the thermo-regulatory centre in the hypothalamus, the part of the brain that controls body temperature.

This means that the nerves between the brain and skin transmit 'red alert' messages via the blood vessels to the skin to sweat when, in fact, there is no need. You can see it working the other way too: in tests where ice was applied to the skin of menopausal women, it was found that the blood vessels which would normally contract at the touch of the ice did not do so.

Some women don't seem to suffer at all for reasons we don't really understand. It may be that they do get them but hardly notice because the sensitivity of their thermo-regulatory system and blood vessels is lower. Also, because external factors can influence hot flushes, it's possible that women with less stress, who don't drink stimulants such as coffee or alcohol, are not stimulating the hot flush mechanism. It may also be that some women produce more oestrone (the type of oestrogen in menopausal women). It's known that plumper women tend to suffer less and this makes sense because oestrone is produced in fat tissue.

Additionally, as we mentioned earlier, the adrenal glands, which release stress hormones, also produce androgens – the male hormones that women have too in lesser quantities – and these can be converted into a form of oestrogen. The main androgen used in this way is called androstenedione. Exercise kickstarts this process (see page 279).

Hot males!

Men can have hot flushes too. If the man's testicles are removed, which decreases testosterone level and gives a high LH and FSH level, as happens with menopausal women, then they can get severe hot flushes.

Another form of flushing

Some women mention 'blip-outs', which they describe as nanosecond losses of consciousness. This is probably due to the same mechanism as hot flushes but in a much less extreme form, according to Thomas Marshall-Manifold, a natural health practitioner in London who specialises in hormonal problems. He suggests that the regulation of blood vessel dilation and constriction becomes volatile, producing sudden dips in blood pressure especially in the brain, which would account for the sudden blips in consciousness. In Traditional Chinese Medicine, the cause would be considered to be an imbalance between heart (fire) and kidneys (water). Another possibility is an imbalance in the kidney energy, which could produce an interruption or sudden change in the cerebral spinal fluid pressure.

Related to this may be another rare symptom where menopausal women drivers report feeling the car they are driving overtaking their bodies. If this happens to you, stop your car as soon as safely possible. This symptom can be alarming and the only immediate remedy we have heard of is deep breathing.

What do you do if nothing seems to help?

If you clean up your lifestyle, adopt the simple measures we suggest below and still nothing works to stop your hot flushes, you need to consider whether they are bad enough to warrant your considering HRT or other drugs for a short time. Read the chapter (page 129) and discuss it with your doctor. Alternatively, you could consider consulting a homeopath, herbalist, Traditional Chinese Medicine (acupuncture and/or herbal medicine) or Ayurvedic practioner, all of whom may be able to help. See Chapter Six for more information.

If you have, or have had, breast cancer

Many of the lifestyle measures below should help but before you take any herbs or embark on phytoestrogens in any form do consult your doctor. However you may like to know that a study published in the *International Journal of Oncology* in November 2003 showed that black cohosh does not have oestrogenic activity and does not promote breast cancer cell growth. There are also research studies showing that therapies including acupuncture and hypnotherapy (where you learn self-hypnosis) can help hot flushes. (If you want to check on all these yourself, go to www.nlm.nih.gov/nccam/camon

pubmed.html: this is the US government website listing all the entries in peer-reviewed medical journals worldwide to do with complementary and alternative medicine (CAM).

SOLUTIONS: hot flushes

Self-help

First things first: don't panic! There are lots of simple things you can do to help yourself. Do remember that different women respond to different remedies. You can combine most of the suggestions below, for instance breathing, the menopause cocktail, smoothie, vitamin C and E supplements, yoga and lifestyle tips. But please don't mix up all the herbs without professional advice – they are potent and may upset your body and mind.

In rare cases, hot flushes can be due to other problems such as thyroid dysfunction, a histamine reaction (which triggers a reaction similar to a hot flush) or, very rarely, a tumour on the adrenal glands. There are usually other symptoms of these conditions but if you are at all worried you should talk to your doctor.

Many of the remedies below are not targeted just at hot flushes: they should help virtually all your menopausal symptoms.

Simple things to do first

Cut out known triggers
Hot flushes usually occur out of the blue but there are some common triggers and you may find a pattern. Keep a diary of your flushes and see if you can identify any triggers. If you do, try to avoid them. Here are the most usual:

- hot spicy foods.
- chocolate.
- alcohol.
- hot drinks: particularly tea and coffee which contain caffeine.
- smoking tobacco.
- sudden changes of temperature, e.g. coming in from the cold and going into a hot room.

Minimise anxiety and stress

Suzie: *"I think my flushes are mainly caused by stress. I was at home for a week before Easter and I had hardly any during the day although night-time is always a pain with the sweats – dancing in and out of the covers. But as soon as I was back at work, the daytime flushes were back on the attack!"*

- feeling worried makes everything in your life worse, including hot flushes. So try to minimise pressure in all areas of your life.
- practise saying 'No' – nicely – to extra jobs of all kinds at home and work (literally, practise in front of the mirror, or with a friend, to get you in the habit).
- take up relaxation techniques such as yoga, meditation and visualisation and practise breathing (see below) so that you can calm yourself before any anxiety takes over.
- reward yourself every day with at least one nice thing, which could be anything you enjoy – lying on your back in the grass, watching your favourite video, having a long scented bath with the radio on or phoning a friend.
- play relaxation tapes in bed; listen to soothing music such as Gregorian chants any time (research shows that it slows your brain waves).
- turn to the chapter on complementary and alternative

therapies, page 184, for ideas like work/life coaching, laughter therapy and so on.

• massage will help, particularly if your state of mind is causing tension in your body – have a professional one or trade massages with a friend or partner; also consider healing, acupuncture, chiropractic or osteopathy (see Aches and Pains below).

• biofeedback, where you learn to regulate your brainwaves and your physical responses, is also useful (see page 216 for more details).

• if these measures don't work, do consider consulting a counsellor, a psychotherapist or a doctor.

If you feel a hot flush coming on

• immediately drink a glass of cold or iced water (take some in a vacuum flask if you're out and about), or cold herbal tea (try keeping a jug of your favourite brew in the fridge).

• if you're at home, put a bag of frozen peas (or any other handy veg or fruit) on your forehead – it's a great flush-buster. When you go out, take a cold face cloth with you: try wrapping it round an ice cube in a sealed plastic bag. Or keep a couple of packets of facial wipes in the fridge, then take the chillier packet with you on the next outing.

• spray your face pronto with a mister (you can buy handbag-sized mineral water sprays such as Evian) and then blot gently. Spraying reduces the temperature on and around the face and so despatches the flush more quickly.

Tip: Nutritionist and bestselling author Kathryn Marsden: 'I fill a small atomiser with spring water and a drop each of essential oils of juniper, clary sage and geranium to spray on my face and neck if I have a flush; shake before each use.'

- sniff essential oil of chamomile (Roman or German).
- if possible (i.e. you're at home and can escape for five minutes) have a cool or cold shower – this was Indian health and beauty guru Bharti Vyas's 'lifesaver' through the menopause.
- open the nearest window and/ or get out in the fresh air as soon as you feel the flush coming on.
- breathe deeply! See below.

BREATHING WELL

Deep abdominal breathing can reduce the frequency of hot flushes by 50 to 60 per cent, according to extensive studies by psychologist Robert Freedman, professor of psychiatry and behavioural neurosciences at Wayne State University School of Medicine. By deliberately trying to slow your breathing rate with deep, slow inhalations that fill up the belly and long, smooth exhalations, you can learn to breathe just seven to eight times per minute (compared to the average rate of 15 or 16). His research shows that when a women begins this kind of breathing as soon as she feels a hot flush coming on, she can interrupt the flush, eliminating it entirely or reducing its severity.

Not only can you stop a hot flush in its tracks, but practising this breathing twice a day or more also helps to limit the number of flushes and sweats. It will also help you to deal with anxiety and stress.

You can learn this type of breathing in a yoga or t'ai chi class or follow our simple guidelines below. The aim of yoga breathing is to slow the breath to about eight breaths a minute so that the pituitary gland, which controls your body thermostat, is working at its best, according to Dr Mosaraf Ali of the Integrated Medical Centre in London.

This form of breathing can also reduce body temperature. (Think of the Tibetan lamas and other yogis who control their body temperature at will through respiration.)

Doing these breathing exercises in the middle of a meeting or dinner party could look a mite strange: the trick is to practise them so that they become second nature. Then if you feel the rising tide heralding a hot flush and you can't slip off to the loo or behind a large pot plant to do alternate nostril breathing, just let someone else do the talking while you breathe slowly and deeply as described in the retention breathing exercise below (it makes you look fantastically relaxed).

Breathing exercises

Retention breathing
This is a deeply calming and stabilising exercise, which is particularly useful for hot flushes, according to Dr Ali. It may seem complicated to start off with but once you get used to it, you'll find that you can do it unnoticed if you're with people.

Stand or sit with feet planted on the floor – or sit cross-legged on the floor.

Inhale slowly and gently through your nose to a count of three, feeling the air travelling down to your abdomen and inflating it like a balloon.

Hold the breath for a count of three, then exhale very slowly through your mouth to a count of six, feeling your abdomen pressing against your spine.

As you get more practised at this, you can extend the counts to four, four, eight, then six, six, twelve and so on.

> **BE CAREFUL**
> If at any point you feel woozy or your heart rate goes up, breathe naturally until calm is restored then try again.

Tip: Visualisation While you're practising retention breathing, imagine you are on the seashore. Feel the wind on your face and the sun on your back. As you breathe in, see the waves coming up the beach and hovering at the top before, as you exhale, they ebb away.

Alternate Nostril Breathing

This exercise directly helps to control the heating and cooling mechanisms in your body so you can regulate your thermostat. (This is impossible to do unnoticed, though Michael claims he does it during meetings!)

Sit on a straight-backed chair, feet planted in front of your hips, or cross-legged in lotus position if you're very supple.

Place your thumb on your right nostril to close it and breathe in deeply through your left nostril.

Now close your left nostril with your index finger and release your thumb.

Breathe out completely through your right nostril.

Feel your chest muscles relaxing and your shoulders dropping away from your neck as you exhale.

Now breathe in through your right nostril with your finger over the left one.

Close your right nostril with your thumb, release your finger and breathe out through the left nostril.

That is one cycle.

Repeat for ten minutes if possible.

For calming and un-tensing purposes, you will find that even a few cycles make a real difference and also re-energise you.

Lifestyle tips

* ditch any polyester and nylon or other manmade fibres in your wardrobe – manmade fibre traps the heat and makes flushes much worse. Wear easily removable layers of natural fibres: cotton, silk and wool are good.
* carry facial blotters in your make-up bag (for more beauty tips, see pages 328 to 348).
* carry a fan with you always, either an old-fashioned one (elegant and romantic for day and evenings) or a battery-operated, handbag-sized mini-fan.
* if you are blow-drying your hair with hot air, have an electric fan on near you to cool down the air.
* have an electric fan in your bedroom.
* never get dehydrated. Drink plenty of still, cool water – at least eight glasses a day between meals – and unsweetened cool drinks; keep a jug of water by your bed at night. Keeping well-watered is vital for the functioning of the whole body and brain, particularly if you suffer from headaches or constipation.
* keep your blood sugar levels stable by eating every three hours.
* make sure all rooms are well ventilated.
* have pure cotton bed linen; use layers of blankets or coverings, which you can cast off one at a time, rather than duvets.
* if you are sharing a bed and you're casting off the bed-clothes while your beloved freezes, consider separate coverings (it can save a trip to the spare room ...)

* for night sweats, try sleeping under a giant pure cotton bath towel and a lightweight blanket. Towelling insulates without retaining too much heat and also soaks up sweat without feeling cold and clammy.
* keep wet face flannels in the fridge at home and have one by your bed at night; take facial wipes out with you and a facial spray.
* for a bit of pampering, wring out the face flannels in cold water mixed with a drop of essential oil of chamomile or lavender, or rose water.

Longer term

You read it here first! These two easy-to-make-at-home drinks have literally changed the lives of some women. Of course, there is no single panacea for everyone's problems, but they may help your hot flushes and they're certainly good for your health in general. You can drink them both on a daily basis.

Daily Menopause Cocktail

We say longer term because this delicious drink may take about 14 days to work although some of Michael's patients have reported instant relief. The recipe comes from Californian-based aromatherapist Ixchel Susan Leigh, who did lots of research and developed this potion when she was hit by severe hot flushes and night sweats. It stopped them 'dead in their tracks' within two weeks, she says. Ixchel recommends taking it daily until you are certain the symptoms have gone for ever. If you stop and they come back, just start again.

> Ixchel: *"At 51, all of a sudden, MAJORRRR night sweats hit! Such severe hot flashes, averaging nine to eleven*

*per night! And the sweating, not just a dribble but what
seemed like buckets and soaking sheets. For the first
time in a couple of years, I was actually grateful that I
did not have a man in bed next to me! That was only
night-time … Imagine them again at no notice during
the day: meeting a friend for lunch; in line to buy gro-
ceries; getting up in front of hundreds to teach a class –
that didn't make me nervous, but the hot flashes did."*

Recipe

- ¼ cup (about 60 ml) aloe vera juice
- 1 small glass raw organic apple juice
- 200 mg powdered elemental magnesium citrate (take as
  capsules if you can't get the powder or substitute magnesium taurate which Kathryn Marsden considers the best
  formulation for the menopause: her preferred brand is
  Biocare)
- 1 g black cohosh capsule/s

Mix juices together then stir in the magnesium citrate.
Swallow the black cohosh capsules with the drink.

BE CAREFUL
If you are taking black cohosh in this form, don't take it
in another way too unless you've consulted a medical
herbalist.

Daily Menopause Smoothie

There is considerable evidence that plant oestrogens (known
as phytoestrogens) can help ease menopausal symptoms and
particularly hot flushes. Soya (e.g. tofu) may help about
half of women with hot flushes. This smoothie, devised by

naturopath Roderick Lane, is based on organic tofu and berries. It is delicious and nutritious, takes only a few minutes to make and is a perfect labour-saving breakfast or replacement meal any time.

The secret of success with soya is consistency, consistency, consistency! according to Roderick. So try hard to have 35 to 50 g of organic soya (tofu or tempeh) daily, rather than lots once a week. (For an HRT cake recipe containing soy and other menopausal goodies, turn to page 267.) If you are vegetarian and using tofu as your only protein source, go for 100 to 125 g daily. If you don't manage to consume your soy during the day, take a supplement containing the same amount. The particular antioxidants (proanthocyanidins) in red and black berries can also help. Roderick emphasises that any milk you drink should be organic whole milk, not skimmed: this is because whole milk contains vital nutrients including Essential Fatty Acids, in the form of conjugated linolenic acid or CLA. (If your blood lipids are abnormally high, however, you may be advised to use skimmed milk.)

Recipe

* 35 to 50 g organic tofu, cut into small chunks
* 1 cupful of red and purple fruit (you can buy frozen packs at supermarkets)
* 1 banana
* a little organic milk, yoghurt or apple juice to help the mix blend more easily
* whizz up all ingredients in a blender and drink slowly

Nutritional supplements
Generally, we believe it's always better to get nutrients through food rather than supplements if possible: they are

better absorbed and it's much more difficult to overdose. However, researchers in Israel have published studies showing that a soy product marketed as Tofupill, which they call a phyto-SERM (selective estrogen receptor modulator), significantly helps the range of menopausal symptoms, including hot flushes, vaginal dryness, low libido, aches and pains and insomnia. It may also improve bone mineral density in the hip and spine. Importantly, it does not appear to increase the risk of breast or womb cancer, unlike combined HRT and some other pharmaceutical drugs.

As well as the menopause cocktail and/or menopause smoothie, you can try taking daily supplements of vitamin C with bioflavonoids (up to 1 g daily) and vitamin E (up to 800 to 1,000 ius daily), which have been shown to help with several menopausal symptoms including hot flushes. Vitamin C also helps skin (as well as a multitude of other factors), and vitamin E improves vaginal dryness and has been shown to help prevent heart disease and cancer.

Gamma oryzanol, an antioxidant extracted from rice bran oil and found in whole grains, fruits and vegetables, has been shown in research to help hot flushes. In two studies, women were given 100 mg three times daily, and 70 per cent showed decreased hot flushes. It may also help reduce the risk of heart disease.

Herbs

If hot flushes persist, you may want to add in herbs. Scientific research is throwing up several herbal superstars, notably black cohosh, which is accepted as useful by many conventional doctors. A systematic review of herbal medicinal products designed to treat menopausal symptoms says that the available evidence for black cohosh is promising and that red clover may help with more severe menopausal problems. However, there is so far no hard evidence for other herbs or for evening primrose oil although many herbalists and traditional health practitioners are clear that they are effective.

Sage (which was not included in the review above) is another time-honoured remedy, which also shows promise with memory loss. But, as we've said before, don't mix them up yourself and always *always* read the contraindications. Try one product at a time, or one of the suggested combinations below, for at least a month. If your budget allows, we suggest consulting a registered medical herbalist or natural health doctor.

Choices

* the proprietary brand Meno-Herbs, which Michael suggests to his patients, contains nine herbs including wild yam, black cohosh, dong quai, agnus castus, red clover, Siberian ginseng and nettles, which are known to act synergistically in helping with menopausal symptoms. Combining this with Woman Essence by Australian Bush Flower Remedies is working well for a significant number of women in Michael's practice, although a proper research study is still required (Woman Essence is also helping regulate periods in some younger women we know).

* Dr Marilyn Glenville, nutritionist, psychologist and author of several excellent books on natural alternatives to HRT, recommends Femarone 40+, which has a combination of agnus castus, dong quai, false unicorn root, blessed thistle, squaw vine, black cohosh, ginseng, barberry, cayenne, cramp bark, ginger, raspberry leaf, uva ursi, sarsaparilla and liquorice.

* extract of sage has also been shown to help reduce hot flushes by 50 per cent in a small study. Alternatively, you

can make sage tea: cover two level teaspoons of dried sage leaf (heaped if fresh leaf) with half a litre / one pint of boiling water, infuse for an hour, then drain. When cool, take one tablespoon every hour or two until sweats go. You can also combine this with black cohosh.

"Sage drops helped me the most and also someone saying, 'Love your hot flushes, go with it, feel the pleasure of the heat coursing up through your body'. Very zen, but it works. I reckon that when you fight it and tense up, everything gets worse. As soon as I began to love my flushes, they stopped bothering me!"

Hilary Boyd, nurse and writer

- herbalist Andrew Chevallier recommends taking a combination of black cohosh, wild yam and/or agnus castus for hot flushes and to promote hormonal balance. (Don't try to mix them up together; take them separately in the doses suggested. Remember to read the contraindications first.) Try black cohosh and liquorice for hot flushes with extreme tiredness. Remember: if you're drinking the menopause cocktail daily, you won't need to take extra black cohosh unless it's recommended by a qualified herbalist.
- the combination of black cohosh and St John's wort works well for some women, especially when the flushing is combined with poor sleep, low mood, nervous exhaustion and/or long-term stress. Scientific research backs up this use. A new product called Black Cohosh & St John's Wort by MedicHerb has been launched on the market in the UK and other countries. It contains a low amount of black cohosh (42 mg) and a standard 300 mg of St John's wort.

Mind/life problems

Hot flushes can make life hell for some women and their partners and family. If this rings a bell with you, do consider some kind of talk therapy, such as counselling, just to help tide you over the worst. Also make sure that you are getting plenty of relaxing healing therapies, which can enable you to cope better.

SYMPTOM: period changes

Over the three (or so) years leading up to the menopause, most women find that their menstrual cycle becomes irregular – with longer or shorter cycles – and periods may become unusually heavy. Over a third of women in their late 40s have shorter cycles which skip ovulation, leading to heavier bleeding. Heavy bleeding can also happen when the cycle is longer than usual and the period is delayed.

Oestrogen and progesterone, the hormones that decline at the menopause, are of course the same reproductive hormones that control your periods. So it stands to reason that the changing hormones of menopause will involve changes to your periods. The upset is virtually certain to have some effect on your cycle before periods finally cease but exactly how it will affect you is unpredictable. Some women have very few changes, others find that cycle lengths career madly from short to long as changing hormones dictate.

The upside about menopause-related period problems is that they can't last forever – after your last period they vanish! Also remember that improving your diet, exercising and relaxing will help.

But it's important to know that heavy and painful periods can also occur due to other complaints. Most are benign (that means non-malignant) and include:

- fibroids: these are benign growths of the muscle of the womb.
- endometriosis: where some of the lining of the womb grows outside it.
- adenomyosis: where some of the lining of the womb grows in the muscle of the womb.
- pelvic infection (aka pelvic inflammatory disease or PID): this is an often forgotten but well-recognised cause of period problems; your partner will also need to be checked for this.
- other hormone problems including thyroid disorders.
- bleeding/blood clotting abnormalities.
- side effect of the copper-containing coil IUD.

There is the outside possibility of something more serious, such as cancer of the womb: endometrial or cervical cancer, so don't forget our favourite maxim: 'If in doubt, give a shout!' In other words, go to your doctor if you're worried.

You should expect your doctor to take a full history and carry out an examination including an internal investigation, which takes a good look at your cervix. Depending on the findings, you may then be referred for further investigations and/or to be seen by a gynaecologist.

The following tests and investigations may be done by your doctor or gynaecologist.

- full blood count to check if you are anaemic.
- thyroid function test.
- ovarian hormone analysis.
- transvaginal ultrasound scan to include ovaries and uterus.
- cervical smear.
- swabs to see if there is infection.
- endometrial sampling (sample of lining of womb with very fine tube): usually done as outpatient.
- hysteroscopy, where a small camera is put into your

womb, sometimes with an anaesthetic, and a small sample is taken; this is an update of the rather rough and ready old technique called D&C (dilatation & curettage).

SOLUTIONS: period changes

Heavy periods

Western medicine
If you have heavy vaginal bleeding, there are several options. If any abnormality is found after the tests above, this would obviously be treated. Often, however, no actual cause is found. The medical treatments that need to be considered in that case include those outlined below but doing nothing is an option too. Remember: having regular check-ups is very important.

Drug therapy

- **Non-steroidal anti-inflammatory drugs (NSAIDs, such as mefenamic acid)**: these can help to decrease the amount of bleeding as well as the pain. Ideally they should be started 48 hours before you bleed, which is not always easy if you have irregular bleeding. Side effects: mainly gastrointestinal problems, occasionally headaches and/ or dizzy spells.
- **Antifibrinolytic drugs:** e.g. tranexamic acid; these can help to decrease blood flow. Side effects include: nausea, dizzy spells, abdominal cramps.
- **Hormone therapy**: in the past, progestogen therapy was considered beneficial for heavy periods but this advice has changed although it may still occasionally have a role with irregular periods; standard HRT may be considered or possibly the Pill. Side effects: see pages 144 to 146.
- **Levonorgestrel-containing coil (the Mirena coil)**: this can be very effective for reducing heavy menstrual blood loss

and should be considered as an alternative to any surgery; see page 380. Information on side effects is also on page 380.

Surgical treatment

- **Ablation of the endometrium (removal of the lining of the womb):** this used to be done by a method called trans-cervical endometrial ablation or resection, when the womb lining is cut out or burnt away with an electric current. This has complications which may necessitate an emergency hysterectomy but is still sometimes used to remove polyps. Generally, nowadays, more modern and safer treatments are used, including balloon thermal endometrial ablation (using heat) and microwave endometrial ablation (using a microwave). Both these methods were endorsed by the UK NHS National Institute for Clinical Excellence (NICE) in August 2003. Other newer methods are also being investigated.
- **Hysterectomy:** this is the final solution if bleeding is uncontrollable by the above methods but may be offered as first line of treatment in very severe cases or if you have large fibroids.

This surgical operation to remove the womb may be done through the vagina, by cutting into the abdomen or through laparascopic (keyhole) surgery. It may include taking out the ovaries and/or the cervix.

Hysterectomy is an established and effective treatment but that must be balanced against its potential risks, which include upsetting bladder function, pain with intercourse, painful scar, and a clot in the legs or lungs which is potentially life-threatening. It's very important that you are fully informed about the procedure and the risks involved. Ask for literature and see whether there is a nurse counsellor at the hospital who you can talk to. Ring advice lines. Do not be afraid to say no if you decide you don't want a hysterectomy.

Irregular periods

These may be longer or shorter cycles, as we explain above. If you are worried you must go and scc your doctor who will take a thorough history, examine you and arrange appropriate tests. If you have not had a period for six months and then you have a bleed, please do go and see your doctor because it's just possible you may have a serious problem, which should be treated as soon as possible for the best chance of a cure. This is referred to as postmenopausal bleeding and many hospitals in the UK have postmenopausal bleeding clinics where you will be fast-tracked for a scan and possibly an endometrial sample or hysteroscopy.

Treatment is not always necessary for irregular periods. It largely depends on the cause: if you are perimenopausal and have no other underlying cause and it's not affecting you too badly then it may be better to take this phase as it happens. However, hormonal drugs such as the Pill or combined HRT may be prescribed to try to help balance your hormones.

Self-help

For period problems in general:

- make sure you don't get dehydrated (can lead to migraines)
- keep your weight under control
- avoid alcohol and other stimulants
- eat every three hours
- take plenty of moderate exercise and do therapeutic yoga

Nutrition

If you are having heavy periods, make sure you don't become anaemic. Talk to your doctor about possibly taking a gentle iron supplement such as Floradix or Spatone+, or one dessert-spoonful of black-strap molasses and a teaspoon of Marmite daily (not mixed together!). Make sure you are getting plenty of vitamin C (from fruit and veg) to help the iron get absorbed properly.

Herbal

For heavy periods, Andrew Chevallier recommends drinking nettle tea, which is good for heavy bleeding and helps prevent anaemia. He also suggests trying the herb agnus castus (not with other hormonal treatment, e.g. HRT or the Pill) plus lady's mantle.

Ayurvedic medicine

A remedy called Qars Bandish Khoon (literally 'blood vessel stop') may be prescribed to help heavy bleeding but only by a registered practitioner.

Flower remedies

We hear reports that Australian Bush Flower Woman's Essence helps in some cases of irregular bleeding.

Stress

Make sure that you keep your stress and anxiety levels as low as possible. Get plenty of rest and relaxation. Do yoga and meditation. Have therapies such as massage, aromatherapy and/or reflexology. Also consider homeopathy to help balance your mind and body.

If your period problems are triggering a cascade of stress problems with your partner and family or at work, it may be helpful to talk these through with a counsellor or psychotherapist.

SYMPTOM: depression, anxiety and low mood

> Katie: *"The greatest problem for me is my complete lack of motivation. My husband died four years ago at the age of 63. I am comfortably off financially and could afford a nicer home and unlimited holidays but have no inclination towards either. I would be so glad to have more enthusiasm for life if only for the sake of my family and friends. Sometimes I feel as though my life is on hold, waiting for the time I return to my old self."*

A mountain of negative emotions – from anxiety to depression with side helpings of guilt, hopelessness and lack of self-confidence or simply 'feeling low' – can affect women around the menopause. Women report feeling insecure, wobbly, emotional and frightened. (Michael asked one of his patients how she was. Somewhat to his surprise, she replied 'Fine!' Then she explained that 'fine' stood for 'f***ing insecure, neurotic and emotional'.)

According to UK government figures, one in five women suffers 'unwelcome stress' and the peak time is between 35 and 54. One in three women experience a more severe form of low mood at some time (double the figure reported for men). Stress can be positive, of course, the sort of feeling that gingers up life and makes us rise to a challenge. But all too often, women feel that their lives are out of control and too much is expected of them. This can lead to anxiety – where you are wound up too tight – or depression – where you feel yourself sinking into a low state in which you feel pessimistic and often hope-less.

According to counsellor and family therapist Philip Bacon, symptoms of anxiety include:

* feeling wound up and restless.
* thinking and worrying about what might happen tomorrow and what happened yesterday.
* feeling panicky.
* having trouble getting to sleep.
* wanting to avoid people and challenges.
* setting unrealistic expectations for yourself.
* getting indigestion and other gut problems.
* feeling constricted in your throat; hyperventilating.

Symptoms of depression include:

* feeling isolated and misunderstood.
* feeling tired or exhausted.
* sleeping badly; waking too early.
* feeling sad for no apparent reason.
* losing your appetite and losing weight *or* eating much more than usual and gaining weight.
* not wanting to do anything or be interested in anything.
* having no motivation at work.
* feeling worthless and/or hopeless.
* having no self-confidence.
* fearing the future.
* having thoughts of ending your life.

The big question is whether low mood and depression at this time of life can be caused by the hormonal changes of menopause alone. There is no doubt that hormones have an effect on the brain and it's obvious from every woman's monthly cycles that hormones can have a marked positive and negative effect on mood. So it is quite possible that feeling low and unhappy, or having emotional ups and downs, may be connected to falling levels of oestrogen, progesterone and testosterone, which lead to changes in other hormones, notably the feel-good hormones serotonin and dopamine.

Professor Marie-Annette Brown of the University of Washington Women's Health Care Clinic has researched this subject widely. The results are detailed in her book *When Your Body Gets the Blues*, in which she puts forward the theory that anxiety and depression in women can, in many cases, be attributed to the ups and downs of your reproductive hormones. In particular, she says, up and down cycles of oestrogen can affect serotonin levels profoundly. 'Every time there is a dip in the level of oestrogen, a woman may be experiencing a reduction in the dopamine and serotonin activity in her brain, less blood flow to her brain and a decrease in the interconnectedness of her brain cells.' It's the surge and withdrawal of oestrogen every month that accounts for PMS, according to Professor Brown. Then, with the unpredictable nature of hormone production leading up to menopause, women are at even greater risk of the body blues. The answer for Professor Brown and her colleagues is not HRT.

The reasons that some women don't seem to be affected by this oestrogen-related low mood syndrome are twofold, says Professor Brown: genes and lifestyle. Our genes we can't alter but lifestyle we can. That's where getting out in the daylight, regular moderate daily exercise and a good diet with adequate B vitamins, vitamin D and selenium can make all the difference. Expect to see a lot more research on this in the next few years.

However persuasive the hormonal hypothesis is, life circumstances are almost always involved too. We detail a whole list of possibles on page 37, so flip back to that if you've missed it. Then think of a few obvious scenarios, such as tiredness. If you are deprived of sleep due to night sweats, this can set up a spiral where you become so tired that you get low. Everyone knows that when you're exhausted, the glass is always empty and the end of the world is probably nigh. So anxiety or depression could be triggered by lack of sleep due to night sweats.

Another possibility is chronic aches and pains. You may have got so used to them that you hardly notice but long-term pain is depressing. Get it checked out by your doctor or health professional and think about consulting a chiropractor or osteopath. Equally, some drugs can cause depression as a side effect. It's very important that you look at all the factors in your life that could be causing you to feel low: this may be done most easily with a health professional. (Sarah had a bad accident and then took morphine for the pain for some months, which resulted in appalling depression, insomnia and panic attacks: but her reaction to the drug was undoubtedly exacerbated by stress from the accident and a very sick father. The solution was integrated therapy: homeopathy, herbs, nutritional supplements, psychotherapy and chakra therapy; unfortunately Western medicine could only offer sleeping pills and anti-depressants which her consultant advised her not to take.)

What is certain is that the effect of life stresses that often occur around this time, both for women and for their partners and families, can be enormous. If you are anxious or depressed, it could be due to falling levels of oestrogen or the pressures of life, or to a double whammy of both. So remember you don't have to be Superwoman: just do the best you can.

If you do feel depressed continuously and/ or feel like ending your life, you must seek professional help immediately. Never be afraid to ask for help. Self-help solutions may not be able to help you here.

SOLUTIONS: depression, anxiety and low mood

Remember HALT: don't get Hungry, Angry, Lonely or Tired. One nurse says she uses this as a checklist if she feels low. Very often, her bluesy mood is due simply to being exhausted and not eating properly: early nursery-type supper and straight to bed with a magazine or book changes her whole world view by the morning.

Self-help

* exercise daily for at least 20 to 30 minutes. More is better! If you're feeling down, move. Buy a small trampoline – brilliant for weight loss and cellulite (but be careful if you have a bad back). Walk, dance, ride, do anything but don't sit and brood. Yoga is great.
* go out in the daylight for at least an hour a day.
* eat well, every three hours, and take carefully chosen supplements.
* take warm to hot baths with aromatherapy oils for 20 minutes (but not just before bed or you risk insomnia).
* learn relaxation techniques such as meditation (may be part of yoga).
* talk to friends.
* do things you enjoy.
* plan adventures and expeditions.
* laugh.
* cry.
* play your favourite music.
* sing and dance.
* watch your favourite video.

Plan your strategies for black dog days
Sarah's neighbour Kate, a single working mother of two in her mid 40s, came up with this idea and we thought it was

so good we asked her to develop it to put in the book. This is what she suggests:

"When the going gets tough, you need a 'difficult day menu' to get you through. No one single thing will instantly lift your mood or solve life problems but taking care of yourself really can get you through in a reasonable enough way – which is an achievement.

Those days are all about negative feelings: you *feel* powerless to shift a mood, which you *feel* will last forever. Ideally, you need to see the red alert when the feelings are on the horizon and take steps before they set in. If you're still having periods, mark them in your diary and keep a record of how you feel. If you don't catch the black dog in time, you can still apply the same principles.

So don't wait until the bad times roll! Make a list of things that make you feel good or at least okay. It needs to be individual to you but here are some broad guidelines:

- *be very gentle to yourself*: if you're feeling low, very low, even getting out of bed can seem impossible; one friend says she had to fall on the floor and crawl sometimes. Acknowledge the achievement, tell yourself that was a triumph.
- *keep reminding yourself that this state is temporary*: write a big note and stick it up saying, 'This will not last forever', but also know that it's okay not to be okay all the time. Everyone has up and down days: it's not a crime to admit to it.
- *keep life simple*: make a list of what you have to do and what's bothering you; prioritise and do the things you have to do that day – anything else is a bonus. Do not try and solve your life problems, invent a cancer cure or climb Mount Everest. Set your sights low (or what you would normally perceive as low) and make everything achievable. Each thing you complete is a step further on and

away from the black dog. Keep telling yourself how well you are doing even if it's 'Hurrah! I've put the rubbish out!' Anything is good. Remember, you've done it – no one else did – so well done!

- *treat your senses*: when you're low, your sensory world needs TLC. Think taste, smell, sound, sight and touch. So have a bath and slosh on body lotion, fix your hair, put on make-up, wear your fave clothes – look for soft, gentle, cosseting fabrics – and scent, eat food you like and make it look nice (watch the caffeine, sugar, alcohol intake though because they often cause mood swings), light fragrant candles at home and work and put scented pads in your bed and the car, put flowers round the house (or twigs if it's winter), put on the music you like best and so on. You get the picture. It's all about reconnecting with your positive side and you can do this on a very basic level.
- *a 'should'*: there are not many 'shoulds' on black dog days but you *should* exercise – gently. Just the rhythm of moving can help dispel the gloom. If you're lucky enough to be able to combine some inspiring views, go to them. Yoga and dance can really help: if you do yoga with a teacher, tell them how you feel because there are specific poses that can help you feel empowered.
- *give yourself treats*: do something you really like, with people you like; one friend goes to the sea and potters round collecting shells and pebbles, another grooms horses.
- *hug someone and/or stroke an animal*: look for comfort; Kate makes for her neighbour's beautiful cats. If there's no one else to hand, give yourself a big hug.
- *start a Lovely Letters Box or Happy Album*: on nobody-loves-me days you need to know you are worthwhile and precious; so keep all the nice letters and mementoes of lovely times in a file or album to remind you that they will come round again.

- *don't expect other people to sort out your life but do ask for help if you need it*: no one can live your life for you – only you can do that and you decide how you want to. But people can help: draw up a list of friends and professionals who can be your Fear Busting Team. On the whole, it's not a good idea to regularly get on the phone and moan. They need to be people who care for you but will give you tough love if necessary and be straight with you.
- *get outside yourself*: finding someone or something else to care about, or doing an activity you love and can lose yourself in, can make all the difference. So trying looking out rather than in."

Nutrition

- maintain even blood sugar levels – so always eat every three hours.
- cut down or cut out sugar, alcohol, drugs, coffee and quit smoking: all these have been linked to depression.
- cut out wheat and gluten-containing grains: they can profoundly depress some susceptible people; investigate other food allergies.
- eat well but don't overeat.
- eat oily fish (salmon, sardines, pilchards, mackerel, herring, trout) at least three times a week and consider a fish oil supplement (the Essential Fatty Acid contained in fish oil has been shown to help all types of depression). *The Natural Way to Beat Depression* by Dr Basant Puri and Hilary Boyd is full of information on using fish oil to treat low mood. See Useful Books section for details.
- do not try to lose more than one to two lb per week if you are dieting.
- take a multiple vitamin and mineral supplement daily.

Herbs

Take the herb black cohosh (in quantities given for hot flushes) with St John's wort to lift your mood and help you sleep. This may take a few days or weeks to work so try an over-the-counter herbal mixture (such as Kalms or NatraCalm) while you wait for it to kick in. Consult a practitioner if you can.

Light therapy

If it is really impossible for you to get out in the daylight, sit in front of a light box or panel.

Homeopathy and other therapies

Check our list of complementary and alternative therapies in Chapter Six and see what appeals to you. Homeopathy and herbalism can help 'tweak' your mind and body so that you feel better, often very quickly. Healing too can have an immediate and potent effect. Relaxing therapies are obviously helpful but so are 'doing' ones. You might find that, say, doing art or music once a week gives you an outlet for expressing yourself that really helps. Dancing Scottish reels has been shown in research to increase the joy factor more than any other activity, although amateur dramatics came in a close second. The key is to do something you enjoy that allows you to stop thinking about your problems for a bit. Usually, company is good because it shows you that you are an okay human being.

Drug therapy

This must be individually prescribed and is often given in conjuction with 'talk' therapy, such as psychotherapy.

SYMPTOM: weight changes

Hormones and weight simply can't be separated. Think of the intimate connection between weight gain (breasts, hips etc) and puberty. In the same way, menopausal women almost never escape some weight changes when it comes to the hormonal chaos of menopause. Women on HRT seem to be most afflicted by intractable weight gain (see page 182).

Almost everyone, women and men alike, puts on weight as they get older. Research shows that most women put on a significant amount of body weight between 38 and 47 years. There are several reasons, including:

- *changes in the way your body handles food*: simply speaking, everything slows down as you get older. From around 40, your metabolism (the rate at which your body functions, and uses the energy supplied by food) slows down by one to two per cent every ten years so you need to eat less to do the same amount. If you don't adjust your food intake, you could put on 20 to 30 lb per decade
- *decreased amount of exercise*: you may not notice it but you probably do considerably less physical activity as the years go by. Remember: you can add more activity to your life in little ways: always walk up stairs rather than using the lift; don't use the TV remote control, get up and push the buttons; walk every day
- *changes in various hormone levels*: for women, these are oestrogen, thyroid and the recently discovered leptin, which has a role in both the reproductive process and appetite control. Interestingly, it is now being suggested that your weight increases as you go towards menopause to help protect you from symptoms. One form of oestrogen (oestrone) is produced in fat cells so your body reasons that having a few more is better to help protect you against

menopausal symptoms. This absolutely does not mean that it's good to be really overweight or obese.

SOLUTIONS: *weight gain*

Essentially, the solution is always the same – diet and exercise. Your goal should be being fit rather than thin. There is no doubt that being a little plumper is not only natural but helpful for women going through menopause and you should be comforted to know that the weight gain does invariably level out by a couple of years after your final period. See our chapters on food and exercise. We also suggest doing yoga not only because it's a wonderful all-round form of exercise but also because it helps you move gracefully.

If you find it difficult to moderate your appetite, consider the connection between mood and food. When you are bluesy, the temptation is often to eat sugary, fatty, creamy foods – they remind us of our first big security blanket, breast milk. Do see the information above on serotonin levels: very often, low serotonin (the hormone whose lack is associated with anxiety, depression and insomnia) is allied to an instinctive desire for comfort foods. Balance your serotonin levels with more daylight, exercise and adequate nutrients and you may not feel like medicating your low mood with food.

If you are on HRT and experiencing weight gain, do talk to your doctor about this: it may be possible to switch to another preparation.

When it comes to crash dieting, just don't. Crash, or yo-yo, dieting is the most ineffective and dangerous thing to do. It's a hiding to nothing, since the body goes into famine mode whenever it sniffs food: that's the raid-the-fridge-and-stuff syndrome. Virtually all dieters put on all the weight they lose and more within two years. Increasing your exercise levels, while eating sensibly, is the best way of staying fit and shapely. Research shows that acupuncture may help if it's difficult to shed excess pounds.

INSTANT FIX!

This is the ultimate, self-help solution that works instantly! You can appear to lose 5 lb in 5 seconds just by standing and walking taller and straighter.

Take off your shoes, and stand with your feet a hip width apart. (In front of a long mirror preferably ...)

Have your weight on the centre of your feet; roll on to your toes, then back to your heels to see the wrong positions, then find the centre over your instep.

Breathe slowly and rhythmically, in through your nose and out through your mouth; as you breathe, let your chest float upwards and your shoulder blades sink down.

Tighten your buttock muscles, but don't stick your bottom out.

Draw in your tummy muscles – imagine you're sending your navel towards your spine.

Don't forget to breathe! And don't let your shoulders shoot up ...

Now look straight ahead and imagine a thread drawing the crown of your head up towards the sky; let your chin and jaw relax. Remember to let your chest float up and your shoulder blades sink down. (Think back to when you last had some really good news, or were really full of life and joy ... you'll find everything shoots upwards!)

Breathing gently, prowl around the room, swinging your arms, hips and legs gracefully like a cat (think of models on a catwalk). If you can, do this barefoot on the grass. Your feet should face forward, leading with your second toe. When you take a step, let your heel touch down first.

Practise daily!

SYMPTOM: *gut and bowel problems*

Many women complain of a range of different gut and bowel symptoms through the menopause. These include:

- bloating: this is often mistakenly linked with weight increase but is a separate factor
- flatulence
- constipation
- diarrhoea

There is some evidence that hormonal changes may be a contributory factor; for instance, changes in progesterone levels can cause bloating but there are many other possible and likely reasons for these problems. Usually the underlying cause is more to do with lifestyle than anything sinister: stress, irregular mealtimes, processed and sugary foods, plus increased stimulants such as coffee are major culprits. But it's important to remember that there may be something more serious. If you have any concerns or experience a change in your bowel habit or any bleeding, do consult your GP.

Common causes of gut and bowel problems include:

- **dehydration**: not drinking enough water is a huge and greatly underestimated problem, causing constipation and an overall unhealthy effect on the functioning of the whole body. Dehydration at 2 per cent means your body is down about 1 litre of fluid. Likely results are that your energy fails and you feel generally under par. You may also have a headache and other aches and pains. If your urine is dark yellow, you are dehydrated. Aim to pee pale.

- **decrease in roughage (fibre from fruit and vegetables) in your diet**: this can cause constipation (also see page 263 for solutions to constipation).
- **decrease in physical activity**: can cause constipation, bloating and loss of muscle tone, which may make it difficult to evacuate your bowel completely.
- **stress**: can lead to diarrhoea and constipation, also digestive upsets of all kinds such as flatulence and bloating.
- **smoking**: causes excess stomach acid and can lead to a wide variety of gut problems.
- **candidiasis**: can cause a range of bowel problems, particularly bloating (see page 263 for suggestions).

If you have gut and bowel problems, we recommend a recent book by nutritionist Kathryn Marsden called *Good Gut Healing*, which gives you a complete lowdown on gut and bowel problems and solutions. For more information on eating the right diet for your biochemical type, which should help to settle these problems, read *The Adam & Eve Diet* by Roderick Lane & Sarah Stacey.

SOLUTIONS: gut and bowel problems

Quick fixes

- never eat on the run or standing up; eat slowly, chew your food thoroughly until it's almost soupy and sit for ten minutes at the table after your meal; then take a gentle stroll.
- don't chew gum and don't talk with your mouth full – you take in air and the result is anything from hiccups to burps and other explosions.

- don't slouch; sit up straight so your digestive organs are less likely to trap gas.
- try food combining: this means not eating proteins and starchy foods, for example meat and potatoes and pasta at the same meal (see page 265 for chart). Eat fruit as a snack between meals, not with meals except at the beginning if necessary; never eat fruit at the end of meals because it can then ferment in your stomach causing more problems.
- drink plenty of still filtered water between meals; aim for eight large glasses (1.5 to 2.5 litres) daily.
- try to drink less with food and certainly not fizzy drinks; sip a little still water if you wish.
- drink ginger or mint tea as often as you wish (either use a teabag or brew it yourself); for stomach gripes, try stewed black tea of any kind with some grated ginger: the tannins in the black tea (it must be stewed) kill the bugs and the ginger settles your tummy.
- avoid raw cold food in winter; poach vegetables and fruit instead.
- avoid citrus fruits, except for lime juice which is more alkaline and gentle on a sensitive stomach.
- avoid rich food of all kinds.
- avoid creamy, fatty, sugary foods (that includes dried fruits and snack bars); make sure you carry healthy snacks such as oat cakes or rice cakes and hummus with you so that you don't have to snaffle a chocolate bar.
- avoid all processed foods, which may contain additives and preservatives.
- eat live natural yoghurt (sheep's or goat's rather than cow's) to help repopulate your gut with good bacteria. (You could also try a course of probiotic supplements for three months and continue long term if you feel better).
- try herbal supplements containing meadowsweet or

charcoal for reducing gas if you suffer bloating and digestive eruptions (breaking wind etc.).
- reduce stress and take up relaxing therapies such as yoga and meditation.

Longer term

If your symptoms continue, go and see your doctor. Try the following options while you're waiting:

- cut down on cow's milk in all forms because many people are sensitive to it; wherever possible substitute goat's or sheep's milk products and try non-cow's milk in drinks, e.g. soya, oat, almond, rice.
- if that doesn't work, or only helps to a limited extent, cut out the foods below for three days and see if it makes a difference. If it does, reintroduce the food groups singly and see what happens. If you suspect that you have a food intolerance or allergy (which can be very serious, and sometimes fatal), you must consult an appropriately qualified health professional. For more information, read *The Complete Book of Food Allergy and Intolerance* by Professor Jonathan Brostoff and Linda Gamlin.

  - wheat-containing foods, e.g. bread, pasta, cakes, biscuits, pies, breakfast cereals containing wheat.
  - yeast-containing foods and drinks, e.g. bread, pizza, nan bread, vinegar, blue cheese, mushrooms, Marmite, beer and grain drinks including vodka and whisky.
  - coffee and other alcohol.
  - sugary foods of all kinds.
  - citrus fruits.
  - fizzy drinks.

○ beans of all kinds, broccoli, cauliflower, onions, spinach and beetroot.

If you have tried the solutions above, including chewing your food thoroughly, and you still have bloating and other problems, you may need to take a digestive enzyme. If the problems only occur when you eat meat, try digestive enzymes (such as Polyzyme forte by Biocare), and hydrochloric acid supplements (such as Hypo-D by Nutri, or HCL and Pepsin by Biocare) with each meal. Do not take HCL supplements if you have an ulcer. If you have problems with foods other than meat, take digestive enzyme supplements with each meal.

Professional help

Always consult your doctor or health professional if symptoms continue long term.

Traditional therapies that may help include nutritional therapy, acupuncture, Western herbal medicine, Chinese herbal medicine and Ayurvedic medicine.

SYMPTOM: sexual problems

Around the time of menopause, women frequently complain of a range of sexual problems, varying from decreased sexual desire (libido), difficulty in getting aroused, pain with sex and reduced – or almost no – ability to have an orgasm.

Although life factors, including stress and changing relationships, play a significant role, part of the problem is certainly down to hormones. Painful sex is often due to vaginal dryness, which is directly caused by a decrease in oestrogen. It results in reduced production of mucus (lubrication), which is coupled with a loss of elasticity in the vaginal walls, making the vagina thinner and tighter. This makes penetration difficult and painful and also causes discomfort through frictional pain and often bleeding in the vagina after sex. Small wonder that libido can take a nosedive.

If the vaginal problems are sorted out early on, which should be fairly simple (see below), and there are no or few relationship issues, the situation should be straightforward to solve. If, however, sexual problems are caused by both physical and psychological issues, an integrated approach is vital. And remember – it takes two to tango! Men are affected both by their partner's problems and by their own: they may be going through their own insecurities and adjustments to ageing, which may result in erectile problems. Talking about it to each other is the start. You may also need to get some professional psycho-sexual help. Therapist Frances Emeleus, who is accredited by the British Association of Sexual and Marital Therapists, says that while the idea of sexual therapy is still a big taboo, it can help many people. 'I've seen people turn their sexuality around after 25, 30, even 40 years of mediocre sexual relations. Bodies are magnificent things and sex should be a celebration – so spend time and imagination on it.'

It's also important not to see penetrative sex as the be-all and end-all of making love. Tenderness and intimacy – connecting with your lover – are at least as big a part of lovemaking, and often neglected. Cherish yourself and your partner. Spend plenty of time stroking and cuddling. If you are on your own, don't feel that you can't experience sexual sensations: experiment with pleasuring yourself. According to Dr Marilyn Glenville, dry vaginal tissues can be revived by lovemaking and orgasm, so it's a case of use it or lose it.

The art of touching

Sensate focusing exercises, which are aimed at mutual pleasure only – not penetrative sex (important to agree this, because otherwise there may be an underlying anxiety), have proved a successful way to overcome problems for many couples. These can be done to/with another person or by yourself. Remember they are for your pleasure; don't get tempted to give your partner a massage.

TOUCHING WITH A PARTNER

* make sure the room is warm, light candles and put on lovely music. Use body lotion, scented if you both like.
* take it in turns to silently explore all over the other's body with different degrees of touch, hard and gentle, circular or long strokes; spend 15 minutes on the back and the same on the front, caressing everywhere except breasts and genitals. Notice which parts give you the most pleasure – or not.
* you can do the same on your own too. Glory in your own body.
* it may also help to practise slow controlled breathing to help increase the sensitivity of the erogenous zones of the body (hips, breast, lower abdomen and thighs). Twice a day, spend 10 to 15 minutes practising retention breathing, advises Dr Mosaraf Ali of the Integrated Medical Centre in London. (See page 80 for details.) Then when you are touching your partner or yourself, instead of hyperventilating as most people do, you can go into this pattern of respiration, enhancing your sensitivity and pleasure.

Some women notice little change to their sex lives during and after the menopause; others experience significant improvements and some become dissatisfied. If you are looking to keep an already good sex life on track, if you would like to improve one that is a bit of a let-down or even rekindle one that petered out some time ago, you may like to bear in mind the following ten tips which were written for this book by Val Sampson, author of *Tantra: The Art of Mind Blowing Sex* (no half measures there then ...):

1 Never forget that sex (even a one-night stand) is inevitably part of a relationship, however brief. If you and your partner lead distant, unconnected lives, it is unlikely you will experience a flourishing sex life. Take time to talk together before you make love. Spend an hour or so exchanging your views on your lives and your thoughts and feelings: don't interrupt each other and don't descend into talking about routine domestic matters or even your children, if you have them. Stick to talking about yourselves as individuals, as if you were talking to a fascinated stranger. When it comes to sex, communication is the best lubrication. (And laughter is one of the best aphrodisiacs.)

2 That's not to say there aren't times during the menopause when you could do with a little more help to make sex physically comfortable. If your vagina is drier than it used to be, don't suffer in silence or you'll end up looking for excuses not to have sex. Buy a lubricant and use plenty of it (see suggestions below under Vaginal Dryness). Menopausal or not, nearly every form of sex from masturbation to intercourse is greatly enhanced by a decent amount of extra lubrication. Steer clear of using massage oils in intimate areas, as they block the vagina of its ability to cleanse itself and can result in infections.

3 Hormonally speaking, the more sex your body has the more it wants, and the reverse is true as well. Don't worry if your relationship is basically sound but your sex life feels like a dim and distant memory. Begin to build physical closeness by introducing more affectionate touching into the relationship, whether it's giving your partner a hug after you've been apart or holding hands as you walk together. Studies have shown that without regular touch, women become depressed and uninterested in sexual touch while men become more aggressive and uninterested in any touch that is not sexual. So you both need to cuddle and touch often.

4 Some people have a narrow view that regards anything not in the same style as reproductive sex as not being 'proper' sex. In other words, unless penetrative sex and ejaculation take place, it's a waste of time. This is a sad misunderstanding of our complex sexual and emotional natures. For many women, a tender massage or even a long talk and cuddle can be just as satisfying, albeit in a very different way, from penetrative sex. And for a surprising number of men, especially as they approach middle age, discovering they are not always under pressure to perform sexually in intimate encounters can be a welcome relief.

5 While it's easy in our youthful, looks-obsessed culture to worry about signs of ageing, studies have shown that men find their partners increasingly attractive as they grow older. We may be a world away from Aboriginal culture, where older women are highly regarded sexually by younger men, but it is heartening news, nevertheless.

6 Women's sexual problems tend to decrease as they get older, while the reverse is true of men. Hysterectomies, however, can sometimes mean that you experience a

reduced blood flow in the pelvic area. As a result, you may require slightly more stimulation to become sexually aroused and reach orgasm: tell your lover what you need.

7 Women in long-term relationships can experience desire differently from men. They may become aroused *after* they begin to make love, rather than beforehand. So although they haven't felt particularly sexy beforehand, their partner's touch arouses them and triggers a desire to continue. They may choose to make love for an intimate connection with their partner, rather than being driven by lust or feelings of passion, and as a result, desire follows arousal. So ...

8 Don't subscribe to the myth that sex has to be spontaneous or it's somehow lacking. Once infatuation wears off, desiring your partner is a decision. Equally, there isn't only one appropriate kind of sex for grown-ups – the sort of heaving, grunting and gasping you see in movies. There can be cuddly sex; companionable sex; comical sex; and that's just the kind beginning with 'c'. The joy of sex as you grow older is that you can appreciate its infinite variety.

9 Boredom is the number one enemy of a good sex life and one of the reasons why men and women are tempted to have affairs. Novelty, on the other hand, is a powerful aphrodisiac and huge numbers of people think they have to change their sexual partners, with all the personal chaos and upheaval that involves. In fact, you don't need to change your partner, you need to change the sexual routines in your current relationship. If you want to make some changes, but don't know where to begin, you could always buy a couple of sex books and do a little research. Equally, you could do something new with your partner, whether

it's learning to sail or to tango – if you reinvent your lives together in an enjoyable and fulfilling way, you may well find the fun you share spills over into the bedroom. (And tango was designed as sex on the dance floor ...)

10 Don't be too concerned if your partner is not seized with the same desire as you to shake up your sex life. He may be caught up with all sorts of concerns and sex is down the bottom of the list. (Or the boot may be on the other foot and he may want more than you feel able to give.) The most important thing in a relationship is to have a solid core of friendship giving you each strength and succour – and pleasure. If you begin to make small, unthreatening changes in your behaviour – such as just being more demonstrative and more fun! – your partner will inevitably respond. One word of warning though: always put yourself in your partner's shoes and ask yourself what your reaction would be. 'I'm bored with our sex life,' for example, is probably not a good approach, whereas, something like 'It might be fun to try "X" – please will you try it with me?' is practically guaranteed a good response.

SOLUTIONS: sexual problems

Quick fixes for vaginal dryness

* for topical application as a lubricant try V Gel by Higher Nature. This natural product contains aloe vera combined with vitamins, minerals and herbs including comfrey, which help to assist the elasticity of the vaginal walls. We have also heard good reports of a product called Sylk, which is a natural water-soluble lubricant derived from the

kiwi fruit vine. Natural vitamin E oil can also be applied locally (if you use capsules, which should be pierced to release the oil, make sure they're yeast-free). Other options include Replens and Sensel which are over-the-counter products.

Longer term

- take pure organic aloe vera juice daily for four to six months, two tablespoonfuls in a cup of still water. Ideally find a source of pure raw aloe vera pulp (you can grow your own aloe plant and squeeze the pulp or ask at your local health shop for the product) and mix this with a teaspoon of Manuka honey and take it every other day for two to three months. You can continue taking it after that if you wish unless you get loose stools, in which case stop.
- make sure you have a good intake of Essential Fatty Acids in your diet, and consider a supplement.
- soya contains plant oestrogens called isoflavones, which help balance oestrogen levels. Eat organic soya products including milk, yoghurt and tofu (see our menopause smoothie recipe on page 84). Or try supplementing with soya. Also eat crushed linseeds on cereal and/ or yoghurt. These help to soften the vagina.
- try vitamin C (1,000 mg daily), which may help the vagina walls become more elastic, and also vitamin E (800–1000 IU). One study showed that taking vitamin E daily for one to four months improved vaginal dryness in 50 per cent of women.
- adding a pinch of chillies and black pepper to foods such as soups and stews helps the mucous production in the vagina, according to Dr Mosaraf Ali of the Integrated Medical Centre in London. (Don't worry if it causes a slight burning sensation when passing urine or stools).

* do pelvic floor exercises, which help to increase blood circulation to the pelvic region and revive the vaginal tissues (like sexual intercourse and orgasm).

Professional therapies

If all else fails, talk to your doctor about the possibility of using an oestrogen-based vaginal cream or tablet. The usual recommendation is to use this once a day for two weeks and then twice a week for a short period of time: always discuss long-term use with your doctor. You can use this in tandem with vitamin E applied vaginally (remember to use yeast-free capsules) and a natural lubricant for sex.

SYMPTOM: urinary incontinence

Urinary incontinence is a common problem and can affect women of all ages but it's most often found in older women and particularly women around the menopause. About 20 per cent of women in their 50s are thought to suffer. Incontinence used to be a real taboo subject and there was little information, help, advice or support. But the situation has improved dramatically. Now there are several support groups and much improved treatment with specialist physiotherapists to direct it.

Combined HRT may be a contributory factor to incontinence, according to correspondence published in the *New England Journal of Medicine* (January 3, 2002). Two women doctors, Sally E. McNagny and Nanette K. Wenger, suggested that physicians should be cautious about prescribing HRT because it is 'significantly linked with worsening urinary incontinence', according to the findings of the Heart and Estrogen/Progestin Replacement Study, which looked at the use of HRT in 2,763 women aged 65 or older. However, according to the *Journal of the British Menopause Society*, various studies have shown that oestrogen replacement (as opposed to combined HRT) can improve or even cure urinary stress and urge incontinence.

The problem area is the lower urinary tract, a term which refers to part of the bladder and the urethra (the 4 cm long tube that connects the bladder to the outside). This bit comes from the same developmental pathway as the vagina so it's reasonable to suppose that falling levels of oestrogen may affect its functioning as they affect the vagina.

However, hormones aren't the only culprits. Other factors that contribute to urinary incontinence include:

- **age**: the older you get the greater the likelihood of urinary problems for everyone.
- **childbearing**: vaginal deliveries cause damage to the pelvic floor, increasing the likelihood of stress incontinence.
- **previous vaginal surgery**: such as hysterectomy or an operation on your bladder.
- **overweight and obesity**: this is an underestimated but huge problem: pressure on your bladder causes a decrease in its ability to hold urine.

It may be difficult to trace the exact cause of urinary problems and your doctor may refer you to a gynaecologist for further investigations. At that point, full details will be taken and you will have a vaginal examination. You may then need some bladder tests, known as urodynamic studies, to find out exactly what is going on.

The two main types of incontinence are stress incontinence and urge incontinence (medically called detrusor instability). In stress incontinence, you leak urine when you make a physical effort such as laughing, coughing, sneezing or running. With urge incontinence, you have to pee very frequently throughout the day and often also during the night. You may need to go in a rush and in severe cases, you may start to urinate before reaching the lavatory.

SOLUTIONS: urinary incontinence

Self-help

* keep fluid intake to 1 to 1.5 litres daily. If your main problem is getting up at night, have your last drink early in the evening.
* constipation may aggravate bladder symptoms so make sure you're not constipated (see page 263).
* a chronic cough makes stress incontinence worse so, if you still smoke, give it up!
* if you are overweight or obese, get down to a sensible weight.
* check with your doctor for bladder infection or cystitis which can trigger urgency and frequency; any infection detected in a urine specimen can be treated, usually with antibiotics.
* vitamin C is important because it increases collagen production, which can help to retain the elasticity in the urinary tract and prevent incontinence, according to Marilyn Glenville – so take a multivitamin and mineral supplement designed for the menopause (e.g. Biocare Femforte or Lambert's Gynovite) and 1,000 mg vitamin C three times daily.
* useful herbs for stress incontinence are ladies' mantle (Alchemilla vulgaris) and horsetail (Equisetum arvense), recommends Marilyn Glenville.

Professional treatment

Stress incontinence

Treatment is geared to strengthening the muscles of the pelvic floor and improving support to the bladder to prevent it from dropping. This means doing pelvic floor exercises (the bonus is that it's really good for your sex life ... and sports like skiing). These are usually taught by a specialist physiotherapist and involve repeatedly contracting – squeezing – the pelvic floor muscles. You're usually told to hold each squeeze for four to five seconds, five times in a row. You should do this several times daily. Once you get the trick, you can do it wherever you are: easiest when you're standing still – one woman we know tried it on an escalator and got quite carried away.

Pelvic floor exercises are very effective for mild stress incontinence and may cure the problem completely. But you have to do them daily and long term. If you don't, muscle tone will deteriorate and the problem will recur.

Because the exercises are a bit dull, someone dreamt up the idea of using vaginal concs, for 15 minutes twice a day. These small weighted cones are about the size of a tampon and also have a string attached for easy removal. The lightest weight is 20 g, the heaviest 100 g, and they come in sets of three or five. (You can buy them over the counter without a prescription.) The idea is that when you put one in the vagina, the pelvic floor muscles have to work to keep it in place. When you can hold the lightest in comfortably, you move on to the next one. It may be a bit sore at first as the muscles get used to working, but this wears off. They only work for stress incontinence so do make sure this is your problem before buying them.

Women who are unable to contract their pelvic floor muscles because of illness or disability can be given electrical stimulation treatment by a physiotherapist.

Surgery is a possible option if the problem is more severe or if a woman is past childbearing age and wants a permanent cure. Newer, less invasive operations such as a tension-free vaginal tape (TVT) procedure are becoming readily available.

Urge incontinence

This is caused by an overactive bladder muscle (called the detrusor). As this squeezes, it increases the pressure in your bladder and makes you feel you have to go to the loo when in fact there is only a little bit of urine in your bladder. This kind of incontinence may worsen during the menopause, although it's most common in the elderly.

The simplest and most effective way to help treat urge incontinence is by 'bladder drill' – retraining the bladder to hold a normal amount of urine before contracting. This is successful in about 90 per cent of cases and can be co-ordinated as an inpatient or outpatient. The drill involves keeping a record of the number of times urine is passed during each day. Fifteen minutes is then added to the shortest time interval and the patient is not allowed to empty her bladder until then, even if it's painful or she wets herself. It sounds awful but over a period of two to four days, the patient learns to control her bladder and last the allotted time. The time limit is then increased in 15 minute increments until a time of four hours is reached, which is pretty normal.

Drug treatment to reduce the pressure of the overactive bladder muscle is often used for this condition. However there are unpleasant side effects, which occur with varying severity in most patients. One side effect is a dry mouth, which obviously encourages the patient to drink more – not a good idea in the circumstances.

This type of incontinence is made worse by anxiety and

stress so therapies such as yoga, psychotherapy and hypnosis are all used successfully.

SYMPTOM: restless legs syndrome (RLS)

This is a common problem where you feel creepy-crawly, itchy-twitchy, sometimes painful sensations in your legs and possibly thighs. It's rather like having a minor, more wide-spread cramp. The same may happen with your arms. You can relieve it by shaking your limbs, or walking if it's your legs. (Difficult if you're on a long car journey – the times Sarah usually experienced this.) It's not serious but if it happens half an hour into sleep, which it often does, it can cause insomnia. Because of this, RLS is categorised as a sleep disorder.

The exact cause is unknown although there may be some correlation with hormones since 20 per cent of pregnant women experience it and 15 per cent of women over 50 and around the menopause. Because of the link with pregnancy, scientists have investigated nutritional deficiencies and found that folic acid (one of the B vitamins) and iron are frequently deficient in sufferers. There may also be a deficiency in minerals including calcium and magnesium. There is a genetic component too so if you experience it, it may well be that your mother did too. It seems to occur more frequently in older people but also occurs in the young when it's known as growing pains.

Dr Mosaraf Ali of the Integrated Medical Centre in London believes that the condition occurs because the brain misfires and stray electrical currents go to the limbs, triggering invol-untary movements as well as aches and pains. He has found that circulatory problems, caused by sitting or standing still in the same position for a long time, are a prime cause.

It is also associated with medical conditions including

anaemia, diabetes, kidney failure and Parkinson's disease. It a side effect of certain drugs including some antidepressants.

There is certainly a relationship to stimulants, especially caffeine and other compounds that affect the nervous system, such as nicotine and alcohol. Anxiety and stress also appear to be linked to the condition, possibly by triggering the production of chemicals that don't allow your body to relax totally. Dr Ali believes that stress overload causes a massive electrical impulse to the brain, which triggers such involuntary reactions.

Another possibility is spinal misalignment, which may be putting pressure on nerves.

SOLUTIONS: restless legs syndrome

Self-help

- cut out stimulants and all drinks containing caffeine: coffee, tea, hot chocolate, colas, alcohol, nicotine (and any drugs such as cannabis); consider a brief detox diet (see page 277).
- investigate the side effects of any pharmaceutical drugs.
- make certain that you eat enough iron and vitamin B-containing foods; top up with black-strap molasses, Marmite and brewer's yeast if necessary.
- make certain you have enough calcium and magnesium in your diet, or consider a supplement (e.g. Calcium, Magnesium and Boron by Biocare).
- take regular exercise in the evening if you suffer this problem at night.
- practise a meditation technique such as yoga.
- massage your neck and shoulders at night (for details that can be freely downloaded, see Dr Ali's website www.dr-ali.co.uk).

* massage your legs with olive oil and sea salt before going
to bed (don't have a hot bath as this may contribute to
insomnia by overheating your body).

Professional help

Conventional medicine doesn't really have a lot to offer
apart from drug therapy in severe cases. Homeopathy,
acupuncture and nutritional therapy would be good avenues
to explore. Also consider consulting an osteopath or chiropractor to check on any spinal problems. Massage will
decrease stress and help you to relax.

SYMPTOM: aches and pains

You may experience an increase in joint and muscle pains
around the menopause. Fingers, wrists, elbows and shoulders are usually more troublesome than hips and knees,
possibly due to a reduction of collagen in the joints. Backache
is a common problem and migraine a possibility.

Eating plenty of oily food and phytoestrogens will help
but other foods can make the problems worse: Sarah had
awful aches in her pelvis (accompanied by squawks of rage
at getting old) until a biochemist friend suggested she stop
eating her favourite organic ice cream and cut down on
cow's milk – the pains went and have never returned.

SOLUTIONS: aches and pains

Quick fixes

* drink lots of water (again!), at least 1.5 litres of still water
between meals.
* cut out caffeine-containing drinks and other stimulants.

- cut down on dairy foods and red meat, at least for a while
- eat plenty of oily fish, nuts, seeds and plant oils.
- also eat phytoestrogens including soya, chickpeas and lentils.
- consider a supplement such as glucosamine and chondroitin.
- keep warm: a hot-water bottle on a sore place will help.
- take plenty of gentle to moderate exercise such as walking, swimming, yoga, working out at the gym (see Ros's story).

Ros: *"I went through hot flushes and night sweats but by the time I was 53, I was suffering from a much more painful condition which I didn't initially associate with the menopause. Every joint in my body ached. Walking downstairs was a slow process and although I am overweight not only the weight-bearing joints were aching, it was my wrists, elbows and shoulders as well as knees and ankles. The nurse at my GP's surgery suggested that I take part in an 'active health' scheme that they run with the local leisure centre. I've never looked back. Nowadays, I exercise three times a week for 1 to 1½ hours, have better eating habits and have cut back on my caffeine intake. I eat masses of fresh fruit and veg (mostly organic). I have a mug of tea each morning but no coffee or tea for the rest of each day (except at weekends) replacing it with cold tap water. The aching joints are a thing of the past and I feel supple and strong. The flushes and sweats are all gone and life feels really good."*

Herbal

Devil's claw (harpagophytum) is a natural anti-inflammatory, which is very helpful for reducing aches and pains; Bioforce now produce a one-a-day tablet.

Professional help

It's always worth getting a check-up with an osteopath or chiropractor, or your doctor, to see if anything is out of alignment. Acupuncture can help reduce pain greatly on a short- and long-term basis, as well as tuning up your whole body.

5

HORMONE REPLACEMENT THERAPY

The youth drug, the hype, the woman and her doctor

This chapter covers:
- the history of HRT
- the evidence
- our assessment of the pros and cons
- the risks
- if you still want to try HRT
- questionnaire: Is HRT for you?
- talking to your doctor
- how long should you stay on HRT?
- coming off HRT
- different types of HRT with pros and cons
- trouble shooting

"I have been on HRT for ten years and now off it I feel no different. Why was I on it?"   Anon

The way that male doctors have approached female biology and particularly the menopause has been bizarre for a very long time. In the second century AD, the great Greek physician and philosopher Galen decided the ovary was 'the female testicle and a filter for women's semen'. In medieval times, the menopause was thought to be due to tumours growing within the uterus. Later medics claimed that blood was being trapped within the womb and applied leeches to the cervix as a cure ... During the eighteenth century, the menopause was described as a 'catastrophic attack', which ruined women's looks and sexuality. A century later, doctors decided that blood 'not passed' turned into fat.

Leeches weren't the only unpleasant (and potentially dangerous) treatment you might have been given: cures over the centuries have included purgatives, toxic metals, extracts of ovaries and placentas, bloodletting or, more agreeably, trips to take the waters at a spa.

Things got worse again in the early twentieth century with some doctors opining that it was women's own fault they suffered the menopause – heaven knows what you were supposed to have done, but in any case postmenopausal females needed to avoid sexual excitement because it might attract blood to the brain.

Modern medical science entered the picture with the discovery of hormones in 1906. The link then began to be made between the ovaries and female hormones. In 1923, American researchers Edward Doisy and Edgar Allen reported in the *Journal of the American Medical Association* that they had found an ovarian hormone in test animals. Two groups of women's reproductive hormones were named: the oestrogens and the progestogens. Doisy finally isolated an oestrogenic hormone, later named oestrone, from the urine of pregnant women in 1929. Progesterone from the progestogen group was isolated in 1934 by three different teams.

As we've explained earlier, the menopause happens because your ovaries fail and that leads to a decrease in oestrogen production. The logical thing seemed to be to replace it and that's how Hormone Replacement Therapy was born. It was first launched in the 1930s when injections of oestrogen were given to ease menopausal symptoms. It had to be injected because scientists hadn't worked out how to stop oral versions being destroyed by digestive juices. But in 1942, an oral form of oestrogen was developed from the urine of pregnant mares. Around this time, scientists also realised that if a woman's ovaries – her source of oestrogen – were removed at an early age, she had an increased risk of developing osteoporosis (loss of bone density).

In 1946, the first alarm bells rang. Doctors began to suspect that giving oestrogen alone – medically called 'un-opposed' oestrogen – to women with a womb could increase the risk of cancer of the womb (also called endometrial or uterine cancer) up to sevenfold. By the mid 1970s, more and more evidence had accumulated to show that the risk increased over the years. But by then, HRT had begun to gain its legendary status as a panacea for ageing women. Much of this was due to evangelising by a Manhattan gynaecologist called Dr Robert Wilson.

Wilson wrote a book called *Feminine Forever* in 1966, which outlined a doom-laden scenario for postmenopausal women who did not drink at the hormonal fountain of youth. Breasts and genital organs would shrivel. They would become 'dull and unattractive'. Moreover, he said, 'the meno-pause [sic] is both unnecessary and harmful'. But abracadabra! there was an answer: 'The deficiency disease created by ovarian decline with its painful, disabling and even fatal consequences, is responsive to therapy.' In other words, HRT.

Restoring women's oestrogen levels was neither unnatural nor risky, according to Wilson. 'From a purely biologic point of view, estrogen therapy can hardly be regarded as altering the natural state of life ... It is the case of the untreated woman – the prematurely aging castrate – that is unnatural.' He continued: 'The myth that estrogen is a causative factor in cancer has been proven to be entirely false. On the contrary, indications are that estrogen acts as a cancer preventive.'

Dr Wilson's son Ronald later admitted that his father's work and expenses had been entirely financed by the pharmaceutical company concerned, whose oestrogen drug derived from the urine of pregnant mares went on to become America's fifth bestselling prescription drug.

Aggressive marketing tactics have underpinned much of HRT's iconic reputation. Take the same pharmaceutical company's 1972 film on the *Physiologic and Emotional Basis of Menopause*, designed to give doctors information about hormone treatment that they could pass to their patients. According to Joe Neel of the NPR news organisation (August 2, 2002), the commentary includes this: 'The physical alterations that are associated with the menopause may induce emotional changes. When a woman develops hot flashes, sweats, wrinkles on her face, she is quite concerned that she is losing her youth – that she may indeed be losing her husband.' In the film, a woman in a nightgown, sitting in a plaid easy chair in front of a fireplace says, 'My boys are both gone and my husband is away a great deal with his work. The evenings bother me most. And I think we all give thought to the fact that our husbands might become interested in a younger woman, but I don't dwell on the subject.'

We should add here that drug companies are now compelled by legislation to promote their products responsibly. Many also have general and genuine educational programmes for both patients and health professionals.

The uterine cancer scare peaked in 1975 when the *New England Journal of Medicine* published two studies documenting a strong link between uterine cancer and oestrogen therapy. There was panic and the drug's popularity plummeted. Then researchers came up with a solution, which was seized on by the pharmaceutical companies: a progestogen (from the other family of female sex hormones) could be combined with oestrogen to protect the womb lining from over-stimulation. This reduces – but does not entirely negate – the increased risk of endometrial cancer. (In fact, some scientists today are beginning to say that because of the significantly increased risk of breast cancer with combined oestrogen and progestogen therapy, it might be better to give women oestrogen alone and run the lower risk of uterine cancer. The combination of oestrogen and progestogen may be a greater problem than ever anticipated.)

At the beginning of the 1980s, HRT was relaunched on the market with a fanfare. Women without wombs could go on taking oestrogen replacement only, while women with wombs could take combined oestrogen and progestogen replacement. (This is still the advice today.) Most doctors, and of course the drug companies' marketing departments, hailed it as the Holy Grail for middle-aged women, claiming it had a litany of health and beauty benefits in addition to easing menopausal symptoms. The claims were, to some extent, backed up by research published in peer-reviewed journals.

Over the next two decades, however, it became clear that the claims were based on an over-enthusiastic interpretation of the rather scanty scientific evidence. A big study of nurses in North America, published between 1980 and 1994, appeared to show that HRT users had less heart disease. Wyeth, still the leading maker of HRT, asked the Food and Drug Administration, America's regulatory body, to label the drug as protective against heart disease without further research. That was opposed vigorously by women's health campaigners – and with reason. By the mid 1990s, it was becoming clear that the Nurses Health Study was misleading: the benefits were due more to what's called the 'healthy user' effect than to HRT. Researchers found that the HRT group took the drug as part of a healthy lifestyle package: they had more medical check-ups, smoked less, ate more fruit and vegetables, were more physically active and less likely to have diabetes – all major contributory factors to avoiding heart disease. Later studies showed that, far from protecting against heart disease, combined HRT caused more heart attacks, strokes and blood clots in the first year of use.

In the last five years, the emerging scientific evidence has begun to disturb doctors and patients alike. In March 2002, leading scientists, funded by the US government, drew up an 'International Position Paper on Women's Health and Menopause'. In it the authors say: 'Past perceptions about appropriate indications for the use of HRT were based almost entirely on clinical experience and observational data. These perceptions are being questioned as new knowledge emerges from clinical trials.' The only evidence supporting the use of HRT was for hot flushes and urinary symptoms, also prevention of bone loss. (Since then, the European Expert Working Group has advised that HRT should not be the first line of treatment for osteoporosis because of the increased risks of breast cancer and heart disease; see below.)

In May 2002, one arm of the biggest prospective trial of Hormone Replacement Therapy in the world was suddenly stopped three years before the eight-year study was due to end. Over 16,000 postmenopausal American women received letters from Jacques Roussouw, acting Director of the Women's Health Initiative (WHI), telling them to stop taking their medication. The trial was randomised so that half were on combined HRT, half on dummy pills. Five years in, it was clear that the group of previously healthy women taking combined oestrogen and progestogen therapy had more cases of breast cancer, heart attacks, strokes and blood clots. As Dr Roussouw explained to the world's press: 'A drug which was meant to be good for [the women] was, in fact, doing them harm.'

In autumn 2002, the European WISDOM study of combined HRT, funded by the Medical Research Council in Britain (and it had already cost more than £10 million), was halted for the same reason. (For detailed information, see the section entitled What Key Studies Tell Us About the Risks on page 141). However, the Women's Health Initiative continued the arm of the trial researching the effects of oestrogen replacement only on women without wombs. Although this was due to report in 2006, it too was halted early, in March 2004.

As well as heart disease, the significantly increased risk for women on HRT is breast cancer. The latest study, reported in the leading British medical journal the *Lancet*, looked at more than 1 million women between 50 and 64. It concluded that using HRT was associated with a significantly increased risk of breast cancer, which could be fatal. (For more details, see below: Key Studies: Million Women Study.)

In November 2003, the expert working group of the European Committee for Proprietary Medicinal Products, which covers 28 countries, recommended that HRT should not be prescribed as the first line of treatment for osteoporosis, because of the increased risks of breast cancer, heart attacks, strokes and clots. Oestrogen is now listed as a carcinogen by the American Food and Drug Administration (FDA).

In February 2004, a Swedish study of HRT for women who had previously had breast cancer was stopped early because the risk was deemed unacceptable. Women had been randomised to two groups, one receiving HRT, the other a dummy pill. The group receiving HRT had a three fold increased risk of a recurrence of cancer. (HRT is prescribed for breast cancer survivors because treatment for breast cancer may lead to early menopause and severe hot flushes. However, alternative treatments, including acupuncture, homeopathy and hypnotherapy, have been trialled successfully on breast cancer survivors with menopausal symptoms. Herbs may be useful, including black cohosh).

It must be said here that a small number of scientists believe that, on close inspection, some of the research studies are flawed. However, this does not really change the consensus view on HRT, although the debate will doubtless continue.

The extraordinary saga of the rise and fall of HRT is not just down to profit-oriented drug companies employing aggressive marketing. Doctors have been less than rigorous in scrutinising research throughout and in prescribing HRT and monitoring its effects. Some women in Britain have lost legs due to clots, which have occurred because doctors didn't read their records properly and heed the comprehensive safety information given by the manufacturers.

With hindsight, the main problem was the lack of sufficiently rigorous research before HRT was launched, combined with the desire of doctors – and their menopausal women patients – to find a magic bullet to solve every problem at one fell swoop.

But the reality is that, even with a lot of pre-launch research, no drug is 100 per cent safe and should continue to be monitored in the long term. This is why every doctor should keep informed of research and has a duty to tell the Committee on Safety in Medicines of any suspected adverse drug reaction among patients. So if you have problems, make sure your doctor does do that. (Equally, if you have complications with any complementary preparation, you should tell your practitioner.)

WHAT'S THE TRUTH?

Here we list the claims that were made for the use of HRT in menopausal women and the current knowledge. (Remember it's a different issue for younger women under 50 with premature menopause for whom HRT is an important protection against bone loss.)

- **Claim**: prevents hot flushes and night sweats.
  Evidence: effective in most cases.
- **Claim**: improves urinary problems.
  Evidence: oestrogen improves urinary frequency and helps some types of stress incontinence; recurrent urinary tract infections may also be prevented. But combined HRT may make matters worse.
- **Claim**: improves vaginal dryness and tightness.
  Evidence: effective in most cases.
- **Claim**: prevents osteoporosis in the short and long term.
  Evidence: now not recommended as first-line treatment because of risks; however the WHI study did show a reduction in the risk of fracture and it may have a role in the management of osteoporosis; the downside is that any benefits reverse to start point shortly after HRT is stopped.
- **Claim**: improves low mood.
  Evidence: may help hormonally related low moods.
- **Claim**: improves insomnia.
  Evidence: may help hormonally related sleep problems directly or by alleviating sleep disturbance due to night sweats.
- **Claim**: protects against heart disease and strokes.

Evidence: research shows that combined HRT may increase the risk of heart disease, stroke and blood clots in leg or lung; oestrogen-only replacement increases the risk of strokes.

- **Claim:** improves hair and skin.
  Evidence: may help but may equally cause hair thinning and acne if an unsuitable progestogen is prescribed.
- **Claim:** prevents memory loss and retards the progress of Alzheimer's disease.
  Evidence: past studies have shown an improvement but others differed including the WHI study which showed that both combined HRT and oestrogen alone may cause significantly more cases of Alzheimer's disease and other dementias in women over 75; the Royal College of Physicians has said that there is no role for the use of HRT in the prevention or treatment of Alzheimer's disease.

BE CAREFUL
Always ask for full information about any drug – and read it!

OUR VIEW ON HRT

We have now spent years reading all the research on HRT and listening to women's experiences of it. Its use is controversial but one thing is clear: it is not a wonder drug that should be taken by all menopausal women. Evidence shows that the benefits are much fewer and the risks far greater than the manufacturers and doctors initially claimed – and women hoped for.

But you should remember that all drugs (even aspirin) have potential risks and side effects so the baby shouldn't be thrown out with the bath water. Anecdotally, many women say they feel well and happy on it: equally, however, many report feeling better when they come off it.

What has largely been left out of the medical equation until now is that there are effective alternatives to HRT, as we detail in this book. Unfortunately for their patients, few doctors have made themselves aware of these, although this is beginning to change. While this scientific limbo persists, the most useful thing women can do for themselves is to follow an integrated approach and to keep aware of all the issues.

Michael says: 'I'm the first to admit that I was, in the past, an oestrogen evangelist. Now I feel that although it has an important role, especially for women who go through the change early, it is not my first line of treatment for most patients. Women need to be fully informed of the risks and benefits, kept up to date with new research and offered a full range of alternative options, as well as counselled about the crucial role of diet, fitness and stress management.'

Here is our conclusion based on the available information:

- hormone replacement therapy has some benefits for some women.
- there are definitely risks but in absolute terms (see What Key Studies Tell Us About the Risks on page 141) these are smaller than they may seem from headlines: women must always be counselled individually and the risks and benefits explained so that they can make up their own minds.
- unless contraindicated, HRT is very important for women who have premature menopause, either due to premature ovarian failure or surgical menopause, because of the risk of bone loss. Diet and weight-bearing exercise are crucial too. If you have had a subtotal hysterectomy, you may or may not need HRT.
- While HRT is not essential for women with menopausal

symptoms, HRT is effective at helping hot flushes and night sweats (medically called vasomotor symptoms) within 4 to 12 weeks of starting; if you take HRT for hot flushes, continue for a year because the symptoms will likely return if you stop.

- HRT helps to relieve hormonally related mood changes and insomnia.
- HRT can help vaginal problems including painful sex but it may take several months: systemic HRT (oral, patch, implants or nasal routes) or oestrogen cream or tablet form applied to the vagina may improve vaginal irritation, dryness, soreness and itching not due to infection or other skin problems; may also help painful sex, bleeding after sex, reduced sexual arousal, vaginal discharge or infections.
- HRT may help urinary problems, including urgency (rushing to have a pee), frequency (peeing a lot) and nocturia (getting up in the night to pee). It may also help some types of urinary incontinence in tandem with drugs or surgery. But again it may take several months for symptoms to improve.
- HRT may also help skin and hair loss in some women and may improve wound healing, age-related macular degeneration (the most common cause of blindness in older people) and tooth loss, but all these areas need more research.
- for women with menopausal symptoms there are alternatives to HRT, which must always be discussed and offered by the doctor.
- if HRT is prescribed, it must be in the smallest effective dose for the shortest time.
- the routes of delivery must be tailored to individual women: some routes (see below) may be as effective and carry fewer risks than the traditional oral route.
- if HRT is offered, the option of adding in a progestogen must be fully discussed, together with the benefits, risks and

side effects, plus their routes of administration (see below).

- regular follow-up of HRT users is essential, not only for monitoring but also to keep up with the latest research.
- if you are on HRT and have concerns, do NOT stop abruptly unless there is an emergency (see How should you come off HRT? page 157); see your doctor as soon as possible to discuss the situation.
- if you are not on HRT and want to discuss its possible benefits for you, consult your doctor. Regular check-ups are essential whether you are on HRT or not.

HRT: THE RISKS

Absolute versus relative risks

To understand the increased risks of illness for postmenopausal women with HRT so that you can make an informed decision, it's important to understand the difference between *relative* risk and *absolute* risk, and put it in the context of the period of time.

Relative risk is the increased percentage: so, for instance, the risk of getting a clot in your leg around the age of the menopause is one in 10,000 for non-HRT users, which increases to three in 10,000 if you take HRT. That is a 200 per cent increase in your relative risk, which sounds terrifying. But the *absolute risk* is in fact an extra two cases of blood clots per 10,000 women.

There is still an increased risk, which is a personal tragedy, but the risk is not as vast as it's often portrayed.

What key studies tell us about the risks

The Women's Health Initiative (WHI) study in America (published in the *Journal of the American Medical Association*

2002 and 2003), where about 8,000 healthy postmenopausal women took combined HRT and the same number a dummy pill, was halted in May 2002 just over five years into the eight-and-a-half-year trial.

One in every 100 women experienced an 'adverse event' of some kind over the five-year trial. The additional yearly threat to 10,000 women taking combined HRT compared with placebo (dummy pill) was shown to be:

- seven more coronary heart disease events (heart attacks)
- eight more strokes
- eight more pulmonary embolisms (PEs) – blood clot in the lung
- eight more invasive breast cancers

On the plus side, they would be likely to have:

- six fewer colorectal cancers
- five fewer hip fractures

There were quite a few different areas of the WHI study. The Women's Health Initiative Memory Study (WHIMS) was a randomised, double-blind, placebo-controlled trial involving 4,532 postmenopausal women over 65, who were assessed as free of probable dementia at the start. Half took combined HRT, half a dummy pill. Over four years, it was shown that there were an additional 23 cases of dementia per 10,000 women per year, with Alzheimer's disease the most common in both HRT users and non-users. It was also found that HRT did not prevent mild cognitive impairment.

Two months after the WHI combined HRT study was halted, the multi-million-pound European WISDOM Study (Women's International Study of Long-Duration Estrogen after Menopause) was stopped because of the risks. Then, in March 2004, the oestrogen-only arm of the WHI trial was stopped early because of an increased risk of stroke, and, in women over 65 on enrolment, an increased risk of probable dementia and/or mild cognitive impairment. There was no increased risk or benefit for heart disease or breast cancer. (Oestrogen in this trial was given orally: it is possible that other routes would give different results.)

The Million Women Study, published in the *Lancet* in 2003

This observational study, carried out in Britain, looked at 1,084,110 women aged 50–64 years for links between HRT use and breast cancer. It found that HRT (both combined oestrogen and progestogen, and oestrogen-only products) increased the risk of breast cancer. The risk rose the longer HRT was taken but returned to normal five years after stopping.

HRT resulted in an estimated 20,000 extra breast cancers in the last decade, 15,000 associated with combined HRT. Ten years' use of HRT was estimated to result in five additional breast cancers per 1,000 users of oestrogen-only preparations, and 19 additional cancers per 1,000 users of combined oestrogen and progestogen. Tibolone, a once-daily tablet (for details see page 165), was taken by fewer women but that risk was second to combined HRT (greater than oestrogen-only HRT).

The greatest increased risk by route came from HRT implants, followed by oral (mouth) then transdermal (skin patch). In the past, breast cancer linked to HRT has not been fatal but this study did not confirm that, although the number of extra deaths has not yet been assessed.

Other risks

HRT may also increase the risks of:

- ovarian cancer (this is still being researched).
- endometrial cancer (as we've detailed above).
- gallstones (mostly with high doses of oestrogen).
- fibroids – these may increase in size.
- endometriosis (HRT may reactivate this, causing pain).
- migraine (oral HRT appears to worsen migraine in women who already have the condition, particularly if associated with menstrual cycle, but some HRT users report fewer headaches).
- asthma (slight risk of worsening symptoms, and very small possible increase in late onset asthma).
- osteoarthritis (evidence is mixed but suggests higher risk with long-term use although there is some contradictory research showing benefit).

Side effects

With all the publicity about the risks of HRT, the side effects often go unmentioned. In fact, over half of HRT users come off it in the first year, and 74 per cent within three years, because they can't cope with these. (This type of statistic is not unusual for any long term drug use.) The most troublesome are breast tenderness, unbudgeable weight gain, headaches, mood swings and rattiness. The list below is taken from the *British National Formulary* (*BNF*) and includes some of the risks above which the *BNF* lists as side effects.

Possible side effects of HRT

- abdominal cramps
- bloating
- changes in libido – increase or decrease
- gastrointestinal upsets
- nausea and vomiting
- weight changes
- premenstrual syndrome
- breast tenderness and enlargement
- breakthrough bleeding
- heavy menstrual bleeding
- raised blood pressure
- thrombophlebitis (inflammation of wall of a vein)
- headaches or migraine
- dizziness
- leg cramps
- fluid retention
- depression, irritability, mood change
- jaundice
- increase in the size of fibroids in the womb
- intolerance to contact lenses
- skin irritation (especially with patches) and rashes
- hair loss
- runny nose and, rarely, nose-bleed with nasal spray

So how do you decide whether HRT can help you?

The first thing to consider is the difference between giving oestrogen to women under 50 and women over 50:

- women under 50 would *naturally* produce oestrogen so when doctors prescribe it they are usually replacing what has been lost *unnaturally*.
- if you are going through a premature menopause, because you have had a hysterectomy, oophorectomy or a non-surgical premature menopause, oestrogen replacement is important for you, unless there are good reasons not to take it; also make sure you are regularly monitored by your doctor.

145

- if you have had a hysterectomy but your ovaries are left intact, you still need to have an annual blood test (FSH levels) to check they are working.

But ...

- women over 50 would *not* naturally be producing the amount of oestrogen they are receiving with HRT.
- the risk of taking oestrogen is greater for women over 50 than for women under 50.
- the risk is usually linked to the length of time you take HRT, but it must be mentioned that studies have shown the risk of heart disease and stroke rises in the first year and no-one knows when any risk starts.

QUESTIONNAIRE: IS HRT FOR YOU?

With the changing view on HRT, it's wise to reassess the situation every year if you are taking it. If you're not taking HRT, but have menopausal symptoms and are interested in it, keeping up to date with your doctor on the issues may be helpful for you. If you don't like the idea of taking HRT, don't let anyone convince you that you should take it – one study showed that up to 30 per cent of women don't even pick up the prescription. And, as we keep repeating, there are plenty of effective alternatives for menopausal problems.

If you are still interested in HRT, start here:

Q Do you have menopausal symptoms?
A NO → Take our lifestyle advice on food and fitness
A YES → Continue

Q Have you had your ovaries removed?
A YES → Talk to your doctor about oestrogen replacement

A NO → Have FSH blood test to see if oestrogen levels are falling; if they're not, investigate other causes of symptoms; if they are, continue ...

Q Do you really want to consider HRT?
A NO → Investigate alternative treatments and look at our advice on food and fitness
A YES → Continue to the Traffic Light check list below

Q Are you already on HRT?
A Yes → If you're reaching 50, discuss pros, cons and alternative with your doctor; if you come off HRT, do it gradually (see page 157)
A No → Continue

Now go through the Traffic Light check list below for any contraindications to HRT.

Traffic Light Check List

Red alert

Some women should not take HRT because of the following:

* **active or recent arterial thrombosis, e.g. heart attack or stroke.**
* **active blood clot in leg or lung:** once this has been treated and the acute phase is over, you may move to Amber.
* **undiagnosed breast mass:** this must be investigated first.
* **recently diagnosed breast or uterine (womb) cancer:** you need to have comprehensive discussions with all your health professionals – it is unlikely they will recommend HRT unless you have menopausal symptoms that cannot be helped in any other way.

- **active breast or uterine cancer**: women who have had these cancers and been given the all-clear after several years may be able to take HRT if they really want to. But they should discuss the issues with all their health professionals and be fully informed.
- **acute liver disease**: it's best to avoid HRT until liver function tests are normal.
- **undiagnosed vaginal bleeding**: the causes should be investigated by examination and appropriate investigations, which may include a scan and, if that's abnormal, taking a sample of the womb lining (endometrium) via a hysteroscopy.
- **pregnancy or breast-feeding**: it would be inappropriate to give HRT after conception (unless this was through assisted conception or egg donation).

Amber alert

If you have any of the following factors, discuss them thoroughly with your doctor:

- **strong family history of breast cancer**: there is not much evidence in this area about the use of HRT but since you have an increased risk if you have two or more first-degree relatives (mother, sister or daughter) with breast cancer under the age of 45, you may not want to take the additional risk of HRT; also talk to your doctor about genetic counselling.
- **personal or strong family history of blood clots in the leg or lungs**: the biggest risk factor is personal history. If you've had one clot then you have about a five per cent risk of recurrence per year. It's important to investigate the cause, which could be pregnancy or post-operative. You can be screened for risk factors if you have a personal or

family history: if you have either antithrombin III deficiency or acquired antiphospholipid syndrome, you may be best to avoid HRT. If the screen is negative, you are still at risk of a clot but if you really want to use HRT, a transdermal preparation is advisable.

- **previous history of benign breast lumps**: there is no evidence that HRT changes benign lumps to malignant; but the incidence of benign breast lumps can increase with HRT (breasts become denser and more lumpy) and obviously needs investigation – they are not *per se* a contraindication to HRT.

- **heart (cardiovascular) disease**: HRT should not be used to help prevent heart disease (whether you have had a heart attack or not); if you have heart disease, or risk factors for heart disease, most doctors would advise you not to take HRT but to follow lifestyle changes including healthy diet, no smoking, regular exercise, treatment of high blood pressure if necessary, treatment of abnormal blood lipids if necessary.

- **other cardiovascular problems**:
  - **raised blood pressure**: conjugated equine oestrogens may in very rare instances raise blood pressure, which returns to normal once stopped, but there is no evidence that HRT in general does. (NB If you are on conjugated equine oestrogens, have your blood pressure checked regularly.) However, it is important that if you have high blood pressure you have a cardiovascular risk assessment and that any risk factors for heart disease or stroke are managed and monitored. After that, you can discuss with your doctors the appropriateness of HRT for you, in the light of the evidence.
  - **valvular heart disease**: HRT is not contraindicated. If you are on anticoagulants, you may get heavy bleeding.

If so, a sample of your womb lining (endometrium) may be taken.

- ○ **abnormal blood lipids – hyperlipidaemia**: abnormal blood lipid levels are not a contraindication but again you should have a cardiovascular risk assessment first and proceed in the light of the findings; if you do decide to take HRT, you should make sure you are prescribed the most appropriate route of oestrogen and type of progestogen.
- **previous history of gallstones**: HRT has been shown to increase the risk up to fivefold; women who have already had gallstones but still have their gall bladder may take a non-oral (e.g. transdermal) form of HRT. Taking oral HRT may reveal pre-existing gallstones.
- **any previous liver disease, even mild**: a non-oral route is advisable but close monitoring is essential; a liver function test should be done before you start HRT and, if you take it, three months later.
- **migraine and migraine-type headaches**: migraine is more common in women than men, and can be related to hormone activity – too much oestrogen can be a cause, as can fluctuating levels. Migraine can improve with HRT or get worse: transdermal patches are probably the best route. However, progestogens can also be a problem so changing the route or type of progestogen may help.
- **endometriosis**: this condition, in which bits of the lining of the womb migrate and lodge in other parts of the body, ceases at menopause but may be reactivated by replacement oestrogen; a continuous combined HRT or tibolone may be most appropriate if HRT is required. If you have any return of symptoms, go to your doctor immediately.
- **fibroids**: these may be stimulated by oestrogen so regular pelvic examinations are advisable if you already have

fibroids; any symptoms, including bleeding, pain, bloating or pressure symptoms should be discussed with your doctor.

- **bad varicose veins:** varicose veins are associated with an increased risk of post-operative deep vein thrombosis (clot in leg); a non-oral route of HRT may be more appropriate; if you have to have surgery, discuss the issue with your doctor as long as possible before the operation.

Other conditions that you should discuss with your doctor before taking HRT:

- **epilepsy:** HRT can be taken if needed; however some anti-epileptic drugs increase the activity of the liver and break down oestrogen so the transdermal route may be best (NB Some anti-epileptic drugs increase the risk of osteoporosis).
- **diabetes:** HRT can be taken if needed, provided that glucose levels are monitored closely to ensure they stabilise and insulin levels are then adjusted accordingly. HRT used to be thought an essential part of managing post-menopausal diabetes because it protected against heart disease and bone loss. In the light of current evidence that HRT does *not* protect against heart disease, and is no longer recommended as first time treatment for osteoporosis, the only indication is for controlling symptoms, in which case transdermal or low-dose oral preparations may give the most benefit. The role of progestogens for diabetics is unclear but certain types may have an adverse effect on blood lipid levels. Dydrogesterone may be the best – but discuss it with your doctor.
- **multiple sclerosis:** there is no evidence that HRT causes deterioration but as MS patients are often immobilised and thus at greater risk of osteoporosis (but also at risk of blood clots), this needs to be discussed with your doctor.

- **asthma:** this is not a contraindication but the slight reported increase in attacks and incidence of late-onset asthma should be considered.
- **otosclerosis (inherited deafness):** although no data currently shows a deterioration with HRT, it has been reported to get worse during pregnancy and with the oral contraceptive, so caution is advisable.
- **thyroid disease:** if you are taking thyroxine, your thyroid levels should be checked and possibly adjusted if you go on HRT (NB An overactive thyroid carries an increased risk of osteoporosis and of hip fracture).
- **lupus – systemic lupus erythematosus:** HRT can cause a flare-up of lupus and needs to be used with caution.
- **kidney disease:** there are varying risks to your health, some associated with medication, so discuss all the issues with your doctor.

BE CAREFUL
If you are taking any pharmaceutical drugs, or natural products, discuss the situation with your doctor before taking HRT.

If it's not safe for you to take HRT because you come into the Red category or you come into the Amber category and your doctor does not advise it, go to our sections on Alternative Treatments (start with Solving Your Symptoms on page 66).

If you don't come into either the Red or Amber categories, continue. You may feel strongly that you want to go on HRT and, if you do, you should feel free to pursue it. But you should make sure that you have the most appropriate product for you. Get as much information as you can and read through our summary of the current research on HRT above. Remember the information may change in the future, so you must keep up to date with your GP annually, or whenever you feel concerned.

Discuss your individual situation and symptoms with your doctor, ask questions (see below for suggestions) and find out what the options are. Some doctors are still very keen that all women take HRT, despite the possible risks. If you feel under pressure, remember you don't have to decide immediately. There are lots of helplines available (details on page 439), although do remember that the quality of the information may vary. You may also want to consult a natural health practitioner to get their views.

Talking to your doctor

Around this time of your life, it's important to have a general discussion with your health professional about your all-round health and wellbeing. During this you can discuss the possible role of HRT. Turn to Chapter Three for suggestions on general health check-ups.

Questions to ask about HRT

- what are the benefits of HRT for me?
- what do you think are my long-term health risks, based on my own and my family's medical history?
- why should I start HRT now, rather than waiting until I'm older?
- what product do you suggest? Does it contain oestrogen and/or progestogen and/or testosterone? And what method of delivery?
- why do you suggest this particular preparation?
- is this the lowest dose I can have?
- how long would I have to take HRT?
- what side effects could I experience? Do you have patient

153

information leaflets? May I see the manufacturer's information? (NB This is usually available on the Internet).

- if I decide to take HRT, what tests would I have first, and what kind of follow-up would I receive?
- what alternatives to HRT are there for me, both conventional and natural?
- is there a specialist nurse, or a dedicated (unbiassed) helpline, I can talk to before I decide?

What tests should you have before you start taking HRT?

- **Blood tests**
  - **FSH (follicle stimulating hormone):** useful if the diagnosis of menopause is in doubt, but only of very limited help in the perimenopause because FSH levels fluctuate so much. If you have had a hysterectomy leaving your ovaries, have your FSH checked six months after the operation and then annually to find out when your ovaries stop working.
  - **oestradiol:** one of the most common questions is whether there are any blood tests to decide what dose of HRT is appropriate. The simple answer is 'no' because of the huge fluctuations in levels of hormones: blood tests may simply not be able to measure the exact oestrogen level. However, oestradiol blood levels may be of some value in measuring dosage for non-oral routes, especially if you have an implant.
  - **thyroid function test (TFT):** abnormal thyroid levels can cause tiredness, weight gain, hair loss and even hot flushes. So if the diagnosis of menopause is in doubt or you are not responding to HRT, talk to your doctor about having a TFT.
  - **blood clotting test:** may be appropriate if you've had a

clot or have a strong family history (see page 148).

- ○ **blood lipids**: not done routinely but should be considered if you have a family history of high cholesterol or heart disease.
- ○ **urine hormone tests**: these are done on the very rare occasions that hot flushes don't stop to check for a condition called phaeochromocytoma or carcinoid syndrome.
- **pelvic examination**: this is only done if the doctor thinks it necessary, but if you do go on HRT and have large fibroids initially, this should be done regularly.
- **mammogram and cervical smear**: these should be part of your general health check and should be up to date before you go on HRT.
- **body mass index assessment**: it's important that you are within the recommended BMI range (20–25) for your general health.

How long should you stay on HRT?

- **for women with premature menopause**: you should consider staying on it until you are 51, i.e. the average age of natural menopause.
- **for women taking HRT for menopausal symptoms**: unless you experience potentially risky side effects (see list), do give your body three months to get used to it. If you have problems, or don't feel you are responding well, talk to your doctor.

After 12 months, reassess the reasons you are taking HRT with your doctor. The recommendation is to take HRT for the shortest possible time, which has not been precisely quantified but is usually taken as under five years. It's always wise to have a health check every year (whether or not you are on HRT) and reassessing whether you stay on HRT should be part of that.

You need to talk about:

- why you took HRT and whether those reasons are still valid.
- any side effects, e.g. bleeding problems or changes in bleeding patterns.
- breasts: lumpiness, cancer risk or any other problems.
- any changes in weight.
- your libido.
- general health: diet, exercise, smoking.
- stress levels and stress management.
- latest evidence on HRT.
- in the light of the above, whether you should continue or stop taking HRT; remember you can always come off it (see page 157) for a few months and see how you get on. Like having an umbrella, you need to take it down to see if it's still raining; you can always put it back up.

BE CAREFUL

Stop taking HRT (or the Pill) immediately if you experience any of the following. See your GP or ring an ambulance and go to your nearest A&E.

- sudden severe chest pain (medical advice is always to dial emergency services and go to hospital immediately)
- sudden breathlessness
- unexplained severe pain in calf
- severe stomach pain
- unusual headache
- loss of vision, hearing or ability to speak
- jaundice

- severe depression
- high blood pressure

How should you come off HRT?

The short answer is slowly – unless you have one of the severe complications listed above. Do not just stop one day. You must tail it off gradually, just as you would go through the menopause naturally. The usual time frame is three to four months during which you reduce the dose as your doctor suggests. If you have a womb and are taking a combined oestrogen and progrestogen product, you need to talk about how you have a final bleed.

TYPES OF HRT: WHAT YOUR DOCTOR MAY OFFER YOU

Originally, HRT simply meant replacing the oestrogen your body stopped producing. Later, as we explained above, progestogens were added. Now HRT has become an umbrella term for a huge range of different products with some 70 different combinations on the market as we write. The choice can seem mind-boggling but the message is that there *is* choice. They come in different types and different doses, are used at different times for different things, and taken in a variety of different ways.

Because of the confusion, the International Menopause Society proposed in 2003 that the following terms should be used. If you are British, you will note a further small confusion: we spell it oestrogen and pronounce it 'eestrogen'. In America, it's spelt estrogen and pronounced the same way. (British specialists are now considering dropping the 'o' so we're in line with America.)

Quick Guide to Hormones used in HRT

Oestrogens and progestogens:

	Oestrogen group	*Progestogen group*
Natural	oestradiol	progesterone
	oestrone	
	oestriol	
Synthetic	ethinyloestradiol	C19 androgenic types
	mestranol	norethisterone
		norgestrel
		levonorgestrel
		C21 progesterone types
		dydrogesterone
		medroxyprogesterone acetate

Also

SERMs: Selective Estrogen Receptor Modulars – so-called 'designer oestrogens' which have oestrogenic activity in some tissues and anti-oestrogenic activity in others

Tibolone: a synthetic steroid compound that has a mixed oestrogenic, progestogenic and mild androgenic effect

Testosterone: an androgen or male hormone also found in women; currently only licensed as an implant in the UK

Here are the different general types of HRT:

ET	Estrogen Therapy
EPT	Estrogen and Progestogen Therapy
CSEPT	Combined Sequential Estrogen and Progestogen Therapy
CCEPT	Combined Continuous Estrogen and Progestogen Therapy

EAT   Estrogen and Androgen Therapy
SERMs   Selective Estrogen Receptor Modulators

More Oestrogen Confusion!

There's something strange about oestrogen: during the fertile years when women produce oestrogen naturally, they may also take high-dose oestrogen in the Pill to stop conception (lots about this on pages 349 to 386). When oestrogen levels are falling as you approach menopause, it's prescribed again but in a low dose that is natural to the body. Confused? Okay, let's try and clear this up.

Oestrogens

There are two types of oestrogen:

Synthetic (artificial) oestrogens are much stronger than natural hormones and have a greater effect on your metabolism. These include ethinyloestradiol, which is used in the contraceptive Pill.

Natural oestrogens are very similar or identical to the ones you produce in your body. But they're chemically produced, usually from soya beans or yams or extracted from mare's urine (see box). Natural oestrogens have the same names as your own: oestradiol, oestriol and oestrone.

We talked about natural oestrogens briefly on page 28 but just to recap:

* oestradiol, which is produced in the ovary, is the main oestrogen that you produce during your reproductive life and the most potent.
* oestrone, the second most powerful, which is made in fat cells, is the second major oestrogen found in women. During your menstrual cycle, you produce more oestradiol than oestrone. At the menopause, levels of oestradiol fall but not oestrone.

• oestriol is made in fat cells and in the placenta: it is produced in large quantities during pregnancy, and in insignificant quantities otherwise.

OESTROGEN FROM MARES

Conjugated equine oestrogen is used in some HRT products, including Premarin, the product used in the American Women's Health Initiative study that was stopped halfway in because the risks of both combined and oestrogen only HRT were deemed unacceptable. It comes from the urine of pregnant mares and contains up to 60 per cent oestrone (the same as women) plus other equine oestrogen, which has a very similar structure to human oestrogen. During pregnancy, mares produce a high level of oestrogens in about ten forms, some of which – like oestrone – are very similar to humans'. Equine oestrogen has been used for about 50 years but controversy has developed recently because it is obtained from mares especially bred and farmed for this purpose.

At present, the horses are bred in Canada and America by independent family farmers. Their welfare is regularly checked and a strict code of practice has been developed by vets and other professionals. A recent report prepared by three eminent independent bodies (International League for the Protection of Horses, American Association of Equine Practitioners and the Canadian Veterinary Medical Association) concluded that 'the public should be assured that the care and welfare of the horses involved in the production of oestrogen replacement medication is good and closely monitored.' However, many people are

---

unhappy about the practice and particularly the routine slaughter of the foals produced by the continually pregnant mares.

So what's the difference between the contraceptive Pill and HRT?

The synthetic oestrogen called ethinyloestradiol in the Pill works by stopping ovulation – that is it stops the ovaries working. It has to be potent to do that and it is: ethinyloestradiol is 200 to 1,000 times more potent than the body's natural oestrogen and the oestrogen in HRT. Also, the ethinyl part of the compound does not allow the oestradiol to be broken down in your body so it generally remains active for longer.

The similar-to-natural oestrogens found in HRT are prescribed to replace the oestrogen that would normally be produced by the ovaries. So they are much less potent.

Progestogens

Like the oestrogens, progestogens are a family of hormones. The body's own naturally produced progestogen is called progesterone. A bit confusingly, the synthetic (artificial) versions of progestogens are called, simply, progestogens ...

In HRT, progestogen is usually only needed in combination with oestrogen when you have a womb, when it is sometimes needed to lower the risk of uterine cancer. Occasionally, taking progestogen is advised when you have had a subtotal hysterectomy.

Natural progestogens

The term 'natural' needs clarifying. Natural does indicate that it is the same chemical blueprint as that produced by your body but it may be given in amounts that are not natural.

Natural progesterone, now available in a cream, pessary, tablet or vaginal gel (although you may not find these readily available in all countries), sounds as if it should come from your body, or at any rate straight from nature. In fact, most products are made in a lab. They are more correctly called 'nature-identical', which means that the synthetic molecule is exactly the same structure as your body's.

Some progesterone creams are plant-derived, based on diosgenin, a compound found in the Mexican yam and also in soya. The nature-identical progesterone is mixed with vegetable or vitamin E oil and contains other natural products but no animal derivatives.

Progesterone creams may help symptoms such as hot flushes; certainly many women believe they do although hard evidence is thin on the ground. Some health professionals, both alternative and conventional, believe that they help prevent osteoporosis but there is little proof of this so far.

Synthetic progestogens

The progestogens used in HRT are virtually all synthetic, and are structurally different from your own natural progesterone. (This is thought by some experts possibly to be part cause of the risks associated with combined oestrogen and progestogen HRT.)

In a normal menstrual cycle, progesterone is produced in the second half; if pregnancy doesn't occur it stops, leading to a period. Similarly, in HRT, the progestogen causes a withdrawal bleed.

There are two main types of synthetic progestogens: C19 and C21 (the C refers to carbon molecules). C21s are closer to progesterone and tend to have fewer side effects such as spots and skin problems. However, C19s can be given trans-dermally as well as orally and may help libido because they are closer in structure to the male hormone testosterone. (Testosterone is an androgen so C19s are sometimes referred to as more androgenic.)

Androgens

Although androgen means male hormone, they are also found in women, albeit in much smaller quantities. (Conversely, oestrogens are also found in men.) They are produced in fat cells and in your adrenal gland; your ovaries also produce a little when they give up producing oestrogen. The main androgens are:

* testosterone
* dehydroepiandrosterone (DHEA)
* androstenedione

Testosterone is traditionally the hormone of masculinity; women have about one-tenth the amount of men. The amount of active testosterone in women varies, as it does in men. Women with Polycystic Ovarian Syndrome (PCOS) have more active testosterone; this can cause spots or hair growth, and also male-pattern balding.

In both sexes, androgens decrease with age and it's now recognised that women can develop a condition called Female Androgen Deficiency Syndrome, which is still being researched. It is most commonly seen in women whose ovaries have been removed.

The symptoms are:

* lack of libido
* lack of energy
* depression

- lack of self-confidence
- headaches

Although testosterone has benefits for some – such as zipping up your libido and increasing energy – in the UK it is only licensed to be given by implants, which can't be removed. This means that if it causes side effects, you can't do anything about it for the duration of the implant, usually six months. In other countries, testosterone is available in pills, patches and by intramuscular injection. Testosterone gel is now available and some British doctors are willing to prescribe it this way as long as the patient is fully informed that it's not licensed for this use and is closely monitored.

DHEA is much touted by some experts and devotees as the androgen of the future but it does need more research before we can recommend it. It is not licensed in the UK.

SERMs (Selective Estrogen Receptor Modulators)

Dubbed 'designer oestrogens', the basic idea of SERMs was to develop a smart drug with the beneficial effects of oestrogen but without some of the risks and side effects. So SERMs have oestrogenic activity in certain tissues and anti-oestrogenic activity in others. If you think of oestrogen as watering the whole garden, SERMs only water certain plants. So, some experts claim, they may avoid the increased risk of cancer.

One of the earliest and best known is tamoxifen, which was developed for the treatment of oestrogen receptor positive breast cancer. It emerged that tamoxifen also improved bone density and was good for blood lipids (fats). However, the problem with tamoxifen is that it can stimulate the womb lining (endometrium) and cause uterine bleeding, a growth or even cancer.

The most commonly used SERM for menopausal women in the UK and America is raloxifene, now approved for the prevention and treatment of postmenopausal osteoporosis. The advantage of raloxifene over tamoxifen is that it helps to protect the bone and prevent osteoporosis without stimulating the womb lining and increasing the risk of breast or womb cancer. A recent study has also shown a significant reduction in breast cancer incidence after three years. With the new guidelines that doctors should not prescribe HRT as a first line of treatment for osteoporosis, raloxifene stands to have a role for women at risk of vertebral fracture in the age range 60 to 75. Its effect on the heart is not known but it may be beneficial. It can help improve vaginal dryness and tightness (and thus painful intercourse) to a limited extent. The downside is that it may actually increase the risk of hot flushes and calf cramps and has the same risk of causing a blood clot in the leg or lung as conventional HRT.

Tibolone

Originally researched as a contraceptive, tibolone is now taken as a once-daily tablet for management of menopausal symptoms. It has been used in Europe for about a decade but has only recently been licensed in Australia and is not, to date, available in the US.

Tibolone is a synthetic steroid compound that has a mixed oestrogenic, progestogenic and mild androgenic effect. It doesn't need added progestogens and so should not cause a bleed, one of the least popular side effects of combined HRT.

However, tibolone may be linked with irregular bleeding initially; if this doesn't stop within three months, consult your doctor. There are other drugs that can be added to help manage this problem if tibolone suits you otherwise. But it is best to wait until you are one year past your last period before starting it.

Tibolone is useful for women with short-term symptoms of menopause, particularly loss of libido which is improved by the androgens. It also has a beneficial effect on bone and can be prescribed to help prevent osteoporosis. It may also be a useful treatment for women with known endometriosis, even if they have had a hysterectomy, because its progesto-genic features mean it doesn't stimulate the lining of the womb. Its effect on the heart is unknown; it has the same risk association as other HRT with breast cancer (the risk was second to combined HRT in the Million Women Study).

As with all forms of HRT, an annual review is important.

DIFFERENT WAYS OF TAKING HRT

There are all sorts of different forms of HRT – what doctors call 'routes of administration' or sometimes 'methods of delivery'. You may not hear about the options if your doctor is rushed but do remember to ask. Different routes have different effects.

For instance, if your main problem is a dry vagina causing painful intercourse, all you may need is a vaginal tablet of oestradiol or oestriol cream. There is very little absorption of this into the bloodstream from the vagina so this won't improve your hot flushes or benefit your bones but it also should not be linked to an increased risk of breast cancer. (However, Michael finds that some women who are very sensitive to hormones may have some breast tenderness.) If you're only using a vaginal cream twice a week, relatively short term, you shouldn't need a progestogen. But if you find yourself using it daily and long term, your doctor may also recommend adding in a progestogen to protect the womb lining.

If, however, you are taking HRT to stop hot flushes, you will need to take it via a route that will allow adequate levels to get into your bloodstream, for which the most common route is oral.

Questions to ask yourself about ways of taking HRT (routes)

- do I really want to go on HRT? (Remember, if you have had a premature menopause for any reason you are strongly advised to consider HRT.)
- if I still have a womb, do I want to have:

  - regular bleeds
  - no bleeds
  - quarterly bleeds

- what is the main reason I'm going on it and is the route important (see above)?
- do I prefer: patch, gel, cream, tablets, vaginal route, nasal spray, implant?

Routes for oestrogens

Oral:	tablets or pills by mouth
Through skin (transdermal):	patch or gel
Through vagina (transvaginal):	tablet, cream or ring
Buried under the skin:	implant
Through your nose:	nasal spray

Routes for progestogens

Oral:	tablets or pills by mouth
Through skin (transdermal):	cream, patch or gel
Through vagina:	gel or pessary
Intrauterine system:	coil

Routes for oestrogen and progestogen combinations

Oestrogen is given daily; progestogens are either given daily to prevent any uterine bleeding, for 12–14 days every four weeks which causes a monthly bleed when the progestogen is stopped, or over 13 weeks, which causes a bleed every three months. However, if you're at the early stage of menopause and you try a no-bleed preparation, you may get irregular bleeding. So there is an advantage to having regular bleeds initially, then reconsidering the type of HRT a year later.

SERMs and tibolone should not give you a vaginal bleed.

BE CAREFUL
If you take HRT and have any bleeding at a time you're not expecting it, you must go and discuss it with your doctor immediately.

You can mix and match your routes in discussion with your doctor but the commercially available preparations include:

Sequential therapy: oral, patches or patch plus oral

- daily oestrogen
- progestogen for 10–14 days every four weeks
- causes monthly bleeds

Three-monthly cycle: oral

- daily oestrogen
- 14 days' progestogen every 13 weeks
- bleeds every three months

Continuous therapy: oral or patch

- daily oestrogen and progestogen
- no bleed

Which route should you use for oestrogen?

All the methods are good at providing your body with oestrogen. The research at present seems to indicate no method is a clear-cut winner all round. However, there are pros and cons, which we discuss below.

Oral: tablets or pills by mouth

Any drug you take by mouth goes from your gut straight to your liver: this is often referred to as the 'first pass'. Taking oestrogen by mouth means that the oestradiol in the HRT is rapidly converted to oestrone. Once this oestrone is absorbed, it travels to the liver where it is further metabolised and then partially inactivated – a lot is excreted. Up to 90 per cent of the oestrogen you take orally is inactivated by the liver, so you need a much larger daily dose than if you were taking it via non-oral routes. Also your blood levels of oestrogen increase dramatically within three to six hours, then fall off due to variation in absorption. Generally this isn't too much of a problem but blood hormone levels will fluctuate over the day.

Although there's a lot of discussion about 'liver bypass routes', whatever method you use the oestrogen will eventually go through the liver. Much more long-term research is available about the oral route than others and the British Menopause Society has concluded that there appears to be no clear advantage of the transdermal route over the oral. However, non-oral routes, such as patches, tend to give you more of a steady intake over 24 hours, which may help women with conditions like migraine or gallstones.

Advantages
- easy-to-remember calendar packs
- easily reversible
- many different types

Disadvantages

- Must be taken every day
- potential load on liver
- varying levels of hormone in bloodstream
- nausea
- lactose used in pills is not suitable for women with lactose sensitivity

Through skin (transdermal): patch or gel

Oestradiol goes through your skin to your bloodstream either via a sticky patch, which is changed once or twice weekly, or in a gel, which is rubbed into the skin daily. It virtually avoids the liver and gives a much more constant blood level of the added hormone. However, absorption can still be variable partly because some women are 'poor absorbers'.

Patches can cause irritation in some women so it's a good idea to try a dummy patch out first – your doctor will give you one. If you have fragile skin, a patch may not be suitable. Between four and eight per cent of patches fall off, due to poor adhesion or skin reactions where the patch is. They may fall off in the bath, swimming pool or even in bed – don't worry if it sticks to your partner, it won't do him any harm as long as it doesn't happen too often. Just stick it on your body again. If the patch falls off in a hot bath, allow your skin to cool before applying a new one.

Patches should be removed after three to four days, or once a week with a seven-day patch, and replaced with a fresh patch on a slightly different site. Recommended sites are clean, dry, unbroken areas of skin on the torso below the waistline. Don't apply on or near your breasts or under your waistband.

Transdermal is the route of choice for:

- women with past history of clots
- malabsorption syndromes including irritable bowel (IBS)
- migraine sufferers as more of a steady state is achieved
- women with gallstones as theoretically the liver is avoided (evidence of benefit not great)

Advantages
- easy to administer
- easy to stop
- avoids 'first pass' through liver so fewer side effects are likely
- more constant levels of hormone in bloodstream

Disadvantages
- possible skin reactions, e.g. mild redness or itching
- patch can look unsightly
- may fall off
- possible variation in absorption
- more expensive than tablets/pills

Through vagina (transvaginal): tablet, cream or ring

Tablets and cream
These are useful to treat local conditions such as a sore vagina, vaginal dryness and urinary symptoms. Oestriol is used most often because it's much less potent than oestradiol. (Oestradiol applied vaginally is rapidly absorbed into the bloodstream and, if used long term, can cause thickening of the lining of the womb – a risk for endometrial cancer. However this risk can be offset with progestogen; see below.)

The cream is simply applied to the vagina and the tablet is inserted with an applicator. The minimum effective amount should be given. Michael recommends a daily dose for one to two weeks and then a very low maintenance dose. If this is used long term, you may need to take an oral progestogen for 10 to 14 days every three to six months to prevent thickening of the womb lining. You can also have a scan of the lining of your womb. Do remember the risk is very small and only related to long-term use.

Different types of vaginal oestrogen are available, including:

* oestriol 0.1 per cent
* conjugated equine oestrogens
* oestradiol (see above)

Advantages

* local treatment for local problems
* easy to apply
* minimal absorption

Disadvantages

* cream is messy
* long-term use may cause thickening of womb lining

Ring

A silicon ring, rather like a curtain ring, is placed in the vagina and slowly releases a tiny amount of oestradiol. If you have a womb, you need to take progestogen as described above. Although a minimal quantity, it supplies enough oestrogen to relieve symptoms and may also have a role in preventing osteoporosis. The ring needs changing about every three months.

Advantages

- easy to insert
- only needs replacing every three months

Disadvantages

- may interfere with intercourse
- may fall out
- may be forgotten and left *in situ*

Under the skin: implants

Tiny rods, 3 mm in diameter and 4 mm long, containing crystalline pellets of oestradiol are inserted under the skin. They are usually put in the abdomen, below your tummy button or on your thigh or buttock. It takes less than five minutes in outpatients; pain is minimal as you have a local anaesthetic. A stitch or steri strip is used to close the wound and stop bleeding.

These tiny implants slowly release oestradiol over the next six months, or more, so they are particularly suitable for women who have had a hysterectomy. If you do have a womb, a progestogen must be taken every month (to minimise risk of uterine cancer). Progestogens are taken for 12 to 14 days in four weeks; a bleed happens afterwards. Researchers are now looking at the potential of the Mirena levonorgestrel coil (see page 379) to protect the womb lining and avoid bleeding.

The great advantage is that you don't have to remember to take a pill, smear on a gel, or put on a patch. The downside is that they can't be removed and the residual effects can last a long time, sometimes for many years. Some experts believe that implants should not be given because of the difficulty of reversing the procedure.

The biggest problem is a condition called tachyphylaxis, which leads to the recurrence of menopausal symptoms. This happens because the dosage of oestrogen seesaws up and down.

When it comes time to have another implant, at about six-monthly intervals, you must have a blood test to look at your blood oestradiol levels. If the level is above 600 pmol/l (picomols per litre), you do not need another implant yet. Get the blood test repeated a month later and wait until it falls below 600 pmol/l. Women who feel their implant running out before six months should not simply have it replaced as this could have a negative effect: oestradiol levels should be tested and alternative symptom control used.

Advantages
- nothing to remember
- avoids liver first pass
- may suit women who have had hysterectomies
- can give testosterone to help libido with oestrogen (or alone)

Disadvantages
- needs local anaesthetic to insert in small incision
- potential tachyphylaxis: i.e. high dose in bloodstream and you still get symptoms
- difficult to remove
- can take many years to reverse
- women with wombs still need progestogen and will have a bleed
- if you take progestogen you may need to continue for two years after implants stop being replaced to oppose the residual oestrogen

Through your nose: nasal spray

The mucus in your nose provides a good surface for absorption into the bloodstream, avoiding the first pass to the liver. A synthetic form of oestradiol, called 17beta oestradiol, has now been licensed. It's called 'pulsed oestrogen therapy' (PET) because there is a rapid rise in blood oestradiol in the first 30 minutes, which then drops to pre-treatment levels over the next 8 to 12 hours. Perhaps surprisingly, the nasal spray still appears to be effective if you have a blocked or runny nose, but not with severe congestion when you need to spray or rub twice the dose into the gums. Although you take it in the morning, PET is effective against night sweats.

Advantages
* rapid absorption
* simple to take
* quick to stop

Disadvantages
* absorption may be affected by severely blocked nose
* can cause sneezing or prickly feeling in nose (usually decreases with time)

Which route should you use for progestogens?

Women who have a womb need progestogens to counter, or oppose, the increased risk of cancer of the lining of the womb, which occurs if you take oestrogen alone. You don't need to take progestogens if you have had a total hysterectomy, but you may do if you have had a subtotal one.

By giving progestogens in a cyclical way (sequential therapy) – for instance, 12 to 14 days every four weeks – a withdrawal bleed (period) happens when it's stopped. Studies have shown that up to 50 per cent of women stop taking HRT within one year, and one of the most common reasons is vaginal bleeding. To avoid the bleed, progestogens can be combined with the oestrogen and given continuously: it's called the 'continuous combined' method. This is usually given to women who have not had a natural period for 12 months. If it's started earlier, you are more likely to get irregular vaginal bleeding.

Progestogens have many other side effects including weight gain, feeling of being bloated and uncomfortable, PMS, acne, hirsutism (downy hair growth on face or body), or alopecia (hair loss on head).

Remember the family is called the progestogens, like the oestrogens, and the body's own natural hormone is called progesterone. The options are synthetic progestogen or natural progesterone – more accurately nature identical. Natural progesterone cream or gel, also oral micronised tablets, as we've explained above, may have a role in the relief of some menopausal symptoms and you may find your doctor or health professional suggests them. (Not all are available in the UK.)

The routes are more limited with progestogens than oestrogen, partly because less research has been done.

The main options for nature identical progesterone preparations are:
- Oral (micronised)
- Transdermal cream applied on the skin or gel vaginally
- Vaginal or rectal pessaries

The main options for synthetic progestogen preparations are:
- Oral
- Transdermal patch
- Intrauterine

Oral: tablets or pills by mouth

Oral progestogens have the same advantages as oral oestrogens but also have the 'first pass through the liver' effect (see page 169). Doctors need to give the lowest dose that will protect the womb lining and cause the least side effects.

Synthetic progestogens are the most common oral preparations. Natural progesterone can be given orally in the micronised form, where tiny particles are used but due to the first pass effect, a large dose (300 mg) is required and this can have significant side effects. So this micronised form is not used routinely and is not, in fact, licensed in the UK although it is in France.

Through skin (transdermal): cream, gel or patches

Natural progesterone can be given in cream or gel form (as with solo natural progesterone products; see page 162) but the dose needed in this route to oppose the oestrogen and protect the womb lining is unacceptably large and there are few products licensed for this use. Progestogen patches of norethisterone or levonorgestrel are available and can either be given in a sequential or continous mode.

Through vagina (transvaginal): gel or pessary

Progesterone vaginal gel is licensed in the UK and can be used to prevent thickening of the womb lining and given sequentially. Progesterone pessaries, applied either vaginally or rectally, do exist and are used in PMS and infertility but are not licensed to protect the womb lining.

Intrauterine system: coil

The use of the progestogen coil (Mirena) is very helpful in helping to reduce the side effects of progestogens. In the UK at present, the Mirena coil is licensed as a contraceptive and for treatment of heavy periods but not to protect the womb lining. However there is ongoing research into this and the results look favourable for both the Mirena coil which contains levonorgestrel and also a progestogen coil called Progestasert, which is already licensed in America. These also have the advantage of being contraceptives as well so they may be useful for women coming up to menopause.

TROUBLESHOOTING: WHAT TO DO IF THINGS GO WRONG

Going on HRT is a bit like buying a new pair of shoes. You may need to try on several pairs before you find the one that's right for you. Then, even if you get a perfect fit, it takes time for you to wear them in and get used to them. Michael always advises patients to stick with a preparation for at least three months unless serious complications occur (see page 156) – in which case, you must go to your doctor immediately. (As usual, follow our mantra: If in doubt, give a shout! Always go to your doctor, or call a helpline, if you have any concerns at all.)

You may get lucky and find a product that suits you immediately, but you may need to try several before you hit on the right one.

Here are some of the problems and what your doctor may do about them.

* **symptoms continue after you take HRT**

If you have tried the product for three months and nothing changes, this could be due to:

  ○ not allowing enough time – three months – for the HRT to get into your system.
  ○ forgetting to take the tablets.

○ patch not sticking properly or falling off.
○ inadequate dose of oestrogen.
○ poor absorption because of vomiting or diarrhoea.
○ poor absorption because you are taking other drugs such as antibiotics.
○ too fast breakdown by the liver – this can occur if you are taking drugs such as anti-epileptic medications that stimulate the liver so the oestrogen is broken down more quickly; you may need a bigger dose of oestrogen.
○ wrong diagnosis: this is rare but your doctor needs to exclude thyroid problems and very rare cancers (phaeochromocyloma or carcinoid tumour).
○ unrealistic expectations! HRT cannot make you look and feel 20 – it's as simple as that.
○ too much oestrogen, which can be as bad as too little (or none), especially if the route is an implant.

• **bleeding problems**

One of the biggest reasons women stop HRT is due to bleeding problems. In one study 45 per cent of women said this was the significant factor in their decision to stop HRT.

○ **heavy regular bleeding with once a month or once a quarter bleed preparations:** you may bleed heavily for the first few cycles on these forms of HRT. Talk to your doctor about taking tranexamic acid or mefenamic acid medications, which help reduce the amount of bleeding. If the problem continues, you may need to change your HRT preparation, either by reducing the oestrogen, changing the progestogen or changing the route of administration.
It's also advisable to have a blood test to check that

you're not anaemic or have problems with your thyroid. Low thyroid levels can be linked to heavy periods and high levels to untreatable hot flushes. Other possible causes of heavy bleeding include:

- fibroids – benign growths in the muscle of the womb, a common problem
- polyps – outgrowths of the womb lining
- pre-cancer of the endometrium
- cancer of the cervix or endometrium

Don't just sit back and accept heavy periods – if they continue your doctor should investigate, possibly with a scan of your uterus, blood test and sample of the endometrium (lining of the womb)

○ **no bleeding, no withdrawal bleed**

Up to 15 per cent of women taking once a month or quarterly bleed products, especially those who have been on long-term HRT, have no bleeds at all. There's no worry about the lining of the womb but if you have been prescribed it originally for osteoporosis, you might not be getting enough oestrogen – so it's sensible to check this further with your doctor (Obviously if you are on a no-bleed preparation, you shouldn't be bleeding at all.)

○ **unexpected breakthrough bleeding**

This can be due to HRT or unrelated. It's important to check that you haven't forgotten a tablet – this is a very common cause. Also, if the breakthrough bleeding occurred around a time when you had diarrhoea and vomiting or were taking antibiotics, the absorption may have been reduced. If this bleeding occurs more than once you must go and see your doctor. Possible investigations include a scan of the uterus and testing a sample of the endometrium (usually an out-patient procedure). Once any abnormal cause (pathology) is excluded then the dose or route of the HRT may need to be changed.

It's sensible to chart any irregular bleeding and relate this to the HRT. It may be possible to change the dose of either the oestrogen or progestogen.

Stress may cause unexpected bleeding, as can long-distance travel, which upsets your body's hormonal clock.

• **nausea, breast tenderness, leg cramps, migraine headache, change in vaginal discharge, skin or eye irritation**

These may all be side effects of oestrogen replacement. They often go after the first few months. Simple remedies may help overcome them more quickly:

○ **nausea:** try taking HRT at night or with food; if the nausea continues you may need to change the route.
○ **breast tenderness and pain:** don't touch your sore breast because the body thinks it has a baby suckling and produces more hormones which will aggravate the tenderness. Also wear a bra, which gives good support, take vitamin B6, 40 mg daily, and try evening primrose oil containing up to 320 mg of the active GLA in three doses during the day (this may take up to 12 weeks to have an effect).
○ **leg cramps:** these often affect both legs and are worse at night; they usually improve with time but if they occur in one leg, you *must* go to see your doctor immediately to exclude a blood clot.
○ **headaches and migraine:** these increase with age but

HRT can affect them; discuss a different route with your doctor.

○ **vaginal discharge**: as oestrogen stimulates the glands in your vagina, you will get a slight lubricating discharge.

○ **skin irritation**: this can occur with oestrogen; see your doctor who may do a blood test to check your liver and possibly reduce the dose. Patches can also cause irritation which is usually helped by:

* putting it on your buttock rather than lower abdomen and/or
* moving the patch every 24 to 48 hours. If this doesn't work, try a different brand or a different route.

○ **eye irritation**: contact lenses may be uncomfortable initially.

* **weight changes**

You may lose weight on HRT, put weight on – or have no change. Weight gain is one of the biggest fears of women going on HRT and affects many users, according to clinicians and women. (Strangely, however, several research studies have not confirmed this.) We look at solutions in some detail in Chapters Four and Seven. A low-carbohydrate diet and regular exercise invariably help, and there is some evidence that acupuncture may tip the scales when it seems like nothing else can.

* **PMS symptoms, greasy hair and acne**

If you have had a previous history of PMS, you are more likely to get side effects with the progestogens including: bloating, irritability, depression, headache and lethargy.

The greasy skin and acne are particularly linked to the

C19 progestogens (norethisterone, norgestrel or oral levonor-gestrel). Don't worry if these affect you in the first three months as they often get better. But if symptoms persist, see your doctor and discuss whether you need to change the progestogen you're taking or reduce the amount. Taking vitamin B6 or gammalinolenic acid (GLA, found in evening primrose oil) may help.

6

EXPLAINING COMPLEMENTARY AND ALTERNATIVE THERAPIES

This chapter covers:

- do complementary and alternative medicine actually work?
- acupuncture
- Ayurveda
- Chinese herbal medicine
- homeopathy
- naturopathy
- nutritional therapy
- Western herbalism
- manipulative therapies including chiropractic and osteopathy
- physiotherapy
- touch therapies
- aromatherapy
- massage
- reflexology
- reiki
- nature therapies including hydrotherapy and light therapy
- movement therapies including Alexander Technique
- psychological therapies
- flower remedies
- healing
- hypnotherapy
- laughter therapy
- life coaching
- meditation
- music therapy
- psychotherapy
- radionics

In this chapter you will find a short explanation of the complementary and alternative therapies that we have suggested as helpful to consider for your Integrated Menopausal Therapy. We obviously can't describe them in great detail – each would need a book. But you should get a flavour of them, and in the Directory (page 421) you will find contact details where you can get more information.

In comparison with drugs, there is little conventional research on the effectiveness of complementary therapies. This is mainly due to the fact that most research is funded by pharmaceutical companies, who are extremely unlikely to fund studies of complementary and alternative therapies. Even national medical research organisations (such as the Medical Research Council in the UK) allocate a minute percentage of their budget to complementary and alternative medicine (CAM). But with the problems now surrounding HRT, this situation is changing.

In America, there are big government-funded studies ongoing; including one focusing solely on black cohosh, the other comparing black cohosh, red clover, combined HRT or placebo. Other trials are investigating the role of phytoestrogens (like soy) on mental function in women over 55. But these results will not be available for some time. Meanwhile, the research on complementary and alternative therapies indicates that most users find it effective (see below) if they identify one that suits them. In terms of reality economics, you could argue that women would not spend money on therapies that don't work and the popularity of CAM is increasing all the time. The last national survey in America, in 1997, showed that 42.1 per cent of US adults used some type of alternative therapy, spending an estimated $27 billion.

The other interesting factor is that in many trials, both of conventional drug therapies and CAM, the level of success with placebo (dummy treatment) was as high as with the active treatment. Which confirms what we all know: all human beings need to feel cared for and valued, and if that need is met, we feel better.

Does CAM really help?

'When 886 women aged 45 to 65 in Washington State, some of whom used HRT, were asked how helpful they found CAM therapies – stress management, over the counter alternative remedies, chiropractic, massage, dietary soy, acupuncture, naturopathy, homeopathy and herbalism – over 90 per cent rated them helpful to very helpful.'

Obstetrics & Gynaecology, July 2002

You can keep up with peer-reviewed published research on CAM by logging on to the 'CAM on PubMed' database, which is run by the US department of health and covers medical and scientific publications worldwide. Log on to: www.nlm.nih.gov/nccam/camonpubmed.html

Traditional medical therapies

Acupuncture

This is one of the oldest forms of pain relief and healing, which has been used around the world – but particularly in Chinese medicine – for over 5,000 years. Acupuncture, which means needle piercing, can be used to treat and prevent disease, relieve pain and even anaesthetise patients during surgery. Practitioners insert very fine needles into the skin to stimulate specific 'acupoints', which form a complex grid across the body. When the needles stimulate the acupoints, chi (life force) flows through the body clearing energy blockages along its way; this helps the body to re-balance itself and trigger its own self-healing.

Research has shown that when acupoints are pierced with acupuncture needles, naturally occurring pain-killing chemicals called endorphins are released into the bloodstream, which explains acupuncture's clever pain-relieving effects. There is clear evidence that acupuncture can be really useful during menopause for treating heavy periods, hot flushes, stress incontinence, persistent aches and pains and low mood, even depression. Recent research has shown that acupuncture can trigger significant hormonal changes.

Electro-acupuncture has also been shown to be useful in treating psychological distress in postmenopausal women. Acupuncture combined with a calorie-controlled diet, has been shown to be significantly more effective in helping weight loss in obese patients than diet alone.

DIY? Leave your needles in your sewing kit – this isn't a do-it-yourself treatment.

ACUPUNCTURE AND MENOPAUSE-RELATED SYMPTOMS IN WOMEN TAKING TAMOXIFEN

'In a small Italian pilot study of women with breast cancer, which took place over six months, hot flushes and night sweats, also anxiety and depression were improved by acupuncture, which is seen by the researchers as safe and effective for women taking tamoxifen.'

Tumori, 2002

Ayurveda (aka Ayurvedic medicine)

This Sanskrit word meaning 'science of life' is a complete holistic healthcare system, dating from the second millennium

BC and still used in India today. It embraces diet, yoga, breathing techniques and the therapeutic use of herbs and spices. Ayurveda, which is increasingly respected by Western doctors, works on the principle that everyone's physical and mental constitution is determined by the way in which their three 'doshas' or energies are combined. These are Vata (air), Pitta (fire and water) and Kapha (water and earth). Most people have one (sometimes two) predominant doshas that influence their state of all-round health. Your particular combination tends to make you strong in some areas but prone to problems in others, for instance a propensity to gain weight easily, indigestion, insomnia or catching colds.

Vata women tend to be thin and wiry with small appetites and a tendency towards painful periods and constipation. They might be advised to eat Pitta type foods (spicy, oily, sharp flavours) to balance the Pitta element of their constitutions. Sweet-toothed Kapha women, who are often large-framed, a bit tubby and prone to heavy periods, would be treated with Vata foods, which are mostly sweet, sour and salty. Pitta women, who typically have fair skin with freckles, reddish hair and angular chins, tend to suffer mood swings and particularly benefit from balancing their doshas with yoga postures and breathing exercises.

In an Ayurvedic consultation you answer a comprehensive questionnaire about your personal life and daily habits (everything from bowel habits to favourite foods) as well as having your tongue checked for evidence of toxic build-up and a complex multi-pulse diagnosis.

DIY? Once you know your type, you can treat yourself for minor conditions. There is a wealth of simple but effective Ayurvedic home remedies, such as drinking milk with added cinnamon to get you off to sleep or chewing a nub of ginger root to aid indigestion.

Chinese herbal medicine (aka traditional Chinese medicine or TCM)

To understand Chinese herbal medicine, which dates back thousands of years, you need to embrace the principles of Yin and Yang – opposing but complementary forces, which both need to be in balance for a state of perfect health. If your Yin and Yang are out of kilter, a Chinese herbalist can correct it by prescribing specific herbs. There are six other subdivisions within the Yin Yang constitution – cold and heat, external or internal, excess or deficiency – all of which should be working in harmony so that the chi or life force flows freely.

In China, herbs are often used in conjunction with acupuncture to treat and prevent physical and emotional symptoms. Herbs are sometimes used alone for treating conditions such as viral infections, eczema, anaemia and heavy or irregular periods. Herbs are also used to strengthen and nourish patients who might be too weak for acupuncture. During a consultation, a doctor of TCM pays great attention to listening and smelling. As well as noting the tone of your voice (a hectoring tone shows your gall bladder might be playing up), they will ask to smell your breath (for instance, cheesy may mean you're overdoing things) and also your urine to assess toxic overload.

The World Health Organisation has a huge database of illnesses that benefit from Chinese herbs, ranging from PMS and insomnia to vaginitis and allergies. Dang Gui Pian or Dong Quai (a type of Angelica) is the most commonly prescribed Chinese herbal medicine for 'female problems' and is often prescribed to menopausal women with impressive results. There have been a few scare stories about the toxicity of some Chinese herbs over the years but these have mainly been due to prescribing by unqualified practitioners. One in 10,000 people may also suffer allergic reactions to the herbs. Stop taking them immediately if you feel unwell and contact your practitioner.

DIY? Diagnosis is so complex that you should never try to work out what your problem is or how to treat it without consulting a qualified practitioner. Herbs are prescribed individually for you. As with pharmaceutical drugs, they are strong stuff with potential side effects and should be respected.

CHINESE HERBS AND MENOPAUSAL SYMPTOMS

'Ji-Wy Shiau-Yau San (JWSYS) is a famous herbal remedy used for the management of various menopausal-related symptoms. In a randomised controlled pilot study to evaluate the effects of JWSYS compared with a continuous combined HRT on quality of life in postmenopausal women (who had not had hysterectomies), JWSYS alleviated the menopausal symptoms as effectively the HRT without the same side effects (particularly bleeding and breast tenderness). The researchers at the Veterans General Hospital in Taipei, say that this has promise as a safe and efficacious alternative therapy but needs more study to be sure.'

Maturitas, 2002 Jan

Homeopathy

Developed in the eighteenth century by a German doctor, Samuel Hahnemann, homeopathy is based on the ancient hypothesis, first put forward by Hippocrates, that 'like cures like'. This means that a substance that causes symptoms of illness in a healthy person can be used to treat the same symptoms in someone who is ill.

For example, medicines or foods containing sulphur can make your skin itchy but if you have eczema, homeopathic sulphur pills may relieve symptoms. Homeopathic drugs are made from plant, animal and mineral extracts. They are chopped, ground up and soaked in an alcohol and water solution for several weeks to create a liquid known as the mother tincture. One drop of tincture is then diluted in 99 drops of alcohol and shaken, followed by repeated dilutions until there are virtually no molecules left of the original substance. This process is called 'potentising'. There are three different potencies, 6, 30 and 200, depending on their dilution.

Homeopathy looks at the person rather than the illness so a practitioner will not treat headache symptoms as such but the individual person who has a headache. There are specific remedies that work for certain homeopathic types; for instance, pulsatilla types tend to be blue-eyed and cry easily.

You will be asked lots of questions when you visit a homeopath, not only about your health and emotions but also about flavours and textures you enjoy eating and how you respond to certain situations. This builds up a total picture to ascertain your type. Menopausal symptoms often respond very well to homeopathy.

There are homeopathic hospitals in Britain as well as individual practitioners and some doctors are happy to refer you to a homeopath on the NHS.

DIY? Research confirms homeopathy's benefits for menopausal symptoms when prescribed individually by qualified practitioners. However many high street chemists (including Boots) and health food shops stock an array of homeopathic pills and ointments, often with easy-to-read reference charts, which may help to some extent.

HOMEOPATHY ON TRIAL

Sceptics often suggest that the success of homeopathy is down to placebo or suggestion. But when over 100 trials using homeopathy were analysed in 1991, more than 77 per cent were positive. A more recent meta-analysis of placebo-controlled trials, published in the *Lancet* in 1997, showed that the effects of homeopathy were more than placebo, something that users (like the British royal family) and people who dose their animals with homeopathic remedies are quite certain of. In a survey of women attending the Royal London Homeopathic Hospital Women's Clinic, 70 per cent experienced a definite improvement in symptoms.

Naturopathy

Naturopathy is based on the concept that diet, exercise, fasting, hydrotherapy, massage and relaxation help to kick-start the body's own self-healing mechanism – and maintain health – rather than relying on drugs.

It became popular in the nineteenth century with followers claiming that living in harmony with nature and listening to your body was the key to strengthening the 'vital curative force' that keeps us well.

Naturopaths say that illness occurs when we are subjected to factors including pollution, stress and injury. They believe that childhood illnesses such as mumps, measles and chicken pox are vital in building a strong immune system. They also see many symptoms such as colds, coughs and diarrhoea as a natural way of dispelling toxins and re-balancing the body.

If you visit a naturopath they will check out how well your 'vital' force is working by doing normal checks including blood pressure and pulse, also iridology (iris diagnosis) and hair and sweat mineral analysis. Treatment of any problems will probably include diet (whole organic food, eliminating dairy and wheat), juice fasts, alternate hot and cold baths, osteopathy and even counselling.

DIY? You shouldn't embark on a fast for more than 24 hours without professional guidance but apart from that, using naturopathy's best tools – a whole food diet, gentle self-massage, exercise, relaxation and healing baths – is easy, cheap and really worthwhile.

Nutritional therapy

Food and plants were our first medicines and the nutrients contained in them can be used to treat disease and unpleasant symptoms and to restore and revitalise us when we need a boost. Many health experts treating women going through the menopause see nutrients in food called phytoestrogens (soy is the best known) as a valuable way to treat symptoms and promote balance.

Nutritional therapy is based on the idea that the body is composed of certain elements (including iron, copper, magnesium, calcium, potassium), which are vital for our health and are available to us in high quality foods and supplements.

One of the problems with Western diets these days is that most of us are overfed and under-nourished. Many of the fruits and vegetables that we eat don't contain the levels of vitamins and minerals that they did a decade ago because the land they are grown on has become depleted of nutrients by modern farming methods.

Nutritional practitioners build up a profile of your state of health and particular needs by examining your current diet, alcohol consumption, smoking – if you do – checking on any physical symptoms (e.g. bloating, constipation, headaches), and assessing exercise and sleep patterns. Hair, urine and sweat may also be analysed for mineral content to check for deficiencies.

Nutritional therapy can be very successful in treating food intolerances, high blood pressure, mcnopausal symptoms including hot flushes, constipation, PMT, osteoporosis and insomnia.

DIY? Not too difficult as long as you do your homework. There are many books available on dietary needs and how to choose the therapeutic foods and supplements applicable to you. (See Chapter Eight and also *The Adam & Eve Diet*, which Sarah co-wrote with eminent naturopath Roderick Lane; also Useful Books on page 419.)

VITAMIN D AND BONE HEALTH IN POSTMENOPAUSAL WOMEN

'Vitamin D intake between 500 and 800 IU daily, with or without calcium supplementation, has been shown to increase bone mineral density in women around 63 years. In women over 65, there is even more benefit with vitamin D intakes of between 800 and 900 IU daily plus 1200–1300 mg of calcium daily, giving increased bone density, decreased bone turnover, and decreased non-vertebral fractures.'

Journal of Women's Health, 2003

Western herbalism

The power of herbs has been used to treat illness and promote health since ancient times. Well over 50 per cent of modern drugs are plant-based and research is ongoing. For instance, aspirin is derived from willow bark, the cancer drug vincristine from the Madagascan periwinkle, and sage is being used to treat Alzheimer's disease, as well as hot flushes. Nearly every plant growing on the planet has a medicinal use.

Today's herbalists are combining their ancient knowledge of herbs with modern science to treat a range of disease conditions from cancer to constipation.

Herbs contain a vast cocktail of chemicals including vitamins, essential oils, proteins and starches, minerals and trace elements, which can all help restore the body's immune system, improve circulation and soothe inflammation. Herbs also have a clever way of working synergistically – in some ways they are far more sophisticated than laboratory-created drugs. For instance Lime Flower taken for high blood pressure not only helps to dilate the blood vessels but also acts as a gentle sedative – thus doing two important jobs at once.

Western herbalists prescribe tablets, tinctures, ointments, compresses, herbal baths and even suppositories. Herbal remedies usually take longer than conventional drugs to work but deliver gentler effects and are much easier to tolerate long term.

Only visit qualified practitioners because some herbs are extremely toxic and not to be messed with. (See Choosing a Practitioner, page 15.)

DIY? Simple herbal remedies using familiar plants that you know you can actually safely eat are fine; for instance, garlic to fight infections, valerian to help relax, lemon balm tea or chamomile if the world's just turning too fast. Also see page 86 for details of herbs that can help with menopausal symptoms. There are also many good books written by qualified herbalists, which can guide you (see Useful Books, page 419). As we said above about Chinese herbal medicine, herbs are potent so consult a qualified practitioner if possible, or buy standardised preparations from reputable brands and always respect the dosage prescribed.

BLACK COHOSH FOR MENOPAUSAL SYMPTOMS

'The herb black cohosh, or Actaea racemosa (formerly named Cimicifuga racemosa), is native to North America. The roots and rhizomes of this herb are widely used in the treatment of menopausal symptoms and menstrual dysfunction. Studies have demonstrated that this botanic medicine, when standardized properly to the terpene glycoside fraction, appears to be effective in alleviating menopausal symptoms. Adverse effects are extremely uncommon, and there are no known significant adverse drug interactions.'

Dr B. Kligler, Department of Family Medicine, Albert Einstein College of Medicine, New York, *American Family Physician*, 2003

Manipulative therapies

Chiropractic and McTimoney chiropractic

Chiropractic is a relatively new therapy founded by David Daniel Palmer, a Canadian magnetic healer in 1895. Although Palmer didn't have any conventional medical training he was obsessed with anatomy and the mechanics of bones and how they link to the spine. He developed his system for spinal manipulation after healing a friend who had lost his hearing following a back injury. His success in this developed into modern-day chiropractic.

Chiropractic focuses on the role of the spine and the nervous system. Because the alignment of the spine affects all the main nerves, practitioners treat not only back pain but also problems such as migraine, pelvic pain and painful periods, even toe and finger pain.

A treatment will be preceded by an in-depth analysis of how you use your body: how you sit, walk, stand and even sleep. Your spine will be checked for curvatures and abnormalities that may be due to posture problems. During a session, a series of techniques or 'thrusts' may be used. These are movements aimed at specific joints or areas of soft tissue where a bone may be slightly out of place or where joints have become inflamed through disease or injury.

McTimoney chiropractic is a variation that checks out other areas such as shoulders, arms, legs and the skull for misalignment. McTimoney chiropractors use a specific and very gentle technique called 'toggle recoil' where one hand acts as a hammer and the other as a nail – they are used together to free up joints.

Chiropractic sessions are very helpful for any musculo-skeletal problems including lower back pain, menstrual pain and headaches. They may also help low mood by solving chronic pain. Chiropractic is respected by most doctors.

DIY? No. Just lie back and let the experts get on with their work!

Osteopathy and Cranial Osteopathy

Osteopathy has been described as a philosophy of medicine. With considerable research to support its effectiveness, it has gained merited quasi-medical status and is now a mainstream therapy often recommended by doctors and surgeons for putting backs, shoulders – and almost anything – back in the right place. Osteopathy is similar to chiropractic but takes a 'whole body' view of the problem. For example, as well as treating the bone misalignment that has caused a sore back, the osteopath will look at the possibility of negative emotions or long-term trauma being the root of the problem. You might, say, be sitting badly and rounding your shoulders because you are shy and insecure, and this would contribute to your back problem. Some osteopathic physicians are working with psychiatrists in America.

The system was devised by engineer-turned-doctor Andrew Taylor Still in 1874. He realised the link between poor posture, the effects on the body of negative emotions, poor diet and long-term results of physical stresses and strains. His engineer's mind saw the body as a complex structure, which – if all the parts were well oiled and connected properly – should run smoothly and heal any problems itself.

The therapy involves manipulating the skeleton, muscles, connective tissue and ligaments and a lot of emphasis is placed on reducing muscle tension. Osteopaths can diagnose and treat many conditions including digestive and reproductive problems, sore joints, aches and pains.

An osteopath will observe how you stand and sit to see how your joints function in various positions. They will also check to see if your spine is straight. Treatment may involve gentle massaging of soft tissue followed by high-velocity thrusts that can make a loud clunk-click in deep joints. This shouldn't hurt but some people simply can't take it and prefer the gentler approach of McTimoney chiropractic or cranial osteopathy.

Cranial osteopathy was developed in the 1930s and works on the concept that the bones of the skull (which are connected by interlocking joints) can be gently massaged to improve the flow of the cerebrospinal fluid surrounding the brain and spinal cord.

According to cranial osteopaths, this fluid is the most important substance in the human body. It is pumped down the spine in a regular pulse-like rhythm linked to our breathing. Trained cranial osteopaths can detect the cranial rhythm (which should beat at about six beats a minute if you're healthy) and by very gentle and subtle manipulation of the skull regulate the flow and restore balance. The pressure is almost imperceptible.

DIY? Once you've consulted an osteopath, he/she may give you simple exercises to do at home. Never try manipulating your own bones without an expert's guidance.

Physiotherapy

Physiotherapy, which had its original roots in massage, goes back to the nineteenth century. The UK Chartered Society of Physiotherapy was founded in 1894 by four young nurses who were also trained masseuses and wanted to protect their profession from falling into disrepute. The aim of modern physiotherapy is to have you up and running again as soon as possible after any mishap or illness.

Physiotherapy, which is available on the NHS and also privately, uses manipulation, stretching and massage techniques as well as electrical and mechanical equipment to rehabilitate damaged limbs, joints and ligaments after illness or injury.

Although it shares some similarities with osteopathy and chiropractic, physiotherapists tend to work in conjunction with doctors and work in a wide variety of health settings such as intensive care, mental illness, stroke recovery, occupational health and care of the elderly. Physiotherapists usually specialise in different types of problem such as obstetric, orthopaedic, incontinence or sports injury. They seldom approach problems from a whole person perspective.

Before starting a course of treatment they will usually refer to X-rays and medical diagnosis by a doctor and will remain in consultation with your GP or consultant. Your treatment programme will include exercises for you to work on daily between treatments.

DIY? Just do the exercises.

Touch therapies

Acupressure

Acupressure originates from the Far East and is similar to acupuncture but instead of using needles, the pressure is applied to acupoints using fingertips, elbows, arms, feet, palms and knees.

When the acupoints are stimulated, chi (life force energy) flows through the body's energy channels, or meridians. Sometimes this is enhanced by gentle massage along the meridians or manipulation or rotating of limbs.

Acupressure practitioners recommend abstaining from alcohol for a couple of days before a treatment as well as avoiding heavy meals for two hours before a session. To help them diagnose your condition they look, touch, feel and intuitively sense your problem as well as asking you lots of lifestyle questions. Don't be surprised if they suddenly rub or push a finger into the sole of your feet to unblock a meridian or waken a sluggish kidney point.

Acupressure can be good for relieving stress, back pain, insomnia, nausea and constipation.

In a trial at the Royal Maternity Hospital in Belfast in 1988 expectant mums were shown how to press an acupressure point in their wrists to prevent morning sickness. It was a great success and the technique dramatically reduced sickness with no side effects.

DIY? Once you know where to press, you can use acupressure whenever you need it. Or try the range called Seabands, which has a good reputation.

Aromatherapy

For centuries, cultures the world over have used essential oils in a variety of ways to heal, treat illness and restore wellbeing. In recent times, essential oils have been used as antiseptics, to treat snakes' bites, treat burns, soothe period pain and even clear headaches. You only have to smell the peel of a fresh orange to experience the healing effects of aromatherapy. Plant-based essential oils have become the foundation of the most popular complementary therapy in the world.

According to experts including Geraldine Howard of London-based company Aromatherapy Associates, aroma-therapy is more than a feel-good factor. Although the science is still foggy, there is some evidence that oils on the skin penetrate into the bloodstream, subtly changing the bio-chemistry of the body as well as the brain. The value of aromatherapy is now accepted by many conventional doctors and nurses the world over and it is used in many hospitals – for women giving birth, geriatric and cancer patients among other groups. As well as much anecdotal evidence, there is some scientific research testifying to its potency. At a trial conducted in 1985 at the Faculty of Medicine of Bobigny, Paris, 28 women were treated for persistent thrush with tea tree oil (a strong anti-fungal). After three months, 21 women were completely thrush-free.

When you visit an aromatherapist, you will be asked about your medical history and lifestyle plus details of any allergies you may suffer and medicines you may be taking. You should also be asked if you might be pregnant, have epilepsy, heart disease or cancer as certain oils may aggra-vate conditions or trigger a problem. Check that your ther-apist uses only top-quality oils; if, as is believed, they are absorbed straight into the bloodstream, that's important.

DIY? See our recommendations over page.
Never take oils internally.

DIY AROMATHERAPY

Think of the pleasure you get from burying your nose in a bunch of scented flowers. Well, at its simplest, that's what you get from aromatherapy. This ancient healing art, which dates back for millennia, involves using fragrant essential oils made from plants including rose, lavender, camomile, grapefruit, frankincense, sandalwood and hundreds more.

Everyone we know – and that includes chaps – loves relaxing in a bath or even simply sitting in a room scented with their favourite oils. It takes you through a gamut of lovely positive feelings. Just as smelling nasty odours – or ones that you connect with bad memories – makes you want to get out quick. In one study, the participants were separated into two rooms. One room was sprayed with a pretty flowery smell, the other with a stinky rotting fish aroma. Then each group was asked the same set of questions. The difference was marked. People in the flowery room all gave happy responses while the other group harped on negative feelings and bad memories.

Smell is the most primitive of our senses and the only one that is directly connected to the brain. Neurons from the brain actually dangle into our noses. The power of smell is so well accepted in Japan that 'Friday evening' and 'Monday morning' blends are sprayed around car factories to subconsciously encourage the workers. Because smell has a fast track to the hypothalamus, which controls the pituitary gland, which in turn governs our hormones, aromatherapy has a direct relevance to menopause, helping to calm and soothe frayed nerves and more.

There is no doubt that aromatherapy is a great life enhancer. You can of course have aromatherapy massages from trained practitioners but there is much you can do for yourself. Below, Geraldine Howard, who has practised aromatherapy for 30 years, gives her favourite recipes for helping you through the menopause.

How to ...

It's not a good idea to use aromatherapy oils directly on your skin in case it causes a sensitivity reaction of some kind. Always mix with a base. For bath, shower or body massage blends, you can blend with oil of any kind (see below), milk, cream or honey. You can also put the same blend in a spray and spray it on you if you prefer. Or you can make a room spray with vodka (because it has no smell) and water. The details are below.

Recommended base oils

Depending on your skin you can use different oils which vary in richness:

- the lightest: jojoba, grapeseed and sunflower
- middling rich: sweet almond, apricot, peach and sesame (that's quite strong smelling)
- richest: coconut, macadamia, olive, borage and evening primrose oil

Geraldine's favourites are borage, evening primrose oil, peach and coconut because they are 'fantastic' for cell renewal and for restoring suppleness and velvety texture to dry skin. Food-grade vegetable oils such as olive, sunflower and sesame are also good because they're so pure, she says. Choose organic if you can.

Honey is marvellous for improving skin texture. It has a long tradition of use for healing wounds. Manuka honey, which you will see recommended in the recipes below, comes from New Zealand; the bees have fed on the blossom of the tea tree which is a staple of the Maori pharmacopeia because it has many important properties including being antiviral, antibacterial and antifungal. Manuka honey is now used in hospitals in New Zealand, Australia and the United Kingdom. It's widely available in food stores and health food shops worldwide – expensive but worth it.

Milk and cream give a touch of Cleopatra, who was reputed to have bathed in asses' milk to preserve her youthful skin. If asses aren't to hand (or willing . . .), try full-fat organic milk or cream. You can use oils in a burner. China burners with tea lights are widely available, or try electric ones such as those by Aromatherapy Associates, which are more expensive but safer – you can leave them on without worrying.

Bath and shower oil for balancing and reviving mind, body and spirit

- *geranium*
- *frankincense*
- *bergamot (optional)*
- *rosewood (optional)*

For each bath, mix 4 to 5 drops essential oils in total with 5 ml (a large teaspoon) of oil, milk, cream or Manuka honey.

For each shower, mix 4 to 5 drops essential oils in total with 10 ml of oil, milk, cream or soft honey (Manuka, if possible) and rub on to chest and tummy.

Tips: You can also use this as a body oil to massage on your skin, in which case mix nine drops in 30 ml of base oil.

For joint aches and pains, use nine drops of rosemary and lavender in 30 ml of base oil.

Body massage oil for swelling, bloating and puffiness of any kind, including cellulite

* *grapefruit (or orange, mandarin or lemon)*
* *rosemary*
* *juniper*

Mix nine drops in all into 30 ml of base oil and use as needed.

Massage into skin wherever there is a problem, using long firm strokes. Swollen tummies often respond to being rubbed clockwise for a couple of minutes.

Tip: You can also use this body massage oil before a shower.

Dry skin oil for face, hands and body

* *frankincense*
* *rose*
* *patchouli (fab for turkey neck)*
* *geranium*
* *sandalwood (if skin very dry)*

Blend just one drop of each oil, five drops in all, with 30 ml of borage or evening primrose oil. This makes one oz and will last for several applications. Keep in a stoppered bottle in a cool, dark place, but not the fridge because that's too cold. Always massage upwards on face and inwards around eyes.

Face mask

- *frankincense*
- *rose*

Put one drop of each in a teaspoonful of soft honey (Manuka, if possible) and stroke on your face with your fingers, working upwards where possible. Leave for 10 to 15 minutes then rinse off with warm water.

Tip: You can use this on your neck and décolletage, and also your hands.

Sleeping and relaxing blend

- *vetivert*
- *Moroccan camomile (or Roman, but that's more expensive)*
- *lavender*

Put two to three drops of each in a bowl of boiling water by your bedside to help you relax and nod off peacefully.

If you wake up in the night, mix one to two drops with five ml of oil and keep in a bottle by the bed; when you wake, inhale deeply from the bottle or put a drop of oil on your chest and breathe in.

You can also make a room or pillow spray with six to eight drops in total of the oils mixed with one teaspoon of vodka; shake this well to mix and then add one teaspoon of filtered water.

Try frankincense on its own to help breathing and also relax you generally. Lavender is a popular remedy for sleeplessness and it is worth trying a few drops of lavender on a tissue if you are restless but be aware that it may not be powerful enough. The blend above is much more potent.

Massage

When something hurts, it's instinctive to rub it better. This is the principle on which massage is based. The Romans swore by it for rest and relaxation and today it's as popular as ever as a panacea for sports injuries, for relieving chronic tension, for helping patients recover from heart attacks and surgery and even for helping premature babies to put on weight.

Massage can be stimulating or relaxing, depending on which techniques are used. It can boost circulation in stiff joints, stimulate the lymphatic system helping the body to detox, and even release the effects of old emotional issues. So it can trigger healing on many different levels.

Most of us enjoy the sort of massage that dissolves those knotty tense areas at the back of the neck and the top of the shoulders, and works over the rest of the body. In fact a good session can make you feel and look at least ten years younger. If you are going through a stressful time or have general aches and pains, it's invaluable.

Allow 90 minutes for a good massage. Tell your therapist how you are feeling, if any parts of your body feel especially tense (or ticklish), what you want to achieve from the session and what sort of pressure you like. Feel free to keep your undies on if you wish, although many fans say that the best results come when you strip off completely. Most therapists are immensely discreet at folding towels around you, so you are never visibly naked.

DIY? Definitely! Buy a book on basic techniques (one with pictures is best) and ask your best friend, partner or child to practise on you. You'll soon learn what strokes you like best and what pressure you enjoy most. There is also simple DIY massage on Dr Ali's website (www.dr-ali.co.uk), which you can download freely.

Reflexology

Reflexology works by applying pressure to points on the feet (or hands) to stimulate healing in other parts of the body. Imagine that the foot is like a tiny road map of the body. So each part of it corresponds with another area. For example the big toe corresponds with the head and where it joins the foot corresponds to the neck. In theory you can heal a headache or soothe a stiff neck by massaging the big toe and its base, but you can also tackle other areas such as stomach, ears, even teeth by rubbing the right part.

Reflexology is many centuries old but was made popular by an American surgeon Dr William Fitzgerald in the early 1900s. He worked with a physiotherapist and between them they worked out a map of all the pressure points on feet that link to around 70,000 nerve endings.

Therapists are able to treat blocked ears, head- and back-ache, migraine, period problems, gall bladder pain and many other conditions by massaging and pressing their fingers in the right place. Energy blockages, which are said to be the possible underlying cause of a particular pain or feeling of unwellness, often manifest as painful knotted areas. Be warned that it can be quite – or very – sore at times.

Trials involving pregnant women using reflexology have been held in several countries. All of them showed that women having regular treatments during pregnancy not only had the time they spent in labour reduced but also their need for pain relief. Reflexology has also been shown to reduce the pain of endometriosis. Many doctors admit that good reflexologists can also be excellent diagnosticians.

DIY? Although nothing replaces a really good practitioner who is tuned in to you, reflexology is a safe and rewarding therapy to try at home. Read a couple of good books on the subject (again pictures are really helpful) and try it out. Interestingly, just massaging a woman's foot may help dispel menopausal symptoms almost as effectively. A recent study showed that anxiety, depression, hot flushes and night sweats responded equally to sessions of reflexology and to non-specific foot massage. (However, the non-specific massage was given by qualified reflexologists and that could have affected the results.)

Reiki

Reiki is a Japanese word meaning 'universal life force energy'. It is a safe, hands-on therapy, which aims to heal mind, body and spirit. It was developed just over a hundred years ago by a Japanese priest called Dr Mikao Usui who claimed to have discovered a way of channelling an ancient healing energy. Potential healers participate in an 'attunement process' to open their own healing channels to allow the Reiki energy to pass through them so that they can begin to heal others.

Many Reiki healers believe that illness is a message to you from your body and they see a link between physical and mental health and 'dis-ease'. In simple terms they may connect problems with ears as corresponding with an inability to 'hear' and deal with important issues. Problems with eyes may indicate that you are not 'seeing' certain situations and this may be affecting your health.

Reiki sets out to help clear physical and emotional blockages that may lead to disease by charging the aura (an energy field that healers see around the body) with positive healing energy.

During a treatment you either lie down or sit quietly in a chair while your healer places their hands above your head. Some people may feel a tingling sensation of warmth during a session whilst others experience beautiful colours, dreams or pictures, or remember long-forgotten memories. Some people feel nothing at all until maybe a day or two later. Although it is so gentle, it can have extraordinarily powerful results.

DIY? You have to go through the 'attunement process' to practise Reiki but once you have done a course you can practise healing on yourself whenever you need, which many people find very empowering.

Nature therapies

Hydrotherapy

We are naturally water creatures. After all, we swam in our mother's womb, bathed in amniotic fluid, for nine months. In fact, some scientists now believe that human beings originated in the sea – the so-called Aquatic Ape theory – and that when we were developing higher brains, we lived in freshwater lakes and swamps by the savannah. Infants up to six months old have the same diving reflex as aquatic mammals like dolphins; drop a baby into water and it will submerge, stop breathing, slow down its heart rate, then re-emerge, turn its head to the side, breathe and dive again.

The bones that we have in our arms and hands are exactly the same as dolphins' flippers.

What's more, we are actually made of water. Newborn babies are about 97 per cent water, adults about 75 per cent (women contain more water) and our brains consist of about 75 per cent water (some of it contained in the fat cells, which form about two-thirds of the brain). As women, our cycles mirror the waxing and waning of the moon (which governs the tides) because of the water content in our cells.

The Greeks and Romans insisted on bathing daily, Chinese medicine recognised water as a source of chi – or life energy – and Ayurveda sees water as the source of all life, yet somehow along the way we have forgotten how brilliant water is. Our health is entirely dependent on a constant supply of fresh water (see how a headache disappears if you start drinking more water), and extraordinary things can happen when we exercise, or just play, in water. Yet we hardly notice the scope of its healing energies. We simply take it for granted.

Hydrotherapy can take many forms from a day at a spa to swimming in the sea to using naturopathic sitz baths (where you hop alternately from a hot bath to a cold one). All these forms of hydrotherapy help to boost the metabolism, increase blood circulation, lower blood pressure and remove toxins from your body – through perspiration. Being submerged in water also increases kidney activity, helps relieve aching muscles and sends oxygen and nutrients into the skin's tissues to help repair damage. It also relieves mental fatigue, reduces anxiety, improves memory, increases levels of concentration and creativity, boosts mental alertness and helps you sleep.

DIY? Here's a good treatment to incorporate on a daily basis: pour a fistful of Epsom Salts into warm running water (blood temperature is best) for a relaxing and detoxing bath. And don't forget to drink your H_2O too! At least eight big glasses of still pure water daily.

Light Therapy

We all need light. It keeps us physically and psychologically healthy as well as helping to regulate our inner biological clock which tells us when to fall asleep and wake up. But the notion of using light as therapy is relatively new and came about through doctors helping people to beat the winter blues or SAD (seasonal affective disorder), which is caused by lack of sunshine.

As many as one in three people suffer from seasonal depression when the clocks go back but experts have discovered that light boxes or panels (sometimes called light baths) that give out full spectrum or bright white light – the same as a bright spring day but without the UV rays – are often enough to trick the brain into thinking it's still summer time.

Light boxes can be placed next to computers or televisions. There are also special light clocks that can be programmed to come on in the morning and wake you gently. The light activates a chemical in the brain called melatonin, which controls sleep patterns and can also be used to treat jet lag.

Leading British expert Professor Chris Thompson of the department of psychiatry at Southampton University says two hours of exposure to bright light each day could relieve symptoms in 90 per cent of SAD sufferers. His research shows that exposure to artificial light with the intensity of sunlight lifts depression and helps stop people overeating during winter. It has led to some companies in Europe installing light boxes on their employees' desks.

Even if you don't get SAD, having some light therapy in the winter months boosts most people, both physically and psychologically.

DIY? Yes, definitely. Either buy yourself a light box, or make sure that you get outside in the sunshine for at least an hour a day.

Movement therapies

Alexander Technique

This therapy teaches people how to develop better posture and to move more naturally. It was devised by an Australian actor, Frederick Alexander, in the 1930s to help overcome voice problems.

An Alexander teacher will analyse your posture and balance before introducing you to techniques and exercises that can be worked into everyday life. Lessons typically include lying flat with your head propped up and knees raised while the teacher encourages your muscles to relax. You are also taught how to sit and walk correctly. It needs to be learnt over a period of about six weeks or more, with at least one lesson each week, plus homework! Many devotees like to have continuing regular sessions.

Alexander technique is suitable for people suffering from musculo-skeletal disorders or with back pain, whiplash injuries or repetitive strain injuries. It is also good in pregnancy. Teachers believe the technique can ease some emotional disorders including depression.

DIY? You need to have a thorough grounding with a teacher who will tell you exactly what your particular posture is like and what you need to work on. You can then do your homework on your own. But you can't do the initial work from studying a book.

Dance Therapy

Dance therapy is a way of expressing inner thoughts, emotions and thoughts through dance and free-flowing movements. Sessions are organised by trained therapists, both with and without music. The aim is to unlock repressed feelings and raise self-esteem and self-awareness.

Many adults find they can express themselves better in non-verbal ways and that the freedom of dance unlocks deeply held inhibitions. It can be practised on a one-to-one basis or within a group and a course usually lasts for around six weeks.

Some methods such as Biodanza help to overcome inhibitions about getting physically and/or emotionally near to other people.

DIY? Yes, absolutely. Do whatever you enjoy best whether it's jiving down the hall, playing air guitar along to the Rolling Stones, practising ballet steps at the kitchen sink or dancing the rumba round the sitting room. Dancing loosens us up and makes us smile!

Psychological/emotional 'mind and spirit' therapies

Art Therapy

Art therapy was pioneered around 50 years ago to help people who had suffered traumatic experiences during the Second World War. It's now used widely by psychiatrists and psychologists as a diagnostic and therapeutic treatment for a wide range of mental and emotional disorders.

As well as being creatively uplifting, it can be used as a

way of expressing difficult emotions. It can be literally a life-saver for those recently bereaved or traumatised by divorce or relationship problems. Many art therapists encourage their patients to paint or draw what they see or experience in their dreams or to make a painting using colours they 'feel' are important or significant.

Art therapy can be useful in treating eating disorders, alcohol, food and drug abuse, long-term illness and feelings of low self-esteem and loneliness. It's used extensively in prisons, hospitals and respite centres.

During menopause many women long to be creative and to express themselves. This can take many forms, anything from painting in any medium or sewing collages to jewellery or baking.

DIY? Buy some crayons, paints or felt pens and splurge them on paper – go big, small, coloured or black and white. Let your imagination run riot. Indulge in gorgeous fabrics and beads to make collages or simply walk on the sea shore or in a forest and gather up what you can find to bring home and turn into something beautiful. Or paint a room in a colour you love. It will make your heart sing.

Bereavement counselling

Bereavement and grief affects us all during some stage of our lives, particularly at menopause as parents grow old and die, leaving many women with emotional issues they could never predict. The loss of a loved one (or the guilt of *not* loving parents, however dutiful you've been) can be totally devastating. Some people are able to deal with bereavement on their own while others find one-to-one counselling or support groups, where others are in the same situation, invaluable.

Experts agree that it is usually better to confront grief and anxieties during the beginning stages if possible. Letting it manifest unresolved for months, or even years, can lead to serious conditions requiring treatment and professional help.

If you are bereaved and hurting, don't suffer in silence. There is light at the end of the tunnel. Bereavement counselling is available through various organisations. It can help you come to terms with loss in your own way and in your own time. If you do need help, then reach out for it, ask your GP or look in your local library for details of organisations who are there to help. There are now hundreds of bereavement support groups all over the country.

DIY? Don't bottle things up. Simply talking to friends (the ones who are able to share feelings and experiences without fear) can be very comforting. But you have to admit the need for help – and feel entitled to it. You are not being weak.

Biofeedback

Biofeedback is a technique devised in the 1960s that trains you how to control unconscious functions such as your heart rate, blood pressure and sweat gland activity.

By learning what triggers these events in your body you can – in theory – learn how to control them. A biofeedback device is used, which can sense and measure minute fluctuations in skin temperature, heart and pulse rates, muscle tension and brain-wave activity. Electrodes from the machine are clipped on to the skin of the user. With the sensors in place, you are taught how to relax using breathing techniques and muscle relaxation. When you are relaxed, your skin will warm up a few degrees and you will start to perspire; your heart rate will slow down and your brain will emit long slow alpha waves. By learning how this feels and seeing the effects on the monitor, you can train yourself into a state of deep relaxation – but be warned, it may take quite a bit of practice.

Biofeedback can be useful if you have insomnia, stress, anxiety, high blood pressure, asthma and incontinence (urinary and anal). It is currently being used in helping people with the involuntary loss of wind, liquid or solid stools at the London Biofeedback Centre at the London Clinic. Stress is considered a major factor in this condition, which significantly affects women over 65 years. Results are impressive with a 60 to 80 per cent success rate after a six- to nine-months programme. Biofeedback may also help with hot flushes.

DIY? Not a DIY treatment without a machine but the techniques learnt may be useful at home.

Counselling

Sometimes we have problems that are just too difficult to sort out by ourselves. Counselling is a talking therapy that helps when you want to resolve a specific problem, which is making you feel depressed or traumatised.

Sessions take place with a qualified (do make sure of that) counsellor within a safe and confidential environment and usually last for just under an hour. During this time, the therapist gives unconditional positive support and feedback making the client feel listened to and hopefully understood, and able to express difficult emotions and feelings – sometimes for the first time in their lives. The objective is for the client to be able to perceive herself (or himself) as a person with the power and freedom to change (rather than as a passive object), able to come to terms with negative feelings that may underlie emotional problems.

Counselling is good for problems caused by abusive relationships, work difficulties, anxiety, eating disorders and is very effective in curing depression. Most counselling is shorter term than psychotherapy, which tends to look comprehensively at all aspects of the client's experience. However, counselling and psychotherapy are as much about enhancing your life as about problem-solving.

DIY? Sharing problems with friends can be very therapeutic and women are usually good at that. But for big or intractable problems, it's best to consult a professional.

Creative visualisation

Close your eyes and imagine you are in a sunny flower-filled meadow with a river flowing through it. See the sunlight on the water, watch the grass bending in the wind, look up to the the birds wheeling in the sky ...

If you can picture this you are well on the way to learning the technique of creative visualisation. This simple – and completely free – therapy can bring deep relaxation, feelings of tranquillity and even pain relief. It is highly effective and easily learnt.

Sessions, which can be done on your own or in a group, usually begin with closing your eyes and focusing on your breathing for about five minutes. Then the therapist takes you on an imaginative journey, which makes you more and more relaxed.

In some cancer centres and hospices, creative images are used to help patients feel in control of their treatment – they may see learn to 'see' their cancer cells as dragons to be slain, or imagine themselves standing under healing showers of golden light. As well as feeling relaxed you can feel very empowered with visualisation.

DIY? Begin by imagining or remembering a favourite scene – somewhere you have been happy. Remember you can go anywhere, be any size, take any shape. Let your imagination take you where it will, remembering always that you are in control. There are many books and also pre-recorded visualisation tapes available to buy if your mind's eye needs waking up.

IDEAS FOR CREATIVE VISUALISATION

If you are lying awake in bed fretting about problems, put them all into the basket of an air balloon, launch it and watch it float away into the sky until it disappears from view.

If you are worried about people in your life, put them into a sturdy houseboat and anchor it in a lovely place. Make sure all is safe and sound, then step into a beautiful light sail boat and speed away from them across glinting waves in the sunlight.

In iffy situations, where you sense there is animosity or tension, erect a glass wall between you and others, or surround yourself with a cylinder of golden light at least a metre wide. Or wrap a beautiful blue cloak around you, shot with gold; make sure the hood comes well down over your face and that it covers you completely down to the ground.

If you have a joyful experience, store it away in your mind's eye to use as a visualisation when things are more difficult.

Flower remedies

Flower remedies (also known as flower essences) have become one of the most popular alternative treatments in the last few years. Go into any chemist or health food shop on the high street and you'll see a dazzling selection from Australia, the Amazon and Alaska to our own traditional English blends, each with its own unique healing properties.

They are extremely gentle yet powerful and can act as a healing catalyst, immediately lifting your spirits, soothing fears and putting your life back into focus. They have been used for thousands of years across the globe and are one of the simplest but most effective medicines known to man.

Most flower remedies work on an emotional level helping to solve issues at their source. Many therapists believe that long-term emotional problems may manifest as physical illness if left unresolved. The father of British flower remedies, Dr Edward Bach, a Harley Street physician who developed his range of 38 essences in the 1930s, said that negative feelings such as anger, jealousy, grief and despair could be the root of many illness including cancer, migraine and arthritis.

DIY? Yes. You do not need to consult a therapist before taking them – although some people require a mixture of several which can be hard to work out for yourself.

Take between two and four drops of the remedies either diluted in water or neat on the tongue throughout the day. Treatment is taken for as long as the individual needs but can be effective after just one dose. They can ease tension, anxiety, fear and despair and even a fear of change, which is particularly useful at menopause. (See overleaf for more details.)

THE COMFORT OF FLOWERS

Human beings have an instinctive attraction to plants and flowers. Think of the delight when you are given a bunch of fragrant roses or see the first daffodils in spring. We give flowers naturally to people who are feeling poorly in body or mind. Whatever you're going through, these blooms have the power to make you feel better.

But, according to some health practitioners including medical doctors, you can use the vibrational energy of flowers to shift negative emotions and give powerful help through difficult times. Dr Andrew Tresidder, a family doctor in Somerset, England, says: 'Flower remedies or essences are not for any physical symptom. They act as an invisible support tool to support our feelings and emotions, and restore harmony and balance. This can be important through the time of menopause when there are so many emotional shifts going on as well as the physical changes.'

Flower remedies are not the same as the essential oils used in aromatherapy. They are the healing vibrations of a flower or plant, captured in water, and preserved with brandy or vodka. If that seems barking, consider a compact disc. A CD is a round flat piece of plastic, but it contains a vibrational imprint that gives us sounds – and we take it for granted every day of our lives.

Flower remedies help us to use our intuition – to get out of our logical left brain and into our creative right brain. They enable us to feel with our hearts and then think with our heads so that we can access what we really want, rather than constructing what our brains think we want. 'We need both heart and head to be true to ourselves,' says Dr Tresidder. 'The heart first to tell us where to go, then the head to help us do it and learn from the journey.'

The low moods so often experienced by women at menopause may be due to feelings that have never been honoured and have got stuck, sometimes since child-hood. Using flower remedies can help you over these. Sometimes our frame of mind gets locked in negative emotions such as intolerance, frustration, anxiety, being unloving and critical. Flower remedies can help us move out of the block and let our emotions flow again.

There are three main ways of choosing the right remedies for you – remember that there is no such thing as the wrong essence because they can't do you any harm. You can consult a practitioner, or a book, or you can let your intuition guide you. The first two are self-explanatory. The third may seem slightly weird and whacky. Dr Tresidder suggests getting a box of remedies and running your fingertips over them. If you find that one or more feels unusually hot or cold compared with the others, those are the ones to take. If you are famil-iar with dowsing (the same method used for water and oil divining), you can use that method.

When you have chosen your remedies, put three to six drops of each in a little pure water, and sip. You can also make up your own combination remedy (see below for ready-made ones) by putting the various drops into a dropper bottle and topping up with brandy or vodka, then take this in a little water. Remember that your emotional needs may change frequently, even from day to day, so a set of essences is a useful investment.

Dr Edward Bach made up the first range of flower rem-edies in the 1930s. There are now over 40 major brands worldwide (see Directory for details), some of which pro-duce combinations specifically for the menopause or for problems such as sexuality. These include Female Essence by Jan de Vries, Menopause Essence by South African Flower Combination Essences, Woman Essence and Sex-uality Essence by Australian Bush Flower Essence.

As well as healing yourself, you can create a peaceful

environment around you, which can help others to heal themselves. Although it's not honourable to treat other people without their permission, it is common sense to help yourself and the people who share your space. 'That is neither judgemental nor are you patronising someone by setting out to rescue them,' explains Dr Tresidder. The simplest way to help an environment is with a room spray. There are increasing ranges of these, including specific remedies for children (such as Indigo Essences). You can of course also make up your own sprays too.

One menopausal patient was under a lot of stress from her husband's moodiness. The situation was transformed by flower remedies, according to Dr Tresidder. 'Foot and mouth had stopped them following their favourite hobby, which was walking for long distances. They moved house but he was moody, withdrawn and generally low. My patient dowsed a combination for their living space, which she made up and sprayed in the bedroom and sitting room. By the seventeenth day, he had changed and was back to his former jolly self.'

Flower essences are completely non-invasive and can be taken with any other preparations, including Western drugs and homeopathic remedies.

If you are new to flower remedies, Dr Tresidder suggests the following ones may be particularly helpful for feelings associated with the change of life:

- Rescue Remedy, also known as Emergency Essence: this combination contains five essences which help you cope with acute stress of any kind. Put six drops in a glass of water and sip frequently over an hour or two. If you have a major life event such as the death of a parent, put a couple of drops in every drink for as many weeks as you feel you need. Remember however that you may need other help too (such as homeopathy, counselling or Western drugs).

- agrimony: if you put a brave face on things and find it difficult to share underlying worries.
- centaury: if you have difficulty saying no to demands of all kinds.
- heather: if you have lost your outward interest in life and become introspective and turned in on yourself.
- holly: if you have negative emotions including jealousy, suspicion and greed.
- red Chestnut: if you care and worry about other people too much, this will enable you to care with compassion but without anxiety.
- walnut: gives support through changes of all kinds, e.g. birth, death, house move, job change and also acute problems such as exam or interview nerves; helps you move from one phase to another. You can take for up to two months or until the stress has passed.
- willow: if you have any form of self-pity, resentment or bitterness: 'Why me? It's not fair ... '.

Any flower essence that you have chosen can also be used as a spray. Any Emergency Remedy is useful, because places carry feelings as well as people. Make up a spray by choosing your combination of essences for the situation, placing some of each into a plant or clothes mister, along with some water, some alcohol (to stop it going stale) and aromatherapy oils to your liking. Then just spray!

If you'd rather buy one off the shelf, Australian Bush Sprays are available such as Calm and Clear, Space Clearing, whilst available from the Alaskan Essences are Purification, Guardian and Calling All Angels, all sold quite widely. The Living Tree also make their own Orchid Essence Sprays. For other British-made ones, visit www.greenmanessences.com for a selection of four ready-made goodies!

Healing

Healing, which is sometimes referred to as 'laying on of hands', is a therapy used all over the world and is common among most major religions.

Healers believe that healing energy can be transferred or 'channelled' to sick people (sick in mind, body or spirit) using the power of the mind. Depending on their particular tradition, healers believe this energy comes to them from God (faith healing) or from the universe or cosmos (spiritual healing). The treatment involves nothing more complicated than relaxing while the healer places his or her hands on or near your body. In some forms of healing, you needn't even be present. The healer will simply 'send' healing thoughts to you; this is called absent healing.

Sessions can last up to an hour, although some are much shorter. How often you choose to go depends on whether you feel the treatment is working for you. Many people feel an effect straight away, although others report that they need several sessions for a real difference. Healers, and there are an estimated 20,000 in Britain, claim there is no condition that will not benefit from healing, but most recommend that in cases of disease it is used alongside conventional medicine.

In fact, you could say that healing is part of the interaction between any member of the caring professions and their patient or client.

DIY? Asking God or the universe to receive healing energy can be as effective as going to a healer.

SPIRITUALITY AND PRAYER

In the American SWAN survey (Study of Women's Health Across the Nation), which is following multiethnic women between 42 and 52, spiritual therapies – healing and prayer – were used by over a third (34.7%) in one group. The authors of the report in the *American Journal of Public Health*, November 2002, say: 'Although no clinical evidence exists for the benefits of spiritual methods used for psychological symptoms during midlife, there is growing evidence that the individual practice of spirituality and prayer has positive benefits for physical and mental health.'

Hypnotherapy

Hypnotherapy is based on the theory that the conscious and unconscious minds govern our health. It is increasingly used by the medical profession, particularly to treat phobias, give up smoking, for pain relief and recently for menopausal symptoms such as hot flushes. The hypnotherapist uses deep relaxation techniques to induce a 'trance-like' state in their clients and, during this time, makes suggestions or implants ideas. You are not unconscious and, contrary to popular belief, cannot be forced by reputable hypnotherapists to do anything you do not want to. (If there was a fire alarm, for instance, you would respond immediately.)

Hypnotherapy is thought to work by helping the patient relax and be more positive. Hypnosis induces relaxation, and it is thought that a successful result is brought about by getting the patient to associate strong feelings with the goal of getting over – for instance – the hot flush or desire for a cigarette, rather than focusing on the negative side.

Hypnotherapy is also used to treat problems such as stammering and panic attacks, although some people find only limited success with it.

It is extremely important that you find a reputable hypnotherapist. There is no official umbrella body but you can ask your GP to refer you to a reputable doctor or psychologist trained as a hypnotherapist.

DIY? There are many tapes available for learning self-hypnosis; therapists will also teach you specific exercises.

HYPNOTISM MAY BE A NEW TREATMENT FOR HOT FLUSHES

Doctors who treated a group of women with hot flushes with sessions of hypnotism say that the frequency and severity were significantly reduced. The length of time that each attack lasted was also cut.

All the women in the group were treated with four sessions over a month to see what effect it had. They recorded the frequency, duration and severity of their hot flushes in a diary, and at the end of the trial doctors analysed the results. As well as a reduction in hot flushes, there was an overall improvement of the women's quality of life. They enjoyed better sleep and less fatigue.

'We conclude that hypnosis appears to be a feasible and promising treatment for hot flushes, with a potential to improve quality of life and insomnia,' reported the doctors from the London Regional Cancer Centre, Ontario.

Laughter Therapy

Laughter therapy clinics are springing up in hospitals all over the world as doctors tune into the healing benefits of a good chuckle. Laughter can help in the treatment of various conditions, especially those connected to depression, anxiety, hypertension and diabetes although patients recovering from heart surgery and those undergoing treatment from cancer are also said to benefit. Typically a session involves patients watching funny videos or playing games for up to an hour at a time.

Professor Duncan Geddes, consultant in respiratory medicine at London's Royal Brompton Hospital, says that laughter is an important medicine. 'Laughter is an expression of happiness and happiness is good for all of us. It stimulates the body's defences, reduces pain and helps recovery from illness. Laughter therapy is developing fast and new research is looking into the ways that laughter happens, how it affects hormones, how it stimulates the brain and how it makes us all healthier and happier.'

Psychologists in Scotland at Glasgow's Caledonian University say that comedy could act as a painkiller, after they found that people listening to Billy Connolly show pain tolerance up to three times the normal level.

DIY? Yes! Spend time with friends who make you laugh and enjoy life. Watch funny films, read amusing books, store up jokes for bad days. You can even fake smiling and laughing and get good results. Research shows that 'acting' laughter sends cascades of the same feel-good hormones around your body.

Life/work coaching

If you seem to be stuck in a rut in your life or underachieving at work – bored to tears with life or overwhelmed by it – then a session with a life or work coach could be just what you need.

Just as a sports coach is able to offer better performance strategies, because of his detached perspective and honed psychological skills, so a good life or work coach will boost your confidence, give you greater self-awareness and focus on what you really want to do. They can also help you to discover your choices in life and give you greater motivation to act.

Life/work coaching is available either one-to-one or on the Internet. You will need to discuss the issues you wish to work with and then work out a timetable and plan for change. A good coach will be able to give you lots of support and encouragement along the way and will stop patterns of behaviour or negative attitudes that might be holding you back.

You will usually need at least eight sessions to set you on track but some people find more is better.

DIY? There are many self-help books available as well as organisations like Breakthrough (see Directory). Life coaching is essentially goal setting so try teaming up with a friend and meeting regularly to give each other inspiration, encouragement and support.

Meditation

Meditation is a discipline, rather than a therapy, which aims to give you total relaxation of body and mind. Although there are many different forms, the underlying aim is to clear your mind and become a human being rather than a human doing. Tibetan spiritual medicine describes it as being in the space between moments. You can see it as being at one with the universe rather than buzzing and bustling round in a material world. Once learnt, meditation can be practised anywhere – in the bath, on the bus, or in bed – and will bring a sense of instant calm and wellbeing.

There are many separate schools of meditation in Britain but one of the largest is Transcendental Meditation (TM). This instructs you to sit still with your eyes closed, clear your mind completely and repeat a word or mantra, which is given to you individually. There is quite a hefty charge for learning the technique of TM, which some people object to. The organisation says that people value what they pay for and are more likely, therefore, to practise it. Many other forms of meditation make no charge. In Buddhist meditation, the principle is the same but you are taught to concentrate on positive feelings and breathing, which is common to most Eastern meditative practices.

Meditation is most effective if you do it daily. TM asks that people meditate for 20 minutes twice a day. Regular practice helps relieve anxiety and alleviates many stress-related symptoms such as insomnia and fatigue, migraine, asthma and hormonal problems such as PMS. Fans say that meditation can lead to greater vitality, clarity of mind, creativity and self-belief. There is considerable medical evidence about its benefits and many doctors recommend it.

DIY? Definitely. For suggestions on how to get started, see the section on retention breathing and visualisation on page 80.

Music Therapy

Music therapy can be done on your own or with a group. Either way you will be encouraged to sing, clap, beat out rhythms on drums or improvise using other instruments.

Therapists learn a lot about the way in which people participate with others by their approach to making sound. Emotional and communication problems can be worked through and music can forge a strong link between people who may find using words difficult.

Music therapists work in prisons, schools and hospitals and can help people to shift and articulate difficult issues.

During sessions many people find themselves remembering old memories; this may give them the chance to look at problems that may be the root of new ones or help them lose old baggage.

Another form of music therapy examines the effects that individual sounds have on people and their auras (energy fields); sound healers sometimes work by encouraging people to sing certain notes that help to bring them back into balance. In a similar way, certain pieces of music can have profoundly healing effects on people.

DIY? Most of us are drawn to favourite pieces of music that have the power to transform our moods. Discover which pieces 'do' things for you, record them and have them ready when you need them. Don Campbell, author of The Mozart Effect and leading exponent of music therapy, gets people to integrate with music by playing at conducting it: listen to anything you like and pretend you're directing the orchestra. Or stand on the seashore and conduct the waves and seagulls. You don't need to know anything about real conducting, just let go and pretend.

Psychotherapy

Psychotherapy tends to be a long-term intense programme, which may last from one to five years. However, many psychotherapists are flexible and will be happy to see how things go. It is suitable for people feeling that everything about their life needs working on, rather than just one element.

There arc many different schools of psychotherapy, including Freudian and Jungian, which started to develop as methods in the early twentieth century. If you are contemplating psychotherapy, ask exactly what school a potential therapist is trained by and how sessions will work for you. Some therapists listen in silence – which can be unnerving – while others support you through what may in many ways seem like ordinary conversation with a close friend, the sort where you feel you can say absolutely anything and get a caring, perceptive and intelligent response.

Some psychotherapists will examine your family relationships, others will want to work on specific aspects of your childhood, whereas others may focus on your thinking style and behaviour. An increasing number of doctors employ the services of psychotherapists and also counsellors to work with some patients.

DIY? No.

Radionics

Radionics is a therapy that is both diagnostic and therapeutic. It uses a machine called a 'black box' to analyse hair, nail clippings, blood samples or handwriting from the patient. These samples are called 'witnesses' and can be analysed by a radionics practitioner without ever having to meet the patient. It was pioneered in the early 1900s by an American neurologist Dr Albert Abrahams, who discovered that his diagnoses using the black box were very accurate.

Radionics practitioners say that each of us is surrounded by an energy field which resonates at a certain vibration. The vibration of the 'witness' sample is checked to see if it matches that of a normal well person and if it doesn't, the practitioner can tune in to you via your 'witness' to readjust your energy field using the black box.

Before a consultation you will be asked about your general state of health and whether or not you are on any medication. The practitioner will often dowse across the questionnaire with a pendulum for more clues to the patient's health. (Dowsing is an ancient method of detection also used for water divining.) After diagnosis, the black box is used to 'broadcast' (transmit) healing to the patient. Flower essences and homeopathic remedies may also be recommended as part of the treatment.

DIY? Not for amateurs.

7

BEATING THE LADYKILLERS:

Osteoporosis, Breast Cancer, Heart Disease

This chapter covers:
* essential lifestyle measures for keeping a healthy body and mind
* osteoporosis: what it is
* quick risk test for osteoporosis
* tests for bone mineral density
* treatment for thinning bones: drugs, diet, exercise and supplements
* breast cancer
* heart disease

In this chapter, we look at the main diseases that can affect women as they age: osteoporosis, breast cancer and heart disease. The one that frightens women most – understandably – is breast cancer but, in fact, heart disease is the number one cause of death in women although the rate is falling. The prognosis for breast cancer, which is estimated to affect one in nine women during their lifetime, is also brighter. However, osteoporosis – known as 'the silent illness' because many women are simply unaware of it – has become a health crisis worldwide: it affects one in three women over 50 and the complications following fractures can prove fatal.

These diseases are frightening – many of us have lost friends or family – but the good news is that there is a great deal you can do to help reduce your chances of developing them, or to prevent a recurrence. And far from having to follow different complicated diets or exercise routines, the advice for all of them is simple lifestyle stuff plus regular health checks. Exactly the same as for optimal health and minimising menopausal symptoms.

The essential lifestyle measures that your body and mind need are all in this book but – just to remind you – this is what you should be thinking of:

- eat a good fresh diet with carefully chosen nutritional supplements if necessary.
- graze don't gorge: three meals and three snacks daily is great.
- cut down on red meat (two 3 oz portions weekly is okay) and eat two portions of oily fish a week.
- get five, and preferably more, portions of fresh veg and fruit daily, including lots of green leafy vegetables.
- avoid processed foods and drinks of all kinds.
- drink lots of water – at least eight big glasses daily between meals.
- cut down on coffee.
- cut down on salt.
- don't drink more than 14 units of alcohol weekly (1 unit = 1 small glass of wine).
- don't smoke.
- take regular exercise – half an hour at least daily.
- get out in the sunlight.
- practise stress management strategies such as breathing, yoga and meditation.
- do things you like; be happy.

OSTEOPOROSIS

Unlike our skin, which is on display all the time, we often take our bones for granted. But think of a body without bone – you would be like a jellyfish on land. Bones give the body support and enable you to stand upright. Bone protects vital organs, including your heart, lungs and brain. Every time you move, your bones are involved. Just like your heart or your brain or your blood supply, bone is a wonderful organ that needs to be respected and nourished. From the earliest days of your life, your teeth and skin are fussed over: your bones need the same care. The sooner this begins the better: so please look after your bones and get all the women you know, whatever their age, to do the same – prevention is much much better than cure. (See below.)

Don't think of bone as dead material: it's a dynamic living organ. Your bones consist of two main parts: connective tissue – mainly collagen – which provides the toughness and flexibility, packed around with solid crystals of minerals rather like a honeycomb. These minerals provide the hardness and they include calcium, magnesium and boron: 99 per cent of your body's calcium is contained in your bones and teeth, and 60 per cent of its magnesium. What's more, bone is continually renewing itself. It can grow – as when you break a limb, or it can thin – as with osteoporosis. The bone-making cells are called osteoblasts, which mature into osteocytes. The bone-shedding cells are called osteo-clasts: they actually cause the bone to be 'resorbed' (gobbled up) into surrounding tissues of the body.

Your skeleton grows with you from before birth. The first period of rapid bone growth is from birth to two years. The second is during puberty, roughly from 11 to 14 in girls (13 to 17 in boys). Interestingly, the bone tissue accumulated during that second stage approximately equals the amount lost during the 30 years following menopause. The skeleton reaches its maximum size around the age of 20. The bone mass then consolidates and reaches peak bone density at about 30 to 35. After that, you slowly start losing bone. (That's why it's so important for girls and young women to look after their bones through a good diet and exercise.)

Effect of osteoporosis on bone structure

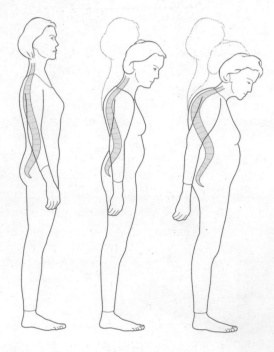

The strength of your bones depends on the fragile balance between bone making and shedding. Disturbing that balance can lead to weakening of the bone. The weaker the bone, the more likelihood of a fracture. The word osteoporosis literally means 'porous bones', from the Greek word *osteo*

meaning 'bones' and *porosis* meaning 'porous'. Imagine a bone as looking like a bath sponge with holes and pores. Now imagine those holes increasing in size so the actual mesh of the sponge shrinks and there are more and more holes and less and less solid material – that's what osteoporotic bone is like. (As someone put it: 'the Swiss cheese look'.)

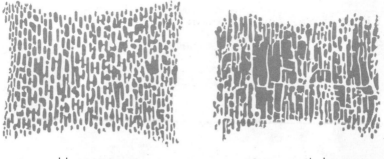

normal bone structure   osteoporotic bone

There are many possible factors that can contribute to bone loss. Each case of osteoporosis is usually due to several different causes, including a genetic susceptibility, poor diet, not enough exercise, some disease conditions and oestrogen deficiency. As we've said in the last chapter on HRT, it was recognised in the mid twentieth century that you need oestrogen to achieve the optimal peak bone density because oestrogen stops bone shedding. That's why missing periods for over six months under the age of 35 is a significant risk factor for osteoporosis, and why falling oestrogen levels at menopause can be a crucial turning point in the life of your bones. (That's why it's important for women who go through premature menopause to consider HRT and to take the best possible care in terms of diet and exercise.)

The current estimate is that one in three women over the age of 50 will develop osteoporosis, which increases their risk of fractures of wrist, hip or spinal vertebrae. (One in 12 men is at risk too so include the men in your life in your bone health prevention strategies.) But all too often, the disease isn't discovered until people have had a fracture and it's too late to put things right.

Spinal vertebral fractures usually happen to women in their 60s, hip fractures in the 70s and 80s – partly because the bones are more fragile and also because women tend to fall more. Although people do not die of the fracture itself, the complications can prove fatal. One in five women die within a year of having a hip fracture. The lifetime risk for women of dying from complications following a hip fracture is the same as dying from breast cancer. About one in five each of hip and spinal vertebral fractures are estimated to lead to death. For survivors, quality of life is hugely impaired with ongoing pain, decreased mobility and increased dependence. One year after a hip fracture, 40 per cent of survivors are unable to walk without help and 60 per cent need help with at least one essential daily activity. Spinal vertebral fractures lead to loss of height, severe pain, reduced mobility, respiratory difficulty and general loss of quality of life. Wrist fractures (known as Colles fractures), which occur when you fall on an outstretched hand, can be very painful and lead to considerable disability short term, as well as making the sufferer dependent on help with everything from dressing to going to the bathroom.

How do you know if you have osteoporosis?

At present experts agree that screening everyone, as for breast or cervical cancer, is not advisable. So we really want you to do this quick questionnaire every year to assess your risk. If you have one or more of the risk factors, please go and discuss the results with your doctor, who may refer you for one of the tests we explain below. If it turns out that your bone density is decreasing, there are drugs to help it if necessary, which we detail below, as well as the lifestyle measures we explain in this book.

Osteoporosis risk test

☐ Have you been through natural menopause and *not* discussed osteoporosis with your doctor?

☐ Has either of your parents broken a hip after a minor bump or fall?

☐ Has either of your parents been diagnosed with osteoporosis?

☐ Have you broken a bone after a minor bump or fall?

☐ Have you had a hip, wrist or spinal vertebral fracture?

☐ Have you had, or do you have, anorexia?

☐ Do you have a poor diet, with little fresh fruit and vegetables and a lot of processed foods, soft drinks, coffee and animal fats?

☐ Is your BMI less than 20 now, or was it less than 20 when you were having periods? (See page 62 to calculate your BMI.)

☐ Have your periods ever stopped for six months or longer, especially before you were 35?

☐ Did you go through menopause before the age of 45?

☐ Have you lost more than 3 cm (just over 1 inch) in height?

☐ Do you have a sedentary lifestyle with little regular exercise, especially weight-bearing (that's when your weight is on your feet, e.g. walking, dancing, running – not cycling, riding, swimming)?

☐ Have you done a great deal of exercise, lost weight and stopped having periods, especially before the age of 35?

☐ Do you regularly drink more than 14 units a week? (One unit = a small glass of wine.)

☐ Do you smoke more than 20 cigarettes a day?

☐ Do you suffer frequently from diarrhoea or constipation?

☐ Have you taken corticosteroid tablets (principally corti-
sone or prednolisone) for more than three months?

☐ Have you used injectable contraception?

☐ Have you had a hysterectomy before the age of 50?

☐ Have you had your ovaries removed?

☐ If you had a hysterectomy and your ovaries were not
removed, have you had an annual blood check to see
how your ovaries are working?

☐ Do you suffer or have you suffered from any of the
following diseases:

☐ rheumatoid arthritis

☐ neuromuscular disease

☐ chronic liver disease

☐ malabsorption syndrome, such as Coeliac Disease

☐ hyperthyroidism

☐ hyperparathyroidism

Tests for bone mineral density

The idea of measuring your bone mineral density (BMD) is
to try to assess the holes in the sponge (or the Swiss cheese)
and thus your risk of fracture. But you have to remember
that bone density is only one contributing factor to bone
strength: bone toughness and flexibility are also important,
so are the internal structure of the skeleton and the rate of
turnover. However, at present, BMD is the most reliable way
of assessing risk.

The main procedures are:

• **DEXA (dual energy X-ray absorptiometry):** this X-ray-
based system uses two different energies to differentiate

between soft tissue and bone. The two main sites tested are the lumbar spine and hip. You lie flat during the scan, which is painless and lasts between 5 and 15 minutes. DEXA is the gold standard but not everyone will be referred for it. However, if you have strong risks and are likely to need treatment, your doctor should make sure you have a DEXA.

- **QUS (quantitative ultrasound):** this uses ultrasound to scan part of the body, usually the heel bone (calcaneum). It's an attractive method because the machine is easily portable and it doesn't use any radiation. Until recently, QUS was not considered an accurate diagnostic test and was only used to indicate where a further test, mainly DEXA, is required. However, new research suggests it may be as reliable as DEXA.

Understanding the results
The way the results of measuring your BMD are presented might well make you feel blinded by science. The World Health Organisation defines categories of bone mineral density compared to an average healthy young adult – which is called 'the mean'. To put it simply:

- if your BMD is 1 SD (standard deviation) below the mean, you are normal
- if your BMD is between 1 SD and 2.5 SD below the mean, you have osteopenia, i.e. your bones are thinning but not badly enough to be diagnosed with osteoporosis
- if your BMD is 2.5 SD or more below the mean, the diagnosis is osteoporosis

Medical treatment for osteoporosis

If your doctor refers you to a consultant it will probably be to a gynaecologist or rheumatologist. Improving bone density is important but what they will aim for is to give you treatment and advise lifestyle changes that will reduce your risk of fracture.

Drugs may be prescribed prophylactically – to prevent the condition developing, or therapeutically – to treat it. But don't forget that diet and exercise are staples throughout your life. Here's how it works:

- up to 35: focus on achieving peak bone mass, through good diet and exercise.
- 35–50: focus on maintaining bone density, through good diet and exercise plus prophylactic drugs if necessary because of risk factors.
- 50 plus: focus on minimising loss of bone density, through good diet and exercise plus prophylactic or therapeutic drug use if necessary.

Remember: All drugs should be reviewed by your doctor annually.

Hormonal therapies

HRT

We know that rapid bone loss occurs as a result of oestrogen deficiency, that is when your ovaries stop working either because of premature or natural menopause. So giving oestrogen replacement therapy (HRT) seems logical. As you know if you've read the chapter on HRT, it is still considered very important for women who go through premature menopause but it is now not recommended as the first line of treatment for osteoporosis in postmenopausal women. This is due to two factors: firstly, although it does help bone to stay stronger (and was shown to prevent fractures in the WHI trial and others), the benefits only last as long as you stay on the drug. Soon after you stop taking it, your bones play catch-up and go back to the state they were in before you started HRT. As long-term HRT is not advisable because of the risks, the maths doesn't work. Taking HRT at 50 for five years won't prevent fractures when you are in your 60s, 70s or 80s, the time they usually happen. Secondly, the European Expert Working Group from 28 countries concluded in November 2003 that the benefits of prescribing HRT as a first-line treatment for osteoporosis were outweighed by the increased risks. (But if you're taking HRT for other reasons, it will have a beneficial effect on your bones during that time.)

SERMs (Selective Estrogen Receptor Modulators)
(see page 164 for more details)
These 'designer' oestrogens have been shown to reduce the rate of spinal vertebral fractures in postmenopausal women with osteoporosis. Raloxifene is now licensed for prevention and treatment of osteoporosis.

Tibolone *(see page 165 for more details)*
This drug, which has a combination of oestrogenic, progestogenic and androgenic actions, is currently licensed for the prevention of osteoporosis, but not treatment.

Calcitonin
This hormone produced by the thyroid is given by injection or nasal spray; it reduces bone resorption but is seldom used because it apparently only decreases the risk of vertebral fractures, not others.

Parathyroid hormone

This is the principal hormone used in the calcium balance in the body. It is now licensed to be given as a daily injection for 18 months and induces a substantial gain in bone mineral density. However, the cost is £5,000 per 18-month course so this will limit its use to women with severe osteoporosis attending specialist centres, who are intolerant of or non-responsive to other treatments.

Other drug choices

Biphosphonates (aka bisphosphonates)

According to the *Journal of the British Menopause Society*, biphosphonates are the most effective group of anti-resorbative drugs (that means they stop the bone being shed and resorbed into the body) currently available for the prevention of bone loss and reduction of fractures. The best evidence of effectiveness is with the two newer biphosphonates Fosamax (Alendronate) and Actonel (Risedronate), which have been shown to reduce fractures at different sites, including the spine and the hip. Weekly doses are as effective as daily.

However there is as yet little evidence about their effectiveness or safety used long term, that is over five years. So the current advice is that it's safe if you come off after five years (some physicians say seven) and have a 'drug holiday' of two years. After that, it may be necessary to start taking the original drug again but there may then be newer options.

For women whose osteoporosis is related to steroid therapy, most doctors would advise continuing biphosphonate treatment long term.

In terms of menopausal symptoms as opposed to osteoporosis, biphosphonates may be less helpful because they don't ameliorate any symptoms. They can also cause unpleasant side effects, mainly digestive.

Future developments include the possibility of monthly or annual injections of a biphosphonate. (At present, zoledronic acid is licensed to be given by four-weekly injections for the reduction of bone damage in advanced malignancies involving bone.)

Calcium and vitamin D supplementation

Adequate calcium and vitamin D, which enables you to absorb the calcium, are essential throughout your life to keep your bones strong and prevent fractures. Your doctor may prescribe calcium and vitamin D, which you get mainly from sunlight but can also be taken as a supplement. Studies have failed to show a significant effect for women in early menopause but there is a clear benefit in older (60-plus), postmenopausal women. In a study of elderly women, 800 iu (international units) of vitamin D and 1,200 mg of calcium were shown to increase bone mineral density. Vitamin D on its own has also been shown to increase BMD. There are also other important minerals for bone strength, which we discuss below.

Other treatments

Strontium ranelate

Research is ongoing into the effectiveness of using strontium, a trace element, combined with ranelic acid to block bone resorption and stimulate bone formation.

Exercise

Experts agree that weight- (aka load-) bearing exercise stimulates the osteoblasts that make bone and is essential to stimulate bone growth. It helps accumulate bone in young women under 35 and helps prevent bone loss in older women.

Additionally, physical activity helps elderly people be more mobile and thus reduces falls and fractures, which enables them to be less dependent. Our chapter on exercise (page 278) gives recommendations. However, excessive exercising is a known risk factor for osteoporosis because of its negative effect on the functioning of the ovaries: a significant number of professional sportswomen develop it at a very young age. So you should do enjoyable exercise regularly (daily if possible) but it's a case where a great deal more is definitely not better.

Diet

DRINKING TEA MAY HELP YOUR BONES

According to researchers in Taiwan, where HRT has not been routinely prescribed, drinking tea may significantly help your bones. In a study of women and men aged 30 and older, drinking tea daily correlated with significant beneficial effects on bone mineral density of the total body, lumbar spine and hip regions in adults. The longer the subjects did this the better: those who had drunk tea habitually for ten years or more had the highest bone mineral densities at all the sites measured. The scientists attribute this to the chemicals including caffeine and phytoestrogens contained in tea. But physical activity was also a determinant, as well as sex, age and BMI.

Epidemiological Evidence of Increased Bone Mineral Density in Habiutal Tea Drinkers. Chih-Hsing Wu and others. *Arch Intern Med*. 2002; 162:1001-1006

Eating a good fresh varied diet is vital to keep your bones healthy, as with everything in your body. The traditional advice has been to drink a pint of milk daily and eat dairy produce with plenty of fresh fruit and vegetables but the point is not just to get calcium into your body but get it absorbed and on to your bones. Some experts say that dairy produce may not be the most effective at actually getting calcium on to your bones and may indeed hinder the process. (See below.) You need to include sources of calcium, magnesium, boron and other minerals that make up your bones, plus the vitamins that help these get absorbed and also nutrients that prevent bone shedding.

Remember too that your bones don't just consist of the hard minerals: they also contain a lot of collagen, which is crucial for strength and flexibility. So you need plenty of vitamin C daily (because your body can't store it) to keep up your levels of collagen, another substance that becomes more scanty as you get older.

Another bone of contention (whoops ...!) is the animal protein debate. Some experts believe that too much protein – which includes milk and dairy products, remember – can hasten bone loss. The Vegetarian Society in the UK cites research showing that a high intake of animal protein increases the loss of calcium from bones. One study published in the *Journal of the American Dietetic Association* in 1980 found that vegetarian women aged between 50 and 89 lost 18 per cent of bone mass, while a control group of non-vegetarians had a 35 per cent bone loss. However, other studies have shown no difference in bone density and bone mineral content between vegetarians and non-vegetarians. Our suggestion is that if you are not a vegetarian or vegan, be careful not to eat too much animal protein and drink too much milk: remember that you can get calcium from other sources (see below). If you are a vegetarian, you may need specific advice, and possibly supplements, to keep your bones strong.

Remember we said at the beginning of this chapter that there are many crossovers with heart disease and cancer? Well, your heart muscle is also dependent on healthy collagen and we know that eating lots of antioxidants like vitamin C and vitamin E (which is also really helpful for vaginal dryness) helps protect against cancer. Equally, high levels of the amino acid homocysteine have now been shown to be a risk factor for increased bone loss, as well as heart disease and dementia. (Homocysteine levels can be lowered with folic acid, so eat plenty of dark green leafy vegetables.)

It's vital to understand that you can only absorb nutrients of all kinds if your digestion is working well (more about this in Chapter Seven). If you have symptoms such as bloating, wind and indigestion, it's a strong clue that you've got problems. Eat live organic yoghurt and consider an acidophilus supplement long term. A food combining diet also helps many people with this type of problem. Again there are more details in Chapter Seven.

Here is a list of the nutrients and foods that you need to include in your diet to keep your bones healthy (and your heart and your skin and your hair and your teeth etc. etc. etc.!).

| **Calcium** | almonds, brazil nuts, hazel nuts, green leafy vegetables, soya, sesame seeds, tinned salmon (including the bones) and dairy produce in moderation (do swop cow's for sheep's or goat's if you prefer; the smaller molecular structure means the calcium is better absorbed into your body and many people tolerate sheep's and goat's milk better than cow's) |

Magnesium	green leafy vegetables, nuts, seeds, whole grains, dairy produce
Vitamin C	berries, blackcurrants, kiwi fruit, green leafy vegetables, potatoes, citrus fruit (but beware too much of this because it brings acid to your stomach, which may hasten calcium loss, and also damages your teeth)
Zinc	pumpkin seeds, fish, eggs, peas and beans (legumes), whole grains
Vitamin D	oily fish, eggs, avocado – and sunlight (one of the reasons why getting out in the light is so important)
Boron	cabbage, dandelion, green vegetables, fruits, nuts, peas and beans, alfalfa
Folic acid	dark green leafy vegetables
Vitamin K	green leafy vegetables, cabbage, alfalfa
Essential Fatty Acids	oily fish, linseeds, avocado
Good gut bacteria	live organic yoghurt (look for ones that contain bioacidophilus)
Cider vinegar	try drinking one tablespoonful of cider vinegar with honey in a cupful of warm water three times daily, which naturopaths say helps digestion and absorption of calcium (it's also said to help arthritis)

Supplements

Nutritionist Marilyn Glenville, who runs a natural health clinic specialising in the menopause, recommends these daily supplements to help bone health before, during and after the menopause. If you have osteoporosis, we suggest you consult a qualified nutritionist or naturopath for an individual programme.

- a good multivitamin and mineral tablet containing boron (e.g. Biocare Femforte).
- B complex (50 mg of each B vitamin per day – including folic acid/folate: but remember to count in the amount you get in your multi-vitamin/mineral).
- vitamin C with bioflavonoids (1,000 mg).
- combined magnesium and calcium citrate supplement (with no more than 500 mg of calcium citrate daily, including the amount from your multi-vitamin/mineral; look for a supplement with a 2:1 ratio of magnesium to calcium).
- zinc citrate (15 mg, including the amount from your multi-vitamin/mineral).
- linseed oil (1,000 mg).

Nutritionist Kathryn Marsden recommends post-menopausal women add:

- 600–800 iu vitamin D
- 3 mg boron (including what's in your multivitamin/mineral)

You may also want to consider taking Ipriflavone, an artificial copy of a soya isoflavone, that has been shown to increase bone density in some women.

BONES MAY BENEFIT FROM BLACK COHOSH

The herb black cohosh was as effective as oestrogen at reducing menopausal symptoms and helping bone metabolism, in a trial at the University of Gottingen. Researchers propose that the black cohosh product, which was equivalent to a daily 40mg dose, acts like a SERM, that is it has good effects in the brain, bone and vagina, without causing changes to the lining of the womb which could lead to cancer. However, the trial was only three months long so research is ongoing.

The Cimicifuga preparation BNO 1055 vs conjugated estrogens in a double-blind placebo-controlled study: effects on menopause and symptoms and bone markers. Wuttke W, Seidlove-Wuttke D, Gorkow C. *Maturitas.* 2003 Mar 14;44 Suppl 1:S67-77

BREAST CANCER

This is now the most common cancer in the UK, and the second most common worldwide (the first is lung cancer). One in nine women will develop the disease during their lifetime. It's most common in older women; four out of five cases occur after 50. Men can also get it but rarely, with around 250 cases in the UK each year. The good news is that the survival rate is going up. You'll find information about breast screening and what you can do to be aware of any changes on page 59.

The breast is made up of millions of cells that are constantly being renewed and replaced. The disease develops when a single cell begins to multiply out of control. As the cancer grows, some cells may eventually break away and spread to other parts of the body.

All breast cancers are caused by faulty genes but that doesn't mean they are all inherited. In fact only about five per cent of breast cancer is triggered by a genetic susceptibility. More often, the damage to the gene happens during the woman's lifetime.

What affects your risk?

Research is ongoing worldwide but here is a summary of what scientists know to date.

Age	The older you are, the greater your chances of getting the disease. Risk of breast cancer by age 30: 1 in 1,900 40: 1 in 200 50: 1 in 50 60: 1 in 23 70: 1 in 15
The Pill and HRT	Taking the contraceptive Pill or HRT causes an increased risk as we've explained on pages 363 and 143. But your risk returns to normal within five years of stopping
Obesity	Being overweight slightly increases your risk
Family history	You have an increased risk if one or two close family members have the disease but most women in this situation will not get it. See page 59 for more details
Having children	The more children a woman has – and the younger she has them, the lower her risk of breast cancer

Breast-feeding	The longer you breast-feed, the lower the risk
Menstruation and menopause	The length of time a woman menstruates affects risk, so starting periods young or having a late menopause increases the risk
Alcohol	Some research suggests that regularly drinking large quantities of alcohol may increase your risk

CARDIOVASCULAR DISEASE
(aka coronary heart disease, referring to heart attack, stroke and embolisms)

As we've said at the beginning of this chapter, cardiovascular disease (cardio refers to the heart, vascular to the arteries) is now known to be the leading cause of death for women in many industrialised countries. However, for many years it was generally thought of as a male disease and women were not included in research of any kind: the results of studying men were assumed to apply to women too. However, it's now recognised that women's bodies – and minds, which have a bearing on heart disease and other illness – work a bit differently from men's.

Women's risk of heart disease more than doubles between the ages of 45 and 65. This appears to be due to falling levels of oestrogen. The answer in the 1980s and 1990s seemed obvious: give postmenopausal women HRT and reduce their risk of heart disease. It's no exaggeration to say that millions of women worldwide were prescribed HRT for this reason. A huge observational study (The Nurses Study, see page 133) seemed to confirm the hypothesis and the drug companies suggested that HRT be licensed for this use without further ado. However, contradictory evidence soon started to come in and in July 2001 the American Heart Association issued guidelines to doctors that HRT should not be given to protect against heart disease. Other expert bodies followed.

Extraordinarily, it seems that combined HRT (at least in some forms) may actually increase the risk of heart disease. Just why this happens is currently a mystery. What is clear is that the oestrogen/cardiovascular connection is complex, undoubtedly involving other hormones and biochemical mechanisms, and so far no one really understands what's going on.

But here's the best bit. What was overlooked by many doctors in the euphoria over HRT is the fact that virtually all the risks for heart disease (see box) can be offset by lifestyle measures – the ones at the beginning of this chapter. The consensus is that even high blood pressure (unless it's dangerously high) should be treated with a year of diet and exercise – and stopping smoking if that's relevant – before drugs are given.

RISKS FOR CARDIOVASCULAR DISEASE

* smoking
* overweight/obesity (particularly if the weight gain is primarily round your waist)
* poor diet
* sedentary lifestyle with little physical activity
* menopause

Also these medical conditions

* diabetes
* high blood pressure

- high homocysteine levels
- unfavourable lipid profile

If you have diabetes or a strong family history of heart disease – or any other concerns – please consult your doctor for specific advice. (And of course, you go for an annual check-up and discussion, don't you?)

8

EATING FOR HEALTH

This chapter covers:
- the Mediterranean diet: simply the best
- phytoestrogens
- your important adrenals
- HRT and weight gain
- anaemia
- gut problems including candida and constipation
- food combining
- basic eating plan
- food rules
- foods to feast on and foods to avoid
- fat free menopause cake recipe
- muesli recipe
- superfruit and veg

After breathing, eating good food and drinking plenty of pure water are the most important things in life. What we put in our bodies (and don't forget that also means our brains) is always important but in times of change and potential stress like the menopause years, it's crucial to support our systems as well as possible.

The essentials of a good diet don't change when you get

to the menopause and beyond. However, eating healthily (if you don't already) becomes even more important because it can contribute so much to your wellbeing, in addition to minimising menopausal symptoms and helping to prevent illness.

Our philosophy is to keep things simple and natural. You could call this the minimalist guide to eating for health, based on consuming fresh wholesome food, little and often. The basis is the Mediterranean diet, which has been shown in research to be top for optimal health.

THE MEDITERRANEAN DIET

Stacks of evidence show that the foods traditionally eaten by people in southern Italy, Sicily and Crete promote optimal health and prevent disease. In a nutshell, the Mediterranean diet is based on vegetables, fruit, fish, a little meat, some cheese and dairy products (often sheep's and goat's rather than cow's), foodstuffs using a range of whole grains, nuts and seeds plus olive and other plant oils. These contain a wide range of nutrients plus vital 'good' fats (Essential Fatty Acids).

What's more, this way of eating is delicious and easily prepared. Think of fish and vegetables, chicken and salad, cheese and celery and olives, wholewheat pasta with tomato and garlic or basil. The marvellous bonus is that it will not only help you through the menopause, giving you balance and energy in all areas of your life, it's also absolutely the best way of eating to help protect yourself against heart disease, cancer and osteoporosis, as well as the other diseases of ageing. Add in exercise and you are on to a real winner.

Helping your body produce its own HRT

As well as stabilising and boosting your whole body function, eating well helps to maximise your supplies of oestrogen. Although your ovaries gradually produce less and less, oestrogen is still produced in your body in the fat cells. As well as safeguarding this source, you can top up supplies (on much the same principle as Hormone Replacement Therapy) by eating foods, such as soya and chickpeas, that are rich in plant (phyto) oestrogens.

Weight gain

Many women find that they tend to put on weight after 35. They notice it particularly in the years leading up to and just after the menopause. In fact, some scientists believe that this is your body being clever. In general, slightly plumper (that does *not* mean fat or obese, it means not skinny) women suffer fewer distressing symptoms of menopause, such as hot flushes. As oestrogen levels from the ovaries fall, it seems that your body helps compensate by producing another form of the hormone from your fat cells. This type of oestrogen is converted from androgens – male hormones that women also have in smaller quantities – produced by your adrenal glands, so it's vital to keep your adrenals balanced.

The importance of your adrenal glands

The adrenals, a pair of glands that sit on top of your kidneys, are the body's primary system for coping with stress. They produce a range of hormones including adrenalin, the 'fight or flight' hormone. If they aren't working properly, they can cause wide-ranging effects on your body's biochemistry, including weight gain on your bottom, hips and thighs, according to naturopath Roderick Lane. As well as compromising the supply of androgens (see above), erratic adrenals can cause blood sugar levels to swing wildly, which researchers are now linking to menopausal symptoms including hot flushes and also mood swings in general.

Keeping your hormones happy

The point of saying all this is that cleaning up your diet, cutting down on stimulants, chewing your food, eating slowly and drinking lots of water plus stress relief such as yoga can help keep your whole hormonal system including your adrenal glands balanced. This makes you feel much better and also helps your menopausal symptoms. (For more information and advice on adrenal function and hormones generally, see *The Adam & Eve Diet* by Roderick Lane & Sarah Stacey.)

HRT and weight gain

Hormone Replacement Therapy may exacerbate weight gain. Although there is no concrete scientific evidence that it piles on the pounds, Michael finds it is a big concern and complaint with his patients. Marilyn Glenville, who runs a women's nutrition clinic, reports seeing many women who take HRT and then put on a significant amount of weight that simply will not budge. She says: 'For many women I've seen, the weight gain can be up to two stone with breasts going up a couple of cup sizes. The medical literature says there is no difference in weight gain for women on HRT and that it is just a product of being menopausal. But a lot of the women I've seen have been menopausal for a couple of years with no weight gain, put on HRT and become completely bloated and fat! Unfortunately it seems to be the hardest weight gain to shift.'

There is some evidence that acupuncture used in conjunction with a low-calorie diet can help. Food combining may also help. Additionally, leading researcher Dr Paula Baillie-Hamilton, author of *The Detox Diet: Eliminate Chemical Calories and Restore Your Body's Natural Slimming System*, believes that unnatural chemicals of all kinds (pesticides, herbicides, colourings, preservatives and other additives) upset the delicate balance of your body's inbuilt slimming system. Her advice is to eat fresh organically produced food, with little or preferably no processed food. Nutritionist Kathryn Marsden says her clinical experience bears this out too and points out that, ironically, one of the biggest sources of these chemicals are low-fat and diet foods.

Anaemia

Anaemia often goes with heavy vaginal bleeding. Telltale signs are low energy, pale lips and inside eye rims. You need a full spectrum of B vitamins plus vitamin C to help you absorb the iron in your food. The simplest old-fashioned remedy for anaemia is a combination of black-strap molasses and Marmite (unless you have candida in which case Floradix, a liquid supplement that doesn't contain yeast and sugar, may be a better option). Take about one dessertspoonful of molasses and a teaspoon of Marmite daily (not together). If the anaemia persists, you must consult a health professional because it may be a precursor of something more serious.

Gut problems and candida

An unhealthy digestive tract is, according to many experts, the main villain underlying a ragbag of modern health problems, including irritable bowel syndrome, food allergies or intolerances (also called sensitivities) and candida. In fact, Kathryn Marsden has noted that many, if not most, of her patients with hot flushes and other menopausal problems have gut problems such as candida. The telltale signs are fatigue, depression, bloating and irregular bowel habits.

These problems usually start when we first put food in our mouths – in other words with chewing or the lack of it, which leads to a chain of disasters in our digestive tract. In brief, the more slowly you eat and the more you chew, the smaller the particles that reach the stomach and the easier they are to digest. Chewing also stimulates the production of stomach acid, digestive enzymes and bile, which allow foods to be processed properly so you get the nutrients.

Gut problems will often resolve if you clean up your diet and treat stress, but Kathryn Marsden also recommends food combining (see box), avoiding cow's milk and all products containing sugar (including fruit for 21 days), yeast and alcohol. Follow the eating guidelines below, cook with garlic and take a garlic supplement. Also take a three-month course of probiotics every 12 months (and always following any antibiotics).

Constipation

Constipation should be tackled immediately. (As one woman said, 'You can't feel gorgeous if you're constipated ...') Drinking lots of water and eating fresh fruit, particularly pears, papaya, figs or compotes of fresh berries (which you can get from the supermarket), usually does the trick. Three tablespoonfuls of golden linseeds (the others won't work) taken with a tumbler of water are also effective. Exercise helps stop constipation: a few sessions on a mini-trampoline are virtually infallible. If that doesn't work, take a dessert-spoonful of olive oil (use in dressing on salad or vegetables if you don't like it neat). Dr Mosaraf Ali of the Integrated Medical Centre in London recommends drinking two glasses of warm water (boiled and cooled, not from the hot tap) in the morning and gently rubbing your stomach in a clock-wise direction (very comforting for any gut problem), then retiring to the loo with a magazine or book: not hurrying is crucial.

For more information on all digestive and related problems, see *Good Gut Healing: The No-Nonsense Guide to Bowel & Digestive Disorders* by Kathryn Marsden.

FOOD COMBINING

This method of eating, also known as the Hay Diet, was devised early in the twentieth century by Dr William Howard Hay, who found it helped patients with chronic ill health. The basis is not mixing foods that are believed to 'fight' in your stomach. So fruit is eaten separately (as is the custom in many Eastern countries) and foods consisting predominantly of proteins and starches are kept separate. It often seems like a fantastic fiddle to start with but the results can be quite staggering for some people.

Kathryn Marsden, who has also written *The Food Combining Diet*, suggests the following basic guidelines, which are specifically designed to reduce your intake of unnecessary chemicals. This will help anyone with allergies or who wants to reduce chemical overload for any reason.

- introduce this way of eating into your diet for one or two days a week to start with, to ease yourself into it.
- if you find it suits you, increase that to three to five days weekly. But don't put yourself under pressure to follow it slavishly. If you fancy breaking out, do just that.
- if you want to lose weight, aim each day for: one protein meal with plenty of fresh vegetables or salad, one starch-based meal with the same, plus one vegetarian meal based on a big salad, vegetable stirfry or fresh fruit salad.

How to Combine Foods

Proteins (A) will mix with anything from Column B.
Starches (C) will mix with anything from Column B.
Don't mix Column A with Column C.

A Proteins	B Mix with A or C	C Starches
Fish/shellfish	All veg except	Potatoes/sweet
Free-range/	potatoes/sweet	potatoes
organic eggs	potatoes	All grains including
Organic poultry	All salads	oats, brown rice,
Lean lamb	Seeds	rye, millet, quinoa,
Cheese	Nuts	bulgar, spelt, kamut,
All soya	Herbs	wholewheat pasta/
products	Fats and oils	bread
Milk (sheep's	including cream,	Sweetcorn
or goat's in	butter, olive oil	Flour products
small quantities)	Natural live	including pastry,
	yoghurt	biscuits, cakes

> NB Pulses/legumes (peas, beans, lentils) combine well with all kinds of veg and salads and with other starches but can cause digestive problems if mixed with protein foods.

Don't diet, get fit

Just to reiterate, if you gain a few pounds – learn to love those curves! But remember to eat a really good diet and exercise sensibly so that you keep fit – you'll feel good and look good that way. Eating well and exercise go together like the proverbial horse and carriage, peaches and cream and so on. Without exercise, our bodies can't function. In fact, leading nutritionist Dr Walter Willetts at Harvard Medical School in America puts exercise at the top of his list of nutritional musts. (Consider this: we start to lose muscle in less than a week if we don't exercise.) Whatever you do, don't try and crash diet. You will put more stress on your body and brain – just what you're trying to avoid – and any weight you lose will crash back again, usually with extra pounds on.

So eat well and move!

FOOD RULES

Basic eating plan

* never let yourself get hungry
* don't eat on the run
* sit down to eat and chew your food thoroughly
* don't leap up from the table the moment you've finished: sit for five to ten minutes to let your food digest
* have a short walk after if possible

EAT LITTLE AND OFTEN

Eat at least every three hours to keep blood sugar levels stable: this is one of the most important things you can do to help prevent hot flushes and other menopausal symptoms as well as helping maintain a stable weight and keeping you more relaxed. Aim to eat breakfast, lunch and supper, with snacks mid morning, mid afternoon and before bed. New research shows that this simple measure can reduce hot flushes significantly.

Tip: Brewers yeast (if you don't have candida) is a good source of protein, packed with B vitamins and high in chromium, which helps regulate blood sugar levels. If you do have candida or don't want to take a yeasty food, try a supplement of chromium polynicotinate.

- good snack foods are a piece of fruit (not citrus), a fruit smoothie, a small handful of nuts and seeds, a rice cake or oatcake with hummus or avocado, raw vegetables.
- also try Kathryn Marsden's recipe for a fat-free, sugar-free carrot cake, which contains a heap of good menopause foods.

KATHYRN MARSDEN'S CARROT CAKE

Use organic ingredients wherever possible:

½ cup soya flour
½ cup spelt flour (from health food stores); use wholemeal if spelt not available
½ cup self-raising flour

1½ teaspoons baking powder
2 dessertspoons oatmeal
1½ – 2 cups grated carrot
1 organic grated apple
1½ cups sultanas or raisins
½ cup chopped dried apricots
2 teaspoons flaked almonds
2 teaspoons pumpkin seeds
2 teaspoons sesame seeds
2 teaspoons sunflower seeds
1 teaspoon mixed spice
1½ cups water

Mix all dry ingredients together, add water and fold together gently with a metal spoon until thoroughly mixed; add more water if necessary; the mixture should be moist enough to be a soft dropping consistency. Pour into a lined or non-stick loaf tin and cook for approximately one hour and 15 minutes at 180°C. This cake works really well without added sugar but you can add one dessert-spoonful of Manuka honey if you like a sweeter taste.

- **skipping any meal is bad but never skip breakfast.** Always make sure you have a good nutritious protein-filled break-fast. Oats, which are recommended by the British Heart Foundation and other experts, are a marvellous medic-inal food: they stabilise blood sugar levels, balance blood fats and reduce food cravings; the vitamin B and calcium in oats help strengthen nervous function and are good for nervous exhaustion, chronic stress and depression; they also improve stamina and may help low libido. (Neuro-scientist and researcher Dr Paul Clayton calls them nature's Prozac because they encourage the production of serotonin, the feel-good hormone.) So good choices for breakfast are classic Bircher Muesli (or make Roderick Lane's version below); millet flakes (for people who find starches upset their stomach) with banana, pumpkin and sunflower seeds and sheep's or goat's milk yoghurt; or porridge with live natural yoghurt (for protein) and stewed mixed dried fruit or berries (packs of red and purple frozen berries are great in the winter).

Other protein-filled starts to the day include fish (sardines, kippers or undyed smoked haddock are great), organic eggs (too many chemicals in the others), organic bacon, grilled tomatoes, mushrooms, full-fat cottage cheese, all served with wholegrain bread or toast and a little butter or olive oil; tofu and berries; soya yoghurt with mixed nuts and seeds; organic nut or peanut butter on wholemeal toast.

RODERICK LANE'S OAT-BASED MUESLI

One serving

Prepare the night before so the fibre content of the grain softens, reducing the impact on the digestive system. Add yoghurt if you wish, and fresh or dried fruit. Swap fruit juice (apple, grape, cranberry) for the milk if you prefer.

1 tablespoon (15 ml) porridge oats
1 teaspoon (5 ml) runny honey
1 dessertspoon (20 ml) full-fat organic milk or soya milk
2–3 small apples and 1 large or 2 small pears, grated (including peel, core and pips), or the equivalent in dried fruit, chopped, mixed with juice of ½ lemon

1 tablespoon (15 ml) walnuts, hazelnuts or peeled almonds, chopped

Mix oats with honey and milk or juice. Add fruit in lemon juice and nuts. Stir and cover, leave in fridge overnight.

---

* **buy fresh, seasonal, locally produced food.** Choose organic products if you can. They are tastier and more nutritious, partly because your body doesn't have to use up energy eliminating unnatural chemicals. Additionally, chemicals may contribute to intractable overweight, according to Dr Paula Baillie-Hamilton.

* **eat at least five portions of fresh veggies and fruit daily.** More is better: American guidelines recommend aiming for eight to ten: try for five portions of veggies and three fruit. Fruit and vegetables should be 75 per cent of your diet.

* **eat good fats:** don't have any truck with fat-free diets but do eat the right 'unsaturated' fats. Experts now say that good fats (which you'll also find called Essential Fatty Acids (EFAs) or omega 3 and 6, with newcomers 7 and 9) should be up there with fruit and vegetables as vital foods to keep us fit. Best sources are oily fish, nuts and seeds, vegetable oils (particularly flax seed and hemp oils which you can use in salads, also olive, rapeseed, soya and sunflower), full-fat organic milk, avocados, sweet potatoes, peanuts and green leafy vegetables. As well as oiling your body and keeping it working well, EFAs help your brain and keep your skin peachy, rather than prune-like. You will also find Essential Fatty Acids in supplement form, including evening primrose oil, starflower (borage) and blackcurrant seed oil, linseed oil, flaxseed oil and hemp oil.

* **eat phytoestrogens:** these plant hormones seem to have a balancing effect on hormones. They help reduce hot flushes, and may also help protect against heart disease, osteoporosis and breast cancer. There are three main types:

  ○ isoflavones: the most beneficial phytoestrogens which are found in soya, lentils and chickpeas; isoflavones have four different groups of chemicals, called genistein, daidzein, biochanin A and formononentin; they're converted by gut bacteria to substances with oestrogenic action (so your gut needs to be healthy; see below).
  ○ lignans: in most vegetables and cereals, with the highest amounts in linseeds and other oil-producing seeds.
  ○ coumestans: found mainly in alfalfa and mung bean sprouts.

  You can take supplements but there is debate about how much you should take. All in all, it's much better to get phytoestrogens in food form, starting with 35 to 50 g soya daily.

  If you have breast or any other hormonal cancer, you may wish to avoid phytoestrogens or discuss the issue with your health professional. There is no evidence to suggest they exacerbate the disease, in fact the reverse, but some physicians are concerned.

* **eat calcium-containing foods:** for many years, the received wisdom has been that a pint of milk a day is the best source of calcium, but over the last decade there has been ongoing debate about whether dairy foods are essential for calcium with many experts pointing out that dairy foods are not the only source of calcium and may not be well absorbed. However, since dairy produce is a staple of the Western diet, it makes sense to have a reasonable

daily intake, including whole organic milk, yoghurt and cottage cheese, and other cheeses – but consider choosing sheep's or goat's milk products rather than cow's because these have smaller molecules and are much better absorbed. Also eat plenty of phyto-oestrogenic foods (soya, lentils, chickpeas, dark green vegetables and herbs). Many nutritionists also suggest eating less animal protein.

Marilyn Glenville recommends anyone with risk factors for osteoporosis, or with diagnosed low bone density, drink a daily cup of herbal tea made from alfalfa herb (medicago sativa), nettle (Urtica spp.) and horsetail (Equisetum arvense), a natural source of silica.

CHOOSING FOOD

Foods to feast on

• go for variety and colour: choose as many different types in the categories below as possible so that you get the widest range of nutrients and are less likely to trigger a food sensitivity. When you're buying fruit and veg, choose a wide rainbow range of colours from deep reds, pinks and purples to the greens, reds, oranges and yellows.
• remember that Public Enemies No. One are pure white and deadly: white sugar, white flour and salt.

Feast on	Portions to aim for
Vegetables (avoid potatoes, turnips, parsnips, swedes) raw or lightly cooked	3 to 5 daily
Fruit (non-citrus)	2 to 3 daily
Peas, beans and lentils (legumes)	1 daily

Soya foods (tofu, soya milk, soya yoghurt)	1 (35 to 50 g) daily
Whole grains (cereals): oats, brown rice, millet, rye, quinoa, spelt, faro, kamut, wholemeal bread, wholewheat or rice pasta	1 to 4 daily
Nuts (fresh almonds, walnuts, hazelnuts, pecan, Brazils, pine nuts)	up to 50 g daily
Mixed seeds (golden linseed, pumpkin, sesame, sunflower)	$1\frac{1}{2}$ tablespoons daily
Live natural organic yoghurt (preferably sheep's or goat's)	1 to 3 tablespoons daily
Organic butter	$\frac{1}{2}$ to 1 oz daily
Extra-virgin, cold-pressed olive oil	1 to 3 dessertspoons daily
Organic poultry (chicken, turkey, guineafowl, game)	3 to 4 weekly
Vegetable protein: tempeh, TVP, Quorn	3 to 4 weekly
Organic eggs (if you have heart disease, stick to 2 weekly)	2 to 4 weekly
Fresh sprouted seeds and beans	2 to 3 weekly
Oily fish (salmon, sardines, mackerel, herring, tuna, trout)	2 to 3 weekly
Cheese (preferably sheep's or goat's)	3 to 4 oz weekly
Seaweed, fresh or dried:	sprinkle liberally on soups, stews and salads
Fresh herbs:	use liberally in cooking and drinks

273

Hummus and avocado spreads: use instead of butter or
                                                          margarine

Still water/organic herbal teas/   1 to 2½ litres daily
    freshly squeezed organic vegetable
    and fruit juices

Tip: Mix nuts and seeds together in a large jar and keep in
the fridge; use on salads or in yoghurt or muesli.

Foods to eat in moderation

Milk: always choose organic milk, the chemicals in conventionally
    produced milk are a concern to many experts. Use cow's milk
    in drinks only; substitute sheep's or goat's wherever possible;
    try oat, rice, soya or almond with cereals.
Red meat, perferably organic: because of the saturated hard fats
    (but a small 3 oz portion of lean beef or lamb twice weekly,
    and a little butter daily can be good for non-vegetarians/vegans).
Organic decaffeinated tea and coffee.
Potatoes, turnips, parsnips, swedes, celeriac.

Foods to eat occasionally

Shellfish, e.g. oysters, scallops, prawns, crab, lobster (NB Make sure
they're very fresh).
Smoked fish.

Foods to avoid (though everyone is allowed the occasional mad bad treat!)

All processed, refined, ready-prepared, packaged and/or canned
    foods (the exception is frozen vegetables and fruit, which can
    be excellent).
Refined white sugar and artificial sweeteners, flour and salt and

any foods with additives, such as colourings and preservatives; sweeten drinks or food with Manuka honey.

Processed, coloured meat/fish/cheese.

Diet foods, including low-fat cheeses or spreads.

Margarine and anything containing hydrogenated (trans) fats (vegetable oils).

Bran and bran-containing foods, which can interfere with calcium absorption.

Fizzy drinks.

Artificially sweetened drinks.

Non-organic coffee and tea.

Beer, lager and spirits.

SUPER FRUIT AND VEG

Red and purple fruits: rich in anthocyanidins, a type of flavonoid, which help protect the eyes from macular degeneration, one of the most common causes of blindness in older people

Mango and red-fleshed melons: rich in carotenoids (vitamin A)

Kiwi: rich in vitamin C

Banana: rich in potassium and other essential minerals

Lemon or lime juice: drink the juice of a fresh squeezed fruit in warm water (boil first then cool, don't take from tap) each morning for the vitamin C and bioflavonoids, and detoxing effect; add a little Manuka

	honey and grated raw ginger if you like
Tomatoes:	contain lutein, which helps protect your eyes, and lycopene, an important cancer-fighting compound
Garlic:	contains about 200 biologically active compounds, many of which help prevent diseases including heart disease and cancer; aim for one clove daily, cooked or raw
Avocado:	rich in Essential Fatty Acids, potassium, B vitamins, vitamins C and E, also iodine; pile high with hummus and a green salad for a perfect nutritious filling meal (and an average fruit is only 190 calories)
Dark green leafy veg, e.g. broccoli, cabbage, Brussels sprouts, cress, kale:	contain folic acid and important cancer-fighting substances, also vitamin K which helps bones
Wild yam:	contains phytoestrogens
Sweet potatoes:	from the same family as yams, contain phyto oestrogens and carotenoids (vitamin A)
Root ginger:	contains magnesium and seems to be naturally balancing for hormones and excellent for digestion; use as tea, and

	in soups, stews and stirfries
Seaweed:	rich in minerals, particularly iodine and calcium; use fresh or as Nori flakes sprinkled over food

---

RECIPE FOR GINGER TEA

Take a one- to two-inch piece of peeled fresh root ginger, grate into a teapot and pour on boiling water; let it stand for five to ten minutes, then strain into a cup; you can add lemon juice and honey or infuse with a teaspoon of Lapsang; continue to top up with boiling water – it gets stronger as it cooks.

DETOXING

If you have been through a time of eating and drinking merrily and are feeling tired and a bit liverish or bilious, give your liver a rest for a few days. Cut out all stimulants including tea and coffee, sugar and alcohol, and just eat vegetables and fruit, in salads, juices and broths, with lots of still water and organic herbal teas to drink. Do this for one to seven days, then add in simple proteins such as fish, organic chicken, yoghurt, cottage cheese and tofu. If you have any health problems at all, do consult your health professional first.

9

EXERCISE

This chapter covers:
- why it's especially good to be fit around the menopause
- how to make exercise work for you
- the types of exercise you need
- what to do if you haven't exercised for years!
- your pick 'n' mix exercise menu
- the baked bean can workout

One thing everybody agrees on: regular exercise is essential if you want to feel and look good. Physical activity keeps you fit physically, mentally and emotionally. It's far more effective at keeping you young, energetic and sparkling than HRT or any other drug – and if it's done correctly doesn't have any side effects. One big American study of postmenopausal women who lifted weights, for instance, showed that after one year their bodies were an amazing 15 to 20 years more youthful. And it's never too late to start – muscles improve with use even when you're 90 plus.

Experts increasingly believe that some of the age-related decline in physical and brain function may be stopped or even reversed by regular physical activity. Conversely, couch potatoes almost invariably age faster in every way.

Research shows that exercise actually stimulates your

body's own production of oestrogen and testosterone. When you're physically active, the adrenal glands produce an androgenic hormone called androstenedione, which whizzes into your bloodstream and is converted to a form of oestrogen called oestrone. Physical activity also stimulates the adrenals to produce other hormones called DHEA (dehydroepiandrosterone) and DHEA-S (dehydroepiandrosterone-sulphate), both of which decline as you get older. DHEA is converted in the body to androstenedione, which you know about, and testosterone, which helps zip up your libido. Dr Miriam Stoppard goes so far as to say that exercise may be more effective than HRT for postmenopausal women: she recommends five 30-minute sessions weekly (minimum) to keep your hormones happy. Because stress can have a negative effect, make sure you do exercise you enjoy.

> *"Being fit is exercising for your own peace of mind and being comfortable with your own body. There are many different theories about how and why to exercise. But for each individual it comes down to just feeling good about yourself."*
> Gillian Boxx, Olympic softball player

Here are just some of the benefits of keeping fit:

* helps keep your weight down (see table on how many calories you can burn doing different exercises).
* helps you have a toned, sleek body.
* keeps you fit – no puffing and panting as you run for a bus.
* helps you sleep well.
* helps your digestive system work better.
* the extra oxygen makes your cheeks pink and eyes sparkle.
* helps headaches and fatigue.

- puts you in a good mood and makes you feel better about life, the universe and everything; lifts anxiety and depression; fights stress.
- helps you think more clearly and focus better.
- helps you maintain your independence.
- has been shown to help reduce the frequency and severity of hot flushes.
- increasing strength, flexibility and co-ordination through regular exercise can help reduce the incidence of fractures through falling or due to osteoporosis.
- helps protect you against coronary heart disease, high blood pressure, diabetes, osteoporosis and several forms of cancer including colon and breast cancer.

'Women who engaged in the equivalent of 1.25 to 2.5 hours per week of brisk walking had an 18 percent decreased risk of breast cancer compared with inactive women. Slightly greater reduction in risk was observed for women who engaged in the equivalent of 10 hours or more per week of brisk walking. Physical activity reduces risk among women who are using hormone therapy, a group that is at increased risk for developing breast cancer.'

Journal of the American Medical Association,
Sept 2003

If you haven't been exercising regularly, remember that change will happen but not overnight. And no one can do it for you! You have to make exercise an integral part of your daily routine. The biggest problem for most women (men too) is keeping motivated. It's easy to start – tough to keep up the pace for a year. So there are three golden rules: have fun, keep within your budget and set yourself goals.

The three golden rules of exercise

* **Do something you enjoy**: see exercise as fun, not a penance. You can make exercise social: go on a picnic hike, for instance, with friends and family, have tobogganing parties in the winter. Or just go for a walk in beautiful countryside with your beloved. Don't be afraid to admit to yourself that you don't like a particular form of activity, or find it too hard: there are lots of others as you can see from our Exercise Menu below.

> *'It's vital to have fun and laugh a lot.'*
> Canadian rower and double Olympic gold medallist
> Kirsten Barnes

* **Make it cost-effective**: getting fit need not be expensive, you don't need to join a gym or health club. Everyday activities from housework and gardening to walking and going upstairs can develop your health and fitness.
* **Achieve something!** it helps most people to have goals – be optimistic but realistic (see below). You may want to team up with an exercise buddy to set your goals and keep each other motivated. You could choose to take up a new sport, maybe something you've always wanted to do but never quite dared – like horse riding. There's a handy acronym – SMART – which sounds a bit like management-speak but it can help you develop a plan.

SMART stands for:

Specific: be clear about your goals. Say, for instance, you want to increase the amount of exercise you do. Just saying, 'I'm going to do more . . .' is unlikely to help. Instead decide what sort of exercise you're going to do – we specify the important types below – and how long you're going to exercise for. So you might say: 'For the next four weeks, I will walk briskly for 30 minutes every day, do two sessions of yoga weekly and lift weights three times a week.' That's being Specific. You can also set medium- and long-term goals too. Don't forget to give yourself a treat/reward when you achieve your goals.

Measurable: your goals must be Measurable. By saying you will walk half an hour daily, do two yoga sessions and exercise with weights three times, that's Measurable as well as Specific.

Adjustable: your goals should be Adjustable. You need to be able to alter them according to factors such as your progress or other commitments. If you find that you can't fit in the type of exercise you had planned, Adjust it!

Realistic: set Realistic goals. If you've never run a marathon before, you won't be able to run one in three weeks. Equally, if you don't have a swimming pool in your neighbourhood, don't include three swims a week in your goal.

Time: include Timing in your goals. That means planning the Time you can commit to, and then keeping to that Time. If you plan to walk 30 minutes daily, do just that. If you want to swim, add in the Time it takes to get dry and wash your hair afterwards, as well as travel Time.

Once you have set your goals, write them down in your diary or day book – or on the fridge. (But not on the back of an envelope!) If you do have an exercise buddy, agree to reassess them at the end of your given Time – four weeks or whatever – and remember to enjoy that too. Award yourselves a delicious lunch or some treat you really fancy.

Lastly, stay positive. Being negative means you won't achieve your goals. Resolve that you will exercise and you will reap all the benefits – feeling great, looking great and staying healthy for the rest of your life.

WHAT SORT OF EXERCISE?

There are three types of exercise that are essential to keep you fit according to David Macutkiewicz MSc, CSCS, sports physiologist at the Olympic Medical Institute, who has devised the exercise programme for this book.

- cardiovascular
- weight (or load) bearing
- resistance

You need to build up to doing some of each of these every week. You will see that some activities, e.g. walking, speed-walking, yoga, racket games and dancing combine two or even three of the types of exercise below. So if you are short of time, you can cover what you need to do in one exercise type. Follow the Exercise Menu to plan your individual programme every week.

Cardiovascular (CV):
(aka aerobic exercise): works out your heart and lungs and starts to burn fat if you do enough

Keeping your heart and lungs fit and healthy will give your body endurance, strength, balance and flexibility so that you can sail through all your daily jobs, and be fit enough to have an adventure if you want to. (Whether that's climbing hills, having a new romance, or swimming with dolphins.) It also helps prevent heart disease and clogged arteries.

You don't have to stick to one form of CV exercise, it's equally beneficial to do a combination such as ten minutes of brisk walking, followed by ten minutes of jogging and ten minutes of cycling. But you should do them at the same time – not ten minutes at three different times in the day.

To ensure you are exercising at the correct level of intensity (that's how hard and fast you're exercising), try the talk test. If you can talk easily during exercise, the intensity is probably too low; if you can't hold a conversation at all, then the intensity is likely to be too high. You're looking to strike the happy medium: you should be able to hold a conversation comfortably but at the same time know that you are exercising.

Weight bearing (WB):
helps your bones

Weight – or load – bearing activities are those where your weight is on the ground. They are of great importance because they help prevent osteoporosis. Continued inactivity leads to rapid loss of bone so exercising prevents this. Also, any physical activity where your feet are on the ground uses the force of gravity to exert a load on your bones that is greater than your weight alone. This stimulates cells in the bones called osteoblasts to form new bone.

Many weight-bearing activities also act as CV and some as RES activities, as you can see in the Exercise Menu below.

Tip: To gain the most benefit from WB exercise you need to feel your whole body working.

Resistance/strength work (RES):
helps develop muscular strength and prevents you losing muscle mass

This is essential in order to prevent vital muscle mass from being lost. Inactivity is one of the main reasons why we lose a large proportion of our muscle mass as we get older. Incorporating resistance exercises into your daily life will help maintain your strength and continue to do everything you want well into old age.

THE EXERCISE MANTRA

ALWAYS warm up, stretch, exercise, cool/slow down, stretch. Allow five to ten minutes each to warm up and cool down, depending on how much activity you have done before starting and the length and intensity you exercise at.

Warm up

Warming up before exercise is important to prepare your body for an increased level of activity. A warm-up is slow and deliberate, designed to increase your heart rate, the rate of blood flow around the body and your core temperature in order to prevent injury to structures like the heart, muscles, ligaments, tendons etc. It's pretty simple: all you need to do is your chosen activity but much slower. For example, a warm-up for a jog would be to start at a walking pace, progress this into a brisk walk and then a steady jog, over about five to ten minutes.

Stretch

After warming up, it is also helpful to do five or so minutes of stretching. Flexibility is a vital component of a balanced fitness programme and you should not overlook it. As well as helping to prevent injury, stretching increases your range of motion, helps you relax, lowers stress levels and keeps your body feeling loose and agile.

It is important that you always warm up first (by walking for instance; see above) to get the blood circulating through your body and into your muscles before stretching. A warm muscle stretches much more easily than a cold one.

One of the most effective ways of stretching is yoga and you will find simple guidelines and postures in the chapter after this one, starting on page 296.

Stretching should be done both before and after exercise. Beforehand, it will help improve the range of flexibility while you're exercising, and also reduce the risk of injury. Stretching after exercise helps relax your muscles, helps remove waste products which might cause muscle soreness, stiffness and/or fatigue and can improve blood flow to joints and muscles.

Cool (slow) down

The importance of cooling down after exercise is often underestimated. In fact the idea of cooling down may be a bit misleading: it's really slowing down so that your body knows it's going to rest. When you exercise, what happens is that your heart rate, the blood flow to the working muscles and your hormone levels all increase in order to cope with the demands the activity is putting on your body. The purpose of the cool/slow down is to reduce those levels gradually and also to allow any waste products produced as a consequence of exercise to be broken down or removed. Cool down in the same way as you warm up, by gradually reducing the intensity and rate of exercise. For instance, after jogging, slow down to a brisk walk, then down again to an ordinary walking pace, over the course of about ten minutes. Then do five minutes' stretching – again you can do yoga stretching. (Your muscles will still be warm enough to stretch easily.)

WHAT TO DO IF YOU'RE DOING LITTLE OR NO EXERCISE NOW

If for any reason you don't do any exercise at the moment, you should consult your doctor for a check-up before starting. Also check what type and level of exercise is safe for you to start with. If you are disabled, we suggest that you check with your health professional for suitable ways of exercising. (See page 292 for a routine for chair, or desk, bound people.) Always be cautious: this is not a competition – the aim is to make you feel better not put you in agony. It's much better to start slowly and build up surely than to risk injury.

How much you do obviously depends on your level of (un)fitness and your health professional should be able to advise you or refer you to an expert. But a reasonable way to start is to walk and/or swim for 10 to 20 minutes at least once or twice each week for two weeks. During the second week, add in a beginners' yoga or Pilates class. Every two weeks, add up to five minutes to the length of time you are exercising for. Once your body has adjusted to your new exercise regime, try increasing the number of sessions per week.

If you're generally fit and in good health, your body will adapt quickly. You may feel tired for the first couple of weeks, but after the first month of exercising regularly, everything will feel a lot easier and you'll begin to feel the fizz of being fit. Progress by adding to the time, and doing the exercise more energetically.

What's the difference? Yoga versus Pilates

People often ask what the difference is between yoga and other Eastern therapies, including martial arts and qigung, and modern Western movement therapies such as Pilates and the Alexander technique. Without getting too complex, Eastern therapies evolved over thousands of years as part of a system of medicine and healthcare that unites mind, body and spirit. Pilates, which was devised by a dancer, and the Alexander technique, which originated to help actors, have a physical basis. However, some people perform yoga purely as a physical therapy and, conversely, others use the Alexander technique as a method of meditative movement.

BE CAREFUL

Stop immediately if you:

- get light-headed
- gave irregular heart beats
- feel sick
- have chest pain
- are excessively short of breath
- sustain any injury

Don't get dehydrated: sip still water continuously

YOUR WEEKLY PICK 'N' MIX EXERCISE MENU

There are lots of different ways of combining cardiovascular, weight-bearing and resistance exercise. With the menu below, you will see that you can do single activities such as yoga, tennis, stair/hill climbing and vigorous housework, which incorporate all three types of exercise so that you can get your optimal quota in four weekly sessions. (You can do more, of course!) Other activities combine two benefits, in which case you should add in the third type for all-round health. If you prefer to do lots of different types of exercise, just make sure that you do some of each type. You can follow the same routine every week or swop around as you wish.

You'll see that there are non-sporting activities in the lists, like hoovering, gardening, car washing and climbing stairs. We want you to see that even if you're very short of time you can integrate exercise into your daily life. The key is to do these things as vigorously and with as much movement as possible. And remember to have fun: put on some dance music and move in time to it while you're doing jobs around the house, or go out for a walk in your lunch hour.

Sessions should be 20 to 40 minutes long plus the warm-up/cool-down period. If you haven't exercised for some time, please see page 287.

If you find your chosen activities are becoming too easy, increase the duration and intensity – exercise for longer and harder, in other words!

Exercise Menu

1. Activity benefit: CV/WB/RES

If you pick one or more activities from this CV/WB/RES menu, build up to four or more sessions weekly

CV	WB	RES
yoga	yoga	yoga
judo/martial arts	judo/martial arts	judo/martial arts
climbing stairs/ hills	climbing stairs/ hills	climbing stairs/ hills
tennis, badminton, squash	tennis, badminton, squash	tennis, badmin- ton, squash

step aerobics	step aerobics	step aerobics
vigorous house-work*/ gardening**	vigorous house-work/gardening if lifting	vigorous house-work/gardening
X-country skiing	X-country skiing	X-country skiing
circuit training	circuit training	circuit training

* pushing/lifting vacuum cleaner, brushing up
** wheeling a wheelbarrow, digging, raking, brushing up

2. Activity benefit: CV/WB

If you pick one or more activities from this **CV/WB** menu, build up to **three** or more sessions weekly plus **two** or more sessions of **RES**

CV	WB	RES
brisk walking	brisk walking	
speed walking	speed walking	
hiking***	hiking	
jogging	jogging	
cross-country running	cross-country running	
aerobics	aerobics	
energetic dancing	energetic dancing	
skating	skating	
circuit training	circuit training	
gymnastics	gymnastics	
handball	handball	

*** striding across country with rucksack etc.

3. Activity benefit: CV/RES

If you pick one or more activities from this **CV/RES** menu, aim for **three** or more sessions weekly plus **three** or more sessions of **WB**

CV	WB	RES
Pilates		Pilates
sailing		sailing
hockey, football		hockey, football
rowing (water/gym)		rowing (water/gym)
canoeing		canoeing
swimming		swimming
aquaerobics		aquaerobics
calisthenics (light benefit)		calisthenics (light benefit)
fast horse riding, e.g. trotting		horse riding

4. Activity benefit: WB/RES

If you pick one or more activities from this **WB/RES** menu, aim for **four** or more sessions weekly, plus **three** or more sessions of **CV**

CV	WB	RES
	weight training in gym	weight training in gym
	free weights	free weights: baked bean can workout

elastic band	elastic band
stretching	stretching
body pump classes	body pump classes
gymnastics	gymnastics

THE BAKED BEAN CAN WORKOUT

Fitness pro Gloria Thomas devised this cheap and cheerful upper body workout which you can do at home. (It was first published in Sarah's book *Feel Fabulous Forever: The Anti-ageing Health & Beauty Bible*, co-written with Josephine Fairley.) Start slowly and do each exercise until your muscles feel tired. If you find it's getting very easy, switch to a slightly larger can of beans – just make sure you can hold them easily.

This is brilliant for anyone who is chair bound for any reason.

Shoulders

Sit in an upright position.
Your abdominal muscles should be pulled in, shoulders back and down.
Relax your head and neck.
Holding a can of beans in each hand, bring your hands to shoulder level, palms facing forwards and arms straight.
Breathe in and take the cans above your head to a count of two, then slowly lower to the starting position.

Biceps

In the same sitting position as before, keep your upper arms by your side and extend your arms from the elbows holding the cans.
Keeping your upper arms close to your body, turn your palms upwards holding the cans, and curl them up towards your shoulders for a count of two.
Lower to a count of four.

Triceps

If you're not used to exercising, do this one arm at a time. If you are fit, do both at the same time.
In the same sitting position, grasp a can of baked beans between the thumb and forefinger of each hand.
Lift your arms behind your head so that the elbows are just above each ear.
Straighten your arms upwards until the baked bean can is over your head.
Take care not to lock your arms, then slowly return to the starting position.

Back

This is great for stiffening the muscles of the back and for posture.
Sit as before, holding a can of beans upright in each hand and take your arms out in front of you at shoulder level.
Now take your arms out to either side in line with your shoulders, pulling your shoulder blades together, and hold for a count of two.
Slowly go back to your original position.

FAT BURNING

The table below shows how many calories you can burn
exercising in different ways. The figures are based on women
weighing between 68 and 80 kg (150 and 176 lb) doing the
particular activity for 30 minutes.

Activity	Calories burnt (kcal) in 30 mins	Activity	Calories burnt (kcal) in 30 mins
Walking		Swimming	
leisure	162–192	*front crawl*	261–306
2.5 mph	132–153	*back stroke*	345–405
3.0 mph	150–177	*breast stroke*	330–390
3.5 mph	183–207		
Hiking vigorously	168–198	Cycling	
		5.5 mph	132–153
Running		*9.4 mph*	204–240
x-country	333–390		
11.5 min mile	276–327	Gardening	
9 min mile	393–462	*digging*	258–303
8 min mile	426–495	*mowing*	228–270
7 min mile	468–537	*raking*	111–129
Aerobics		Household jobs	
easy	201–234	*vacuuming*	132–156
medium	210–246	*dusting*	132–156
intense	276–324	*car washing*	144–171

Exercise

Activity	Calories burnt (kcal) in 30 mins	Activity	Calories burnt (kcal) in 30 mins
Rowing machine		Horse riding	225–264
race	363–426	Judo	357–420
moderate	243–291		
		Fishing	144–168
Circuits		Handball	294–345
universal	237–279		
free-weights	174–204	Sailing	90–105
		Tennis	222–261
Canoeing			
low effort	108–126	Yoga	126–150
moderate effort	249–294		
		Badminton	198–234
Modern dance	147–174	X-country skiing	201–237
Football (structured game)	321–378	Aquaerobics	270–315
		Calisthenics	153–180
Field hockey (structured game)	285–336		

YOGA FOR YOU

This chapter covers:
* why yoga
* a few do's and don'ts
* props
* general tips
* sequences for:
  * hot flushes
  * menstrual pains
  * stress, fear, fatigue and mood swings
  * bladder control

At its most basic, yoga is a system of exercise that keeps your body wonderfully supple and graceful – and gives you energy even when you're tired. But there is much more. The collection of poses – some simple, some more demanding – gives you a marvellous way of calming and relaxing your mind, as well as helping you to use your own natural healing powers to correct health problems of all sorts – physical, mental and emotional. And anyone, any age, can do it. In India, you see women of 70 and 80 entwined in postures that would make most teenagers bleat for mercy. The word 'yoga' in Sanskrit means 'union' – of mind, body and spirit.

On a beauty front, it's absolutely fabulous! It's said that yoga fans, like dancers, never need face-lifts ... or any other nips and tucks (it's very good for keeping the bosom lifted). Just try the warm-up then look in the mirror. You'll see your face softened, eyes sparkling, cheeks pink – with a general brightness and zest. If you're feeling a bit peaky before, say, going to a party or on a hot date – do some yoga and wait for the compliments. Not only will you glow on the outside, yoga releases an inner loveliness that is unbeatable.

> Esther: *"I was exhausted and bony-faced before I went to this big party so I did 20 minutes' yoga – just simple poses. My favourite man told me I looked completely gorgeous and he thought he was falling in love with me ... "*

Although yoga dates back to at least 3000 BC, it really only came to the West with the hippy dippy sixties. Now it's widely respected by the medical profession and research studies show its effectiveness in helping to treat many conditions.

Michael is 100 per cent convinced of the benefits of yoga as a part of Integrated Menopausal Therapy. Yoga is a weight-bearing exercise so it's particularly good for preventing and helping to treat osteoporosis. All the bones of the body, including those in the hands, arms, head and neck, are strengthened. If you read the section on hot flushes (see page 79), you'll remember that simply doing a form of yogic breathing can stop flushing in its tracks. So you can see the potential. Sarah has been a fan for many years and we asked her yoga teacher Hannah Lovegrove to devise simple sequences of poses to help you with common menopausal problems.

There are many different forms of yoga. Hannah practises Iyengar, which is particularly concerned with treating specific conditions. Teachers are trained in therapeutic yoga programmes over many years.

Karen: *"Practising yoga has changed me on the inside as well as outside – I'm not jumpy any more and things don't throw me in the same way. I feel steady, centred ... as well as much fitter."*

You will see that some of the poses involve part or all of your body being turned upside down. These 'inversions' are very important, according to Hannah. 'The body fluids have the opportunity to re-circulate and areas of stagnation can be flushed through. As well as clearing the chest cavity and lungs, the large intestine and pelvic organisation benefit and long-term practice seems to have a regulating effect on blood pressure. Inversions also have a very positive effect on the brain and leave you feeling refreshed and clear-headed.'

Always check with your doctor or health professional before starting yoga, as with any new physical activity.

These sequences are designed for beginners to do at home, although they will work just as well if you are more experienced. Obviously, practising regularly will give you the most benefit, especially with a qualified teacher. We hope that you will start going to classes regularly; look in the Directory under Orange Tree Yoga for details of how to find local Iyengar yoga classes, and web links.

A FEW DO'S AND DON'TS

* always warm up first, and relax afterwards.
* don't practise if you have bronchitis, diarrhoea, during an asthma attack or if you have a viral infection of any kind.
* if you are having period problems, just practise the Warm-up and the relevant sequence below (called 'For menstrual problems') during the days you are bleeding. Don't do any inverted postures or back bends during menstruation because they may affect normal blood flow.

* if you are being treated for high blood pressure, keep your arms down and hands on your hips in standing postures, i.e. don't lift them above your shoulders or head. If you are doing standing postures where you need to bend forwards, keep your head at waist level.
* don't use hand cream or body lotion before your practice – it makes your skin too slippery and your hands may slide on the mat.

PROPS

You can buy yoga props easily from Internet sites (www.orangetreeyoga.com has a list); often there are household items that are fine substitutes. You will need:

* **yoga mat**: buy a good-quality, 'sticky' mat, especially made for the purpose. There isn't a household substitute.
* **foam block**: this is about the size of a fat telephone directory. The best substitute is a folded blanket; use firm cotton or wool, not fleece because it's slippery. Make sure your blanket is evenly folded and smooth with no lumps or bumps.
* **bolster**: buy one, or use a tightly rolled blanket, tied securely top and bottom.
* **yoga strap**: an old tie makes a fine substitute.
* **kitchen timer**: useful for long holds – it's very easy to lose track of time during yoga.

GENERAL TIPS

Breathing

Always breathe slowly, deeply and rhythmically through your nose, keeping your jaw relaxed. Never hold your breath.

Each posture follows on from the last, giving a seamless sequence of gentle stretches – but don't worry if this doesn't happen at first. It will, especially if you take yourself to a class as well as practising at home. Try to synchronise your breath with the movements: breathe in as you prepare for a movement and out as you stretch.

Hands and feet

Yoga is not ballet: you don't need to point your toes. When you stretch your legs, keep your feet at a natural angle to your legs. Similarly with your hands, keep your fingers and wrists in line with your arms; don't overstretch the palms, but don't allow your hands to flop.

Yoga space

If you can put down a yoga mat and stretch your arms up and out, you have space for yoga. Do make it settled and comfortable: try lighting candles or joss sticks and decorating it with flowers and pictures if you wish.

Instructions

Some of the words and phrases used below may be unfamiliar, such as 'lift your breastbone'. This does not mean a big body movement – or getting a 10-ton truck – it's a subtle shift that comes from your brain as much as your body. By being aware of your breastbone, say, and the position it should be in, i.e. floating up rather than falling in, your body will almost do the work for you.

If you are new to yoga, the instructions may sound complicated until you get to know the poses. It may help to read them aloud and tape them, or to practise with a friend so you can talk each other through them. Do each posture slowly and without strain. It's much better to do one well than to rush through a whole sequence. Over time, they will become second nature, especially if you can go to classes. (Ask your teacher to check your postures.)

Which and how often

It's a good idea to practise some yoga every day, particularly if you want to bring about real changes in your body. Ideally, you could do the Warm-up daily and choose one longer sequence – depending on your symptoms – to do at least twice a week. On the days in between, choose a Quick sequence, depending on your immediate needs. If you're still having periods, your practice will vary naturally as you will be including the Menstrual sequence at regular (or irregular!) intervals.

Quick sequences

Once your body is beginning to be familiar with yoga – say, after you've practised the Warm-up sequence daily for a week – you can do the Quick sequences on their own whenever you have a few minutes.

Finish

Finish every sequence by lying quietly on the floor for three to five minutes, legs straight and feet softly falling apart, arms at 45 degrees to your sides, palms up. Put a lavender bag on your eyes and a folded blanket under your head for maximum relaxation. (You can do this any time you need to relax.)

SEQUENCES

Warm-up: 10 to 15 minutes

Try and do this daily. It is a great way to start your day, and a good quick fix in its own right for any physical, mental or emotional problems. We also suggest you use this as a stretching routine before exercise (see page 285).

Posture	No
Full body stretch	1
Drawing up the knees	2
Quick back stretch	3

Always finish by lying quietly on the floor for three to five minutes.

To ease hot flushes: 15 to 20 minutes

Use this sequence at least twice a week if you are prone to hot flushes and night sweats.

Mountain pose	4
Intense leg stretch	5
Downward facing dog	6
Head to knee pose	7
Back body stretch	8
Downward facing hero	9

Quick sequence

With deep breathing, you can stop a hot flush in its tracks

as we explain on page 79 If you're having a hot flush, try these poses after doing the breathing.

Downward facing dog	6
Head to knee pose	7

For menstrual problems (daily when you are actually menstruating) 15 to 20 minutes

Reclining cobbler pose	10
Seated wide-angle pose	11
Head to knee pose	7
Downward facing hero	9

Quick sequence

Reclining cobbler	10

Tip: you can also do this before bed (or even in it) if you suffer from insomnia

To soothe stress, fear, fatigue and mood swings: 15 to 20 minutes

Mountain pose	4
Downward facing dog	6
Downward facing hero	9
Head to knee pose	7
Back body stretch	8
Shoulder stand	12

Quick sequence

Downward facing dog	6
Downward facing hero	9
Head to knee pose	7

To help with bladder control: 15 to 20 minutes

Mountain pose	4

(For this purpose, check the inner edges of your feet are together and hold for one to three minutes. Focus on lifting from the arches of the feet, up through the legs, and strongly lift the pelvic area and the body.)

Head to knee pose	7
Seated wide-angle pose	11
Reclining cobbler pose	10

Quick sequence

Stay in Mountain pose (4) while you're washing up or watching the kettle boil ...

Turn over for descriptions of the poses.

1 Full body stretch

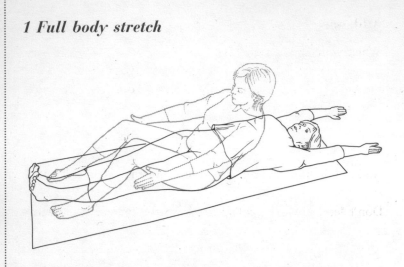

Sit in the middle of your mat, knees bent, and feet on the floor a hip width apart. Lower your upper body in a straight line until you are lying flat. Stretch your legs out straight bringing the inner edges of your feet together, toes pointing up.

Breathe in as you slowly press the backs of your legs to the floor, stretch your arms down your sides then lift them straight over your head to the floor behind. Breathe out as you slowly bring your arms back over your head and down to your sides.

Let your feet fall apart and the backs of your hands lie on the floor.

Relax completely.

Repeat three times, holding the full stretch for a little longer each time.

Add-ons

When your hands are above your head, press them into the broad sides of a block to help straighten your arms.
Lie facing a wall, and press the soles of your feet into it to help straighten your legs.

Watchpoints

Align your body carefully, making sure that both sides are even.
Don't let your chest collapse – keep the breastbone gently lifted and the back of your neck long.
Keep your lower back long by drawing your navel towards your spine. With each repetition, notice how your diaphragm and the side ribs can stretch a little further.

Benefits

Relaxes the body and eases the breathing. Soothes headaches, insomnia, stress and tension. Helps recovery of any sort. Begins to develop stretch, strength and stamina evenly throughout the body.

2 Knees to chest

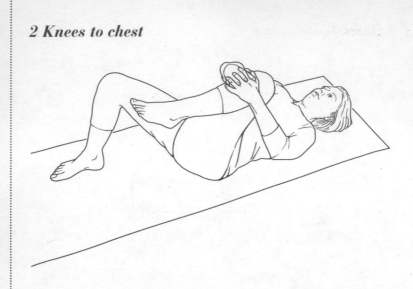

Breathe in and clasp your fingers round your right kneecap.
Breathe out and draw it in towards the chest.
Breathe in and squeeze knee to chest.
Breathe out and lower your foot back to the floor.
Repeat three times alternately with each knee.

Watchpoints

Synchronise your breath – inhale as you prepare, exhale as you move; keep your shoulders on the floor and breastbone lifted.

Benefits

Eases the hip joints, relaxes and stretches the lower leg, thigh, hip, gluteals and lower back.

3 Quick back stretch

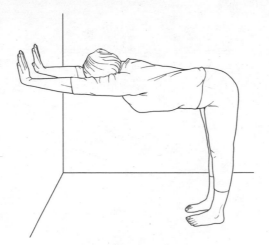

Stand with your feet a hip width apart in front of a wall.
Press your hands into the wall, at hip height.
Keeping your hands pressed in to the wall and arms straight,
walk your legs back until your head is between your arms:
your body should be parallel to the floor at right angles to
your legs, which are straight. (Ask someone to check, or
look in a mirror.)
Breathe in and, keeping the heels of your hands pressed into
the wall, breathe out and stretch your hips back.
Stay for 2–3 minutes, breathing smoothly.
To come up, walk your feet towards the wall.

Watchpoints

Keep your kneecaps lifted and thighs very active to support
the back; press hands into the wall to stretch your shoulders and pull your hips back. Don't drop your head.

Benefits

Stretches the whole back, from neck to tailbone; opens the
sides of the body and the armpits.

4 Mountain pose

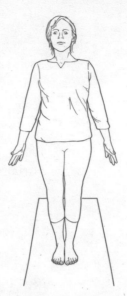

Stand with the inner edges of your feet together, heels and big toe joints touching.

Draw your thighs back and lift your kneecaps to straighten your legs.

Press your tailbone forward and lift the breastbone.

Roll your shoulders back and down, tucking in your shoulder blades.

Stretch your arms and hands down your sides in line with your hips.

Breathe evenly.

Hold for one minute, breathing evenly.

Add-on

Stand with your back against a wall or door. As you lift your breastbone (see above), breathe in and stretch your arms above your head, palms facing.

Watchpoint

Keep your weight evenly distributed on both feet; don't tense your shoulders, neck or jaw. You are aiming to hold the pose but relax your body.

Benefits

Brings your whole body to attention, aligns the skeleton and prepares the muscles for movement.

5 Intense leg stretch

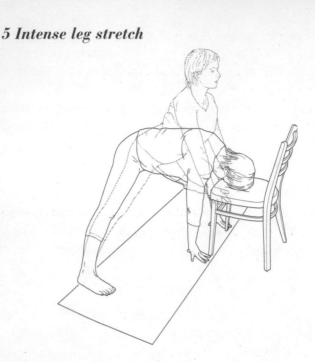

Stand with your feet very wide apart (as drawing) and parallel.
Put your hands on your hips and lift your chest, tucking
your shoulder blades well in.
Lift your kneecaps, draw your thighs back, and push your
tailbone forwards – your legs will feel very active now.
Breathe in.
Breathe out, keeping your back concave (dipping in not
humped), and take your body horizontal to the chair, looking
forwards – not down – all the time. Place your hands on the
chair seat for support.
Pause, strongly stretch both legs up and lift your buttock
bones.
Breathe out, and rest your forehead on the chair; if it feels
comfortable, take your hands to the floor (otherwise leave
them where they are).

Breathe evenly, pulling up the legs strongly throughout. Initially just hold this for as long as you feel comfortable. As your confidence increases, hold it for one to three minutes, breathing evenly.

To come up, breathe in and bring your hands up to the chair seat again, lift the kneecaps again then breathe out and stand up.

Watchpoints

Keep your legs very active and strong throughout; as you go down, don't look down or your back will hump – look towards the opposite wall to keep it concave.

Benefits

Regulates menstrual bleeding. Strengthens the knees and keeps the hips supple. Strengthens the abdominal organs and relieves digestive problems. Is calming for the brain and nerves. Reduces depression and boosts self-confidence. Relieves headaches, fatigue and stress.

Warning

Come up slowly if you have high blood pressure.

6 Downward facing dog

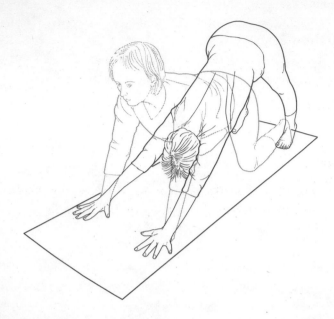

Kneel in the centre of your mat, facing lengthways.

Put your hands and knees on the floor, with plenty of space between them, both front to back and side to side.

Tuck your toes under and breathe in.

Breathe out as you lift your hips high by pressing on the palms of your hands and the balls of your feet.

Squeeze the elbow joints towards each other to straighten the arms.

Lift your shoulders towards your hips.

Lift your kneecaps and the backs of your thighs to straighten your legs.

Let the back of your neck relax completely.

Breathe evenly, lifting the legs, and stretching the body up to the hips. Stay there for three to six breaths.

Gently lower your body back to your knees.

Untuck your toes and sit back on your heels.
Do this twice.

Watchpoints

Put hands and feet parallel to each other on the floor; spread
your palms and soles for support; feel as if you're pushing
the backs of your thighs out more broadly as you lift your
buttocks up.

Benefits

Very calming but gently stimulating posture which checks
heavy menstrual bleeding and prevents hot flushes.

7 Head to knee pose

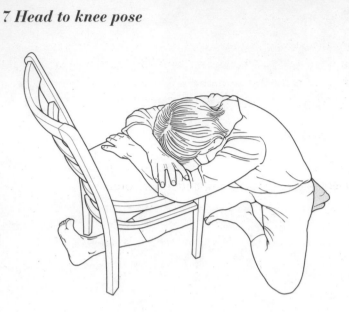

Sit on the floor on a block, legs straight, feet together.
Have a chair with a folded blanket on the seat over your
feet (chair back away from you as drawing).
Stretch the legs forwards, and take your hands to the floor
either side of your hips.
Breathe in and lift your torso.
Bend your right leg, take your knee out to the side and put
the heel of the foot near the groin.
Bending from your hips, allow your torso to come forward
softly over the chair; relax your back, neck and head as you
do so.
Stay down for six quiet breaths.
Come up gently on an out breath, and repeat on the left.

Watchpoints

Do this slowly and take time to relax your bent leg and hip, breathing evenly. Keep your bent knee back and the straight one pressed down. Support the bent knee on blocks if you need to. Don't collapse your lower back.

Benefits

Relieves the effects of stress, and quietens the mind; tones liver, spleen, kidneys and abdominal organs.

8 Back body stretch

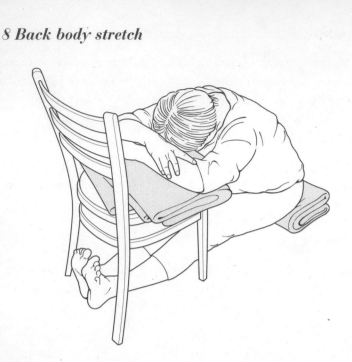

Sit on a block or folded blanket, legs straight, feet together.
Have a chair with a folded blanket on the seat over your
feet (chair back away from you as drawing).
Stretch the legs forwards, and take your hands to the floor
either side of your hips.
Breathe in and lift your torso.
Straighten your legs and press them down.
Lift your chest and press the lower back forwards from the
hips, bringing the front of your body slowly towards the
chair.
Breathe out and reach forwards to the chair with your arms
straight, keeping the backs of the thighs pressed down.
Bring the chair towards you and finally rest your head on
your crossed arms.
Hold this for one to three minutes as your flexibility improves.

Add-on

As you get more experienced, you can dispense with the chair and use a bolster, then finally bring your body down over both extended legs.

Watchpoints

Sit evenly on both buttock bones; stretch your legs forward; keep your thighs pressed down all the time and your lower back lifted.

Benefits

Cools the temperature of the skin, soothes the nervous system, rests the heart, tones and relaxes the whole reproductive system.

9 Downward facing hero

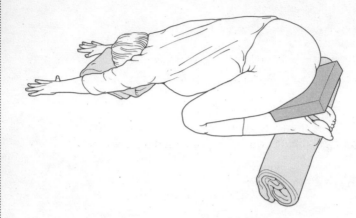

Sit on your heels on a block or folded blanket with your knees well apart, big toes touching.

Keeping your hips and bottom touching your heels, slowly lie the front of your body down over your thighs, pressing your breastbone towards the floor to keep your back flat.

Keep your arms straight, and spread your palms on the floor, a shoulder width apart.

Finally let your forehead rest on a block or rolled-up blanket. Stay there for one to three minutes, breathing evenly.

Add-on

If the tops of your feet are stiff or painful, put a rolled blanket under your ankles.

Watchpoint

If you add a block under your bum, you should add one under your forehead, and vice versa, to keep your neck and spine straight. Try to aim to have your ribs resting on your inner thighs.

Benefits

Alleviates menstrual pain; reduces blood pressure; quiets the mind and lifts depression and headaches.

Warning

Don't do this if you have poor bladder control.

10 Reclining cobbler pose

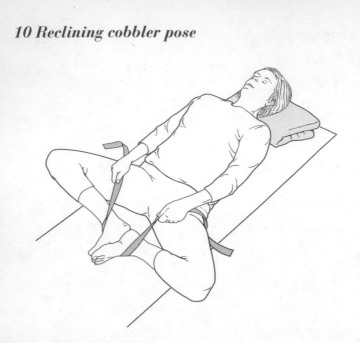

Sit in the middle of your mat on the floor with a bolster (or two folded blankets) under you, where your spine will be. You will also need an extra folded blanket on the end of the bolster to lift your head.

Bend your knees and let them fall to the sides, then bring the soles of your feet together and draw your heels towards your groin.

Lie back carefully over the bolster, with your head on the extra blanket.

Allow your arms to fall to either side, shoulders relaxed, eyes closed.

Stay for five to ten minutes.

Add-on

Wrap a strap round your feet and bottom to pull feet closer to your body. Lay an eye pad over your eyes, if you like.

Watchpoint

Check you are straight as you lie down; don't tilt your head to one side.

Benefits

Relieves heaviness and congestion in the whole pelvic area; relieves pain during menstruation; improves the circulation; quiets the mind and nerves.

11 Seated wide-angle pose

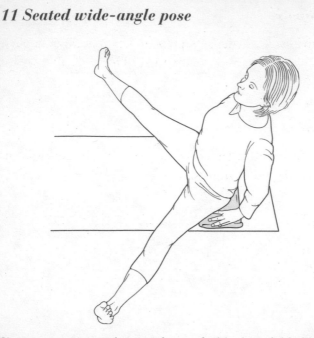

Sit on your mat on the very front of a block or folded blanket and spread your legs wide apart.

Stretch the backs of your legs into the heels and keep the toes pointing upwards.

Put your fingers on the block/blanket either side of your hips and lift up your torso, keeping your elbows bent backwards.

Keep the weight of your body forward on the buttock bones.

Push the backs of the thighs into the floor.

Hold for three to five minutes, breathing evenly.

To come out, place your hand under each knee in turn, bend the leg and lift it back to the centre.

Add-on

Sit against a wall if you need to support your back.

Watchpoint

Keep the back of your legs pressing down and the mid-line of the front of the legs facing the ceiling; your toes should point directly up.

Benefits

Relives menstrual disorders and regulates flow; stimulates and massages the pelvic organs.

Warning

Avoid this pose if you have headache or migraine.

12 Shoulder stand

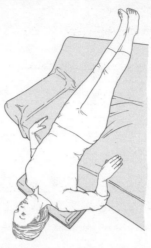

This seems long and complicated but it is simple enough for beginners to do confidently and safely.

Arrange your props as shown in the drawing. Place the narrow edges of the blocks together, fold the blanket evenly and place on top.

Sit on the sofa then swing your legs round and up the back, keeping your buttocks towards the back of the seat.

Allow your upper body to slide towards the floor, keeping your hips on the sofa, settling your shoulders centrally on the blanket and blocks; the back of your head on the floor. (The lump on the base of your neck is on the blanket/blocks.)

Let the back of your neck lengthen and draw your shoulders away from your ears.

Stretch the backs of your legs, pushing the heels away and drawing the toes towards you. Stay for three to six breaths.

Keeping both legs straight, stretch one leg up to the vertical, stretch the heel away, then bring it down and stretch the other leg up.

Repeat this slowly three times on each side.

When you have gained confidence, stretch both legs up together and stay for three breaths.

When you are ready to come down, bring your legs to the back of the sofa.

Push your hips slowly off the sofa and slide the body down on to the floor.

Put a block under your head and lie with knees bent and breathe quietly.

Add on

If you feel constricted in the throat, add another blanket to raise the height of your support. If you feel pressure in the eyes, face or throat, come down and adjust your position, then try again.

Watchpoint

Keep the weight of your body evenly distributed on your shoulders. Take the back of your head, not the top, to the floor. Turning upside down can feel strange at first, so ask a friend to help.

Benefits

Good for overall menstrual health; relieves bloating and trapped wind; soothing to nerves and tonic to body systems; the shoulder stand increases the efficiency of the thyroid and parathyroid glands; aids the whole digestive system, corrects urinary and menstrual disorders, helps recovery from illness; eases stiff neck and shoulders, relieves headaches and prevents insomnia.

Warning

Don't do this if you're menstruating: substitute Reclining cobbler pose.

II

GROWING OLDER GORGEOUSLY

This chapter covers:
- what happens round menopause
- help for hair
- hair colouring
- help for skin
- the products you really need
- your basic make-up bag: make up artist Jenny Jordan's top choices
- making up for hot flushes

One feeling comes over forcibly from many women around the age of menopause: fear that it will mean you lose your femininity. We suspect this may account for much of the taboo surrounding the subject. We found one book advising 'crone sessions' – fine if that's what you really want but the prospect doesn't do a lot for the women we know.

Taking care you look your best is not vain or self-indulgent or any of those negative things that many 40-plus women were brought up to believe. Looking after your appearance is part of valuing yourself. In fact, research shows that improving your self-image helps to conquer stress and anxiety and boost your immune system.

As we've discussed earlier, many women going through the menopause suffer from low mood. Beauty legend Bobbi Brown, the American make-up artist who launched a hugely successful range of cosmetics, describes being in her 40s as definitely the 'Oh shit decade ... ! it's when you first notice that you actually do look older than you used to.'

One woman admitted that although she adored her lovely daughters, walking down the street with them and seeing their effect on passers-by made her feel 'horribly middle-aged, dowdy and gloomy'. While every woman over 40 has to accept that she'll never be a babe again – or roll out of bed looking a rumpled million dollars (although Goldie Hawn is still trying at 50 plus plus) – you must also take on board that you can still look lovely and be as, or even more, alluring.

On a bad day, a bit of so-called vanity can work wonders. However low you feel, doing your hair and make-up, putting on your most flattering clothes and a pair of pretty shoes, spritzing on some scent and switching on the smile light (think of someone/something that you love) can lift your spirits. Everyone you meet responds to it – and your life suddenly cheers up.

We're not talking about complicated stuff here. Bobbi Brown's advice is to stop following trends and aim for a classic look. You could translate that into looking polished, groomed and naturally (well, nearly) gorgeous. Of course, women with lovely features and figures have an advantage but you don't need to start out physically beautiful or even pretty. Taking good care of yourself will give you a glow no babe can better.

The key points are:

- glossy, well-cut hair
- clear, healthy, glowing skin
- well-kept hands and nails

- a little well-chosen make-up
- and most important of all, looking happy and loving

WHAT HAPPENS AROUND MENOPAUSE

There's a temptation to blame every problem on falling oestrogen levels. There does seem to be a connection between dry skin and a drop in oestrogen, as there is with vaginal dryness. The moment your skin starts getting dry, the wrinkles get worse – and more obvious – so there is a knock-on effect. Another significant factor is loss of skin tone ('everything going south' as one woman described it) but that is probably more to do with a natural drop-off in collagen and elastic, the elements that form the matrix of your skin and bone. Your hair condition and growth pattern may also be affected, with drier hair and, possibly, a phase where your hair thins in patches or all over. The good news is that all the simple things we bang on about in this book – good diet, lots of water, relaxation and sleep, plus exercise – will help your appearance enormously. There are also good beauty products especially formulated to help – one bonus from the baby boomers hitting middle age.

Looking after yourself means taking time – not a lot but regularly – and investing wisely. This is about basic beauty techniques, which are simple, enjoyable and need not break the bank. (If you want lots more information, can we suggest you look at *Feel Fabulous Forever: The Anti-ageing Health and Beauty Bible*, by Josephine Fairley and Sarah Stacey.)

HAIR

Dry hair is a particular problem at menopause. It may improve over the years but, meantime, you should use specific shampoos, conditioners and hair masks to restore the shine and manageability. Most labels will distinguish products for dry and very dry hair; look for 'moisturising' on the label; if your hair is flat as a crêpe suzette, look for 'volumising' products.

The one thing you should spend money on is a good cut, particularly if your hair is thinning or in poor condition. Have your hair long by all means if it suits you – though style gurus advise against wearing it loose below the shoulders as you get older – but whatever the length, the ends must be impeccably trimmed and it must look fabulously glossy. Make sure your stylist gives you a cut that you can manage easily at home. Cull all the tricks you can about tools, products and techniques, but remember you will never be able to morph into your hairdresser.

Now to the colour: grey hair, which looks so wonderfully distinguished on men, seldom looks wonderfully anything on women (with a few honourable exceptions). Hair does not in fact go grey but white because the hair stops producing colour. This also affects the condition and texture because the lack of pigment makes it coarser and drier. So if your hair is going grey, look for specific products. Interestingly, white hairs start appearing to many women in their 20s but it's not until the 30s and 40s that you actually start to notice it.

If you want to cover grey, it makes sense to invest in professional colour if possible: either have it done regularly by an expert or stretch your budget to cover one or two sessions (so you get the colour as you want it) and then do it yourself at home. Make friends with the colourist and get as many tips and recommendations as possible. Whatever you do, make sure you can keep it up: it's better to do nothing apart from conditioning than have a permanent all-over different colour and let the roots grow out – nothing is less flattering than, say, an auburn rinse with an inch of salt and pepper on your scalp. (The only answer to that is to go to an expert colourist who will most likely use highlights to soften the grow-out line, or cleanse out and re-colour.)

If your hair is having a nervous breakdown, it's often because you're run down in addition to hormonal fluctuations and it will recover naturally in time. Help it along by taking a good multivitamin and mineral and getting enough iron and oily food in your diet. If you're eating little or no red meat, it may be difficult to get sufficient iron from food in a way that your body can absorb. In that case consider a supplement (such as Floradix, a liquid iron supplement that seems to suit most people). Vitamin C is needed for iron absorption, so make sure you get plenty from fruit and vegetables, and perhaps an added supplement. Evening primrose oil and/or fish oil supplements can also help the condition of your hair.

As with everything, you can't expect an overnight miracle so spend an hour or so playing with your hair and working out a few simple strategies to make it behave when it's feeling bolshie. A spot of serum (less than a 5p piece for most hair lengths) smeared in the palms of your hands and worked through your hair from the nape up to the front hairline can give shine and manageability on the dullest day. (John Frieda's Sheer Blonde Spotlight glosser is fab for coloured hair.) Big rollers can give body but avoid heated ones and hairdriers if your hair is dry; if you have to use either or both, condition even more generously. By the same token, if you're in the sun, keep your hair covered with a big hat and consider a leave-in conditioner to prevent the Desert Storm look. Also practise with kirby-grips (don't try and hide them), slides, barrettes, combs, scrunchies and headbands: a bit of fiddling and perseverance can bring astonishing results.

One quick tip for a Bad Hair Day is to give your scalp a massage: put your fingertips on your hairline at the front and rotate them, progressing slowly backwards. Or, if you have time, wash and condition your hair then finish with a cold rinse. Both will revive your hair – and your brain.

FEED YOUR HAIR (AND SKIN)

Eat lots of

- fresh vegetables, salads and fruit
- live natural yoghurt
- cold-pressed oils – olive, sunflower, sesame, flax
- seeds – sunflower, sesame, linseeds, pumpkin
- fresh oily fish (if you're not a vegetarian) – salmon, sea trout, mackerel, sardines, tuna, herrings
- almonds, figs and dates
- pulses – peas, beans and lentils
- whole grains – oats, brown rice, buckwheat, millet

Drink lots of water

Cut down on

- cow's milk products
- caffeine – coffee, tea, chocolate, cola
- sugar and salt

DIY hair colouring

Colouring your hair at home is inexpensive and can look wonderful – but for good results you must stick to the instructions on the label. (Don't do as Sarah has done in the past and opt for a kind of free interpretation because she couldn't find her glasses ...) Here is a quick guide to hair colouring options from leading colourist Ian Black, Technical Artistic Director for the Aveda Advanced Academy in London. Aveda is a leading natural beauty company and we recommend their products, which include colour shampoos and conditioners for a hint of a tint.

- **Semi-permanent or vegetable colour**: true semi-permanent colour comes ready mixed and will last six to eight shampoos. It is applied to damp hair and left to process for 30 to 45 minutes. It will not cover white hair totally but will give a soft blend. It is a great no-commitment introduction to colouring your hair as the colour will just gently fade out. It gives a feel of what it's like to have coloured hair and is an easy way to play around with different tones to see which you like best. Always opt for tints a few shades lighter than your natural base, which will look natural and give an almost highlighted effect on your white hairs.
- **Demi-permanent (or tone-on-tone colour)**: this is similar to semi-permanent and is mixed with a low-volume peroxide to give results that last up to 24 washes; that's about six to eight weeks. It will darken hair, blend grey and add tone but it will not lighten the natural colour. As this colour fades out over six to eight weeks, your roots won't show too much.
- **Permanent colour**: this chemically based colour needs mixing with peroxide and will give a long-lasting permanent result. Permanent colour will lighten or darken hair and give total coverage to white hair. As the results are permanent it will give a strong grow-out line when covering the grey and the roots will need retouching every four to eight weeks. Think about adding professional highlights to break up the colour and make it more natural-looking.

- **Highlights:** these are created by lifting out strands of hair and applying two or three different shades of permanent colour or bleach, then wrapping them in foil. This will give an overall lighter appearance to the hair. This is a good way of lightening the hair and blending in the white, although it will not give total coverage as only 30 to 50 per cent of the hair is coloured.
- **Lowlights:** these are done in exactly the same way as highlights using either a red or a darker shade. Using a colour the same as your natural colour will give the effect of how your hair appeared a few years previously when there was less white.

SKIN

There are just three vital words to remember: moisturise, moisturise, moisturise ... All over, from top to toe – face and body. Don't forget the especially dry bits such as lips, neck, elbows, hands and feet. As we've said above, everything gets drier as you get older so always look for ranges that are specifically formulated for dry skin, and often for 40-something women – words like 'age defying' in the product name are a big clue. This is a huge market so there's a big choice, which is growing like Topsy, and expensive doesn't necessarily mean better. You can get very good results with budget ranges. That's not to say that the high end of the market brands aren't good but no woman should feel that she has to spend a fortune.

When you're considering a new brand of skincare, always try samples before investing. Any company worth its salt should give them away although you may have to go to a big store and talk to the consultant for each brand. If they don't do trial sizes, ask if you can take some in a pot to try out. Should they be unhelpful, tell them you are sensitive to some products and want to be certain this will suit you. At least half of all women believe they have sensitive skins, so this is entirely legitimate.

In fact, the first thing with any product is to make sure that you don't get a sensitivity reaction. If you do, stop using it immediately. All sorts of ingredients, from high-tech to super-natural, can cause reactions but in our experience AHAs (alphahydroxy acids) which speed up cell turnover are some of the most likely. If the sample product doesn't cause any irritation, give it a trial for at least a week to see if it's effective and goes on suiting you – and, importantly, feels nice. If it does, consider investing in a larger size that will last at least a month so that you can see what happens during your cycle (if you haven't reached menopause). Everything in your body renews itself constantly, even your skeleton, though that takes about two years; your skin turnover starts at about four weeks – one cycle – then speeds up to about three weeks as you get older.

Many people don't think of trying facial oils but they are wonderful for older skin, both face and body. British beauty guru Barbara Daly advises simply putting sweet almond oil straight on your skin before bed if it's particularly dry. You can also cleanse your face at night with oil, and particularly around your eyes. Do the touch test on your face every day to monitor your skin's condition: touch your skin with your fingertips and see how it feels; get used to its different moods and you'll be able to top up the moisture level if you need to. (Michael, who wishes to point out that he has read all this chapter and nearly understood it, also suggests lifting the skin on the back of your hand to see how lax or toned it is and how much hand/body lotion you need to put on.)

You can make your own rejuvenating facial oils by adding essential oils to natural base oils (try Neal's Yard Remedies for supplies). Sarah's website www.beautybible.com, which she writes with Josephine Fairley, has lots of suggestions (look in the section marked Beauty Info, then go to Face Magic). Better to do it when you're having a night at home so that it can soak in – and remember it's not a good base for make-up. Also look at the suggestions for homemade aromatherapy oils on page 202 of this book.

What products do you really need?

The key products you need are cleanser (thorough cleansing is essential night and morning), moisturiser for daytime and night cream, which may be heavier. Skip a toner – most of them contain alcohol, which will dry your skin out even more: if you like to swish your face after cleansing, use pure organic rose water (wonderful for a hot flush, incidentally). Try a rich balm-type cleanser, or pomade, which are made by companies including Eve Lom, Spiezia Organics and E'spa. A non-balm product that suits many skin types is Cleanse & Polish by Liz Earle Naturally Active Skincare, which romped in top in the consumer tests in Sarah's book *The 21st Century Beauty Bible*, co-written with Josephine Fairley. Whatever type of cleanser you like, massage it in well and always finish with a clean flannel rung out in very hot water. (Using a cotton flannel will exfoliate your skin thoroughly without the need for extra products; rub iffy areas like sides of face, nose and chin fairly vigorously.) When your neck and face are dry, stroke on face cream or oil using an upward movement – the warm skin will be very receptive. Don't forget to apply lip balm daily too; you can use the same product on your cuticles (toenails too) for double-duty beauty.

There's a vast number of products nowadays for different bits of you: from eye and neck creams to bust enhancers and cellulite reducers. None is strictly necessary (though some work very well) but an eye gel will help keep the fragile skin moisturised without dragging it down as some creams do. (Tap it on to the bone of the socket and it will find its own way nearer the eye.)

Sun protection products are essential to avoid the risk of looking like a prune. Always apply SPF 15 liberally every two hours if you're in the sun, or even out in the street in the summer. Never ever toast your face, neck or décolletage: use fake tan instead. Protect your eyes with big wrap-around sunglasses. Top it off with a big-brimmed, densely woven hat. (And remember to drink lots of water.)

Have regular salon facials or create your own spa at home and give yourself a facial. Evenings are best, or a weekend when you're not going out. Cleanse your face, then steam over very hot but not boiling water – add essential oils if you like. Put on a skin-nourishing mask and relax with eye pads or lightly squeezed-out, cooled camomile teabags on your eyes. Remove the mask and stroke on your regular night cream.

There are lots of good masks on the market. Again look for products for dry older skin. The B. Kamins Chemist range from Canada includes a 'diatomamus earth masque' (which sounds prehistoric but is amazing), which is designed specifically for menopausal skins and has an extraordinary plumping effect if left on for some time. (It's not cheap but does last for ages.)

For a quick fix, try skin-brightening masks, which can be whisked on and off in a few minutes. Tried and tested favourites include Sisley Express Flower Gel Mask, Laveré's organic Special Effect Anti-Ageing-Energy Gel-Mask and Liz Earle's Brightening Treatment.

If you want to tone up the skin on your body, the cheapest and most effective method is dry skin brushing. Before you have a bath, use a dry brush (available from the Body Shop and other stores) in long sweeping strokes all over your body from your feet, working towards the heart. You soon get used to the slight 'ouch' factor and get to love the tingle of health as everything gets moving. Dry skin brushing has a fantastic effect on cellulite and those funny little goose pimples, which gather on thighs and upper arms. Purists suggest alternating hot and cold showers after, finishing with a chilly one.

Always slather on body lotion everywhere when you've had a bath or shower. Feet need special daily attention: use extra rich products (such as Burt's Bees Coconut Foot Crème with Vitamin E or Liz Earle's Superbalm) and buff regularly with a foot file to smooth rough hard skin. Book regular sessions with a qualified chiropodist/podiatrist, every month if your feet are in a bad way (with lots of dry skin, corns or worse), quarterly or six-monthly when they're back in shape.

Many women have flaking nails, particularly around this time. Moisturing helps hugely: aim to put on hand cream every time you wash your hands – keep a tube by every basin. But what really makes a difference is oiling your nails. Massage Dr Hanschka's Neem Nail Oil or evening primrose oil into the cuticles and nails; Liz Earle's Superbalm also works well. Spiezia Organic's new hand treatment is brilliant for nails too. Protect them with a clear fortifying varnish such as Protein Pro-Growth Hydrating Treatment by Jessica. Some women also swear by the Nailtiques programme.

Once your nails are in good condition, keep them short and well shaped. If you like natural-looking nails, a French manicure with translucent pink nails and white tips always looks elegant. For something more emphatic, try a dark red or plum which will make your hands look longer and flatter the skin.

DAILY BASICS FOR PRETTY, HAPPY FEET

* use a foot file to remove hard skin every day, before bath or shower
* cream your feet afterwards – this is the most effective way to prevent a build-up of tough skin

> * while you're applying cream, twiddle the toes and massage feet and legs.

MAKE-UP

Basic make-up bag

* foundation
* lipstick/lip pencil
* blusher
* lashcurler
* mascara
* eyeliner
* eyebrow pencil
* foundation primer/wrinkle fillers
* loose powder
* concealer

As women age, the colour and vibrancy of the skin tend to dim. So a little make-up can make all the difference between looking well or several degrees under. That doesn't mean hours every morning and evening applying heaps of products: it could just be a sweep of tinted moisturiser and a stroke of triple-duty colour on cheeks, lips and to warm up the lower brow bone. (Make-up artists swoosh blusher over all the bits that stick out, plus neck and bosom.) As supermodel Lauren Hutton, now in her 60s and as alluring as ever, told Sarah: 'Less is much more with make-up as you get older.'

Aim to stock your make-up bag with a few well-chosen items that will lift your whole look – and your day. Below you will find suggestions from leading London-based make-up artist Jenny Jordan who has given us her top tips for the basics, with some of her favourite products and brands.

Before you set off to the make-up counter, it will help

you greatly to know whether your basic palette is warm or
cool. Jenny Jordan has two satin gowns, one in pale butter-
scotch, the other sugar-almond pink. Substitute any scarf,
blouse or length of material in those colours – curtains or
cushion covers are handy too. If you can't find a caramel
colour, substitute an orangey red. Invariably either the pink
tone or the yellow tone will really lift your face, skin and
hair, while the other will make you look a little peaky, less
vibrant, even unwell. Keep them with you while you're
trying out make-up and look for the same tones.

With textures and colours, avoid harsh, dense, matte, over-
glossy and over-pearly: the keywords are soft, natural,
translucent, sheer, shine, shimmer. The wonderful thing is
that modern technology can deliver a marvellous choice of
these nowadays in all prices and colours to suit everyone.
When you're applying any kind of make-up from foundation to eye-shadow, go for small amounts which you can
build up layer by thin layer, rather than sloshing on lots and
having to wipe them off.

MAKING UP FOR HOT FLUSHES

A few tips for women who suffer hot flushes combined
with sweats (hot flushes on their own don't seem to
slough off the make-up):

* opt for fake tan or tinted moisturiser rather than
  foundation – it won't slip off.
* use clear gel blusher, not powder.
* use waterproof mascara and eyeshadow.
* hot sweats don't seem to touch your lippie so invest
  in your favourite brands of lipstick and lipliner: well
  applied, it will lift your face.
* keep facial blotters with you at all times.

Foundation

Foundation – aka base – used to mean a mask-like finish, which was hugely unflattering to older skin. Nowadays you can buy light filmy products that glide over your skin, evening out the texture, disguising tiny flaws and blemishes. Always let your moisturiser settle for at least ten minutes before applying foundation, or it will disappear quicker than you can say hot flush. Alternatively, if you like a sunkissed look you can wear tinted moisturiser; some brands offer a little coverage (try YSL, Dior or Clarins) or make your own by mixing a dab of foundation with your moisturiser. Always test foundation in natural daylight, by applying a stripe down your cheek to the jawline; the one that matches your natural colour is the winner. Apply lightly from the centre of your face out with a damp make-up sponge (do keep very clean), a brush or fingertips – built up gradually, you often need much less than you think.

Favourite Brands
Lancôme Adaptive

Nina Ricci Contouring Complexion Fluid: Luminous Smoothing Foundation SPF 15

Chantecaille Future Skin

For building up to conceal thread veins, try Lancôme Teint Idole Hydra Compact

Day lipstick and matching pencil

To brighten your face in ten seconds, stroke a soft natural-coloured lippie on mouth and cheeks for instant glow. Pinky-brown shades do the trick for pretty well everyone. Look for a silky finish that tends to sheer rather than matte, which is too dense for older skin. Also avoid too glossy and too pearly tones, although a little bit of iridescence or shimmer is flattering, especially for evenings. To take you out straight from work, simply add a little gloss over your day lipstick. If your lips are dry, prep them with lip balm and leave for 10 to 20 minutes to sink in.

Favourite Brands
Estée Lauder Pure Nude Shimmer
Origins Matte Stick in Berry and Cider Apple (these are lovely chubby pencils so you don't need a lipliner; though they're called Matte the texture isn't dense or dull)
Yves St Laurent No 10
Aveda Brilliant Lip Shine

If you like all-natural lippies (because we do swallow a lot of lipstick during our lifetime), look for Jurlique, Dr Hauschka, Annemarie Börlind and Aveda.

Blusher

Look for a soft natural-coloured blusher that you can touch up easily during the day. If you wear foundation, brush on a silky powder blusher; set with translucent powder for the evening. If you put over tinted moisturiser or bare skin, use fingers or sponge to apply cream or gel blush. (Jenny likes to swish cream blushers on with a foundation brush and then blend with fingers or sponge.) Always apply to apple of cheek – you can find them by smiling ... the apples will beam at you.

Favourite Brands
Clinique's Blushwear
Bobbi Brown Cream Blush Stick
Jane Ireland Mineral Cosmetics Complete Colour in Cedar Rose

Lancôme Blush Focus
Lilian by Stila Convertible Colour for cheek and lips

Lashcurler

A quick couple of seconds' pinch on upper eyelashes gives a fresh look; you don't want a folded-up, Barbie doll gaze.

Favourite Brands
Space NK
Benefit
Eyecurl Heated Eyelash Curler

Mascara

Brush mascara on to top lashes and corners of lower ones for a subtle look. Avoid black, dark brown and blue. Aubergine looks wonderful on all hair colours, and makes the whites of eyes sparkle. If your eyelashes seem to be moulting, go for a lash-lengthening effect.

Favourite Brands
Lancôme Flextencils Full Extension and Curving Mascara in Purple (there's also a gorgeous Violet)
Dior Mascara Fascination
Nina Ricci Extension Lashwear 04 Violine Couture
Estée Lauder Magnascopic

Liquid eyeliner

Forget any notion of hard black lines à la Twiggy in the 1960s. We're talking smudgy soft in a dusky metallic heather or bronzy-brown, which suits all eye colours. Trace along the roots, use a cotton bud to take off any wandering splodges, then smudge with a brush.

Favourite Brands

Clinique's liquid liner in Iced Plum, which has a rubber tip applicator and built-in brush

Pop Lash & Line Deep including dark brown mascara and brown eyeliner

Eye shadow

Go for mid-tone, skin-flattering shades such as greeny, sage, grey, silvery, golden, browns in creamy stick formulations. Opt for creamy matte sticks rather than powder and never go glinty – it shows up all the lines and creases. You want to make pale skin look clear and bright, and play up a tan – sagey goldy colours are great for that. (And you don't need to be told that blue eyeshadow is a big Non ...)

Favourite Brands

Origins Single Colour sticks

Dior 5-way compact (powder but non-drying formula)

Eyebrow mousse and brow pencil

Have your brows professionally shaped if possible (or follow guidelines in *The 21st Century Beauty Bible*, or on line at www.beautybible.com). Tweezerman professional Slant Tweezers are the best. Remember you're aiming to remove stragglers between and under your brows – not to look like Bette Davis. Then pencil in the shape with little light strokes, simulating hairs; follow with a tad of mousse to keep the groomed look, pushing the brush right up through the hairs and dabbing down any little spiky ones.

Favourite Brands

Shu Uemura Seal Brown for light to mid brownettes

Virgin Vie Walnut Whip for darker hair and skin
Estée Lauder 04 blonde, a silky greige for blondes and
  redheads
Tweezerman clear mousse (non flaky/crispy) and slant-edged
  tweezers

Foundation primers and wrinkle fillers

A relative newcomer to the cosmetic arena, primers are best
friends for all make-up pros. They give a marvellous velvety
base for foundation (so skin looks softer and dewier), cover
blemishes and last longer.

Favourite Brands
Nina Ricci Contouring Fluid SPF15
Instant Lift Radiance
Estée Lauder Idealist (formulated to also help problems like
  thread veins)

Another amazing advance from the beauty boffins is
wrinkle-filling and/or diffusing products. These either fill the
crevices like cosmetic cement, or deliver moisturising, light-
diffusing ingredients that make lines and wrinkles look softer
and dewier. You usually paint them on (try an eyeliner
brush) over moisturiser, then set with foundation and/or
powder.

Favourite Brands
Nina Ricci Beauty Flash Enhancer
Prescriptives Magic Invisible Line Smoother
Trish McEvoy's Refiner

Powder

To powder or not to powder is usually a lifestyle decision. Most women just keep it for evenings, to ensure a long-lasting finish. But if you have a hectic professional life, there is no doubt that a light dusting of powder will 'set' your make-up so that it lasts from dawn to dusk. Drift it on in the morning with a big brush, then touch up if necessary during the day and to take you into the evening.

Favourite Brands
Space NK Perfecting Powder loose
Chanel Natural Finish Loose Powder
Nars Loose Powder

CONCEALER

If you don't like wearing much make-up, do consider tiny dabs of concealer where you need it. It helps to minimise the need for foundation and gives a lovely canvas for blusher and other products if you choose. Yves St Laurent's cult concealer Touche Eclat Radiant Touch has a place in virtually every celebrity and make-up artist's kitbag for good reason. Light-reflective technology means that it can be dabbed along fine lines, blemishes and dark circles to make them virtually disappear. Experts recommend dotting over foundation for the best result. Touche Eclat romped home top with 9.33 marks out of 10 in consumer surveys for *The 21st Century Beauty Bible*. Testers' comments included: 'Brilliant, especially for frown line and nose-to-mouth lines'; 'Covered dark circles under eyes that nothing else has been able to do – truly a miracle'. Also try Laura

---

Mercier Secret Camouflage and, for more serious camouflage, Estée Lauder Maximum Cover (for thread
veins and some birthmarks), Dermablend (for birthmarks, scars and port wine stains) and Jane Iredale
Circle/Delete (this waterproof range is much favoured
by cosmetic surgeons after facelifts and laser treatment).

We hope you will find all these products on the market, but
beauty products change all the time. To keep up to date, try
logging on to www.beautybible.com

12

CONTRACEPTION AND FERTILITY

This chapter covers:
* contraception and the menopause: how long do you need to use it
* your choices in detail
* fertility: late babies
* the risk of Down's Syndrome: tests for Down's
* if you find yourself pregnant unexpectedly
* if you want a baby but can't conceive
* natural help for women and men
* going to a fertility specialist: investigation, tests, assisted conception

In this chapter, we look at you and babies – after all, that's what your biology geared you to do. The point is that although the menopause is all about stopping having babies, women do get pregnant. Sometimes it happens on purpose, sometimes not. In Michael's clinics, two of the biggest questions from 40-plus women are about contraception on the one hand and fertility on the other.

At the beginning of the twenty-first century, we're at an extraordinary stage in evolution. Over the last few decades, the whole trend of parenthood – over millennia – has changed.

Some things have changed very little: the length of your reproductive life is nearly the same as your great-grandmother's, and even as a woman a thousand years ago. And just as then, the peak time for fertility is in your teens; after that it starts declining. What is changing – and rapidly – is the age at which we have children. In the 1970s, the average age of a new mother was 26. Now, it's 30 and climbing rapidly. And the number of new mothers giving birth over the age of 35 doubled in a single decade – the nineties. (Makes you think the Naughty Nineties wasn't necessarily the 1890s ...)

There's more on that in the fertility section of this chapter, starting on page 386. To start with we'll look at contraception and your choices.

CONTRACEPTION AROUND THE MENOPAUSE

Deciding how long you need to use contraception around the menopause is always tricky because of the difficulty of knowing when you have had your last natural period and also your last ovulation (when an egg is released). As you know, this may or may not be the same date.

Remember, ovulation is crucial for pregnancy: no egg, no baby. Then there's the other essential – sperm! Sexual activity usually declines as you get older and married couples in their 40s make love half as often as married couples in their 20s (maybe that's young lust as well as love ...). Sometimes, however, sexual activity increases, usually because women find a new partner or have more free time (as teenagers leave home, for instance).

WHAT ARE YOUR CHANCES OF GETTING PREGNANT?

Dr Gillian Lockwood, Medical Director of the UK Midland Fertility Services, writes: 'Young couples with normal fertility (and trying quite hard) only have a 25 to 30 per cent chance of getting pregnant with each monthly cycle. When a woman gets to mid 30s, the likelihood drops to 10 to 15 per cent per month. By her early 40s, it's less than five per cent a month and she faces a 40 per cent chance of miscarriage if she does get pregnant.'

Don't forget!

- **You can still get pregnant around the menopause**
- **HRT is not a contraceptive: discuss your likely fertility and contraception needs with your doctor**

As women get older, the number of menstrual cycles that produce an egg decreases. But because the egg is released before your period there are often no signs (see page 33, on menstrual cycle). Without doing elaborate daily tests, therefore, we don't know which cycles do produce an egg and which don't. The big difference seems to be between regular and irregular cycles. One study found that ovulation occurred every cycle in 45-year-old women with regular menstrual patterns but women with irregular periods did not produce eggs in up to one-third of cycles. However, you could have irregular periods, not ovulate for 18 months, and then – abracadabra! – suddenly produce an egg. So it's possible that you could produce an egg at your very last cycle.

Your eggs were formed before you were born and stored

in your ovaries, so they age with you. (Men's sperm, on the other hand, are replenished about every 90 days.) As you get older, the quality of your eggs diminishes and they have a decreasing ability to be fertilised. This means that conception is less likely to happen. Even if an egg is fertilised by the sperm, the likelihood of it implanting safely in the womb is much lower in older women. (Implantation is when the fertilised egg, also known as the embryo or pre-embryo, buries itself in the lining of the womb.) For women between the ages of 25 and 29, the implantation rate is 18.2 per cent of fertilised eggs. This means that, at the time of peak fertility, fewer than one in five embryos actually stick to the womb. By the time you reach 40 to 44 the implantation rate goes down to 6.1 per cent, or about one in 18.

The conception rate per single act of intercourse is another thing altogether and very difficult to estimate. The best guess is that it's around one in 40 for women in their mid 20s and one in 250 by 41 years old. Interestingly, this is completely different from other animals where the conception rate is about 75 per cent per single act of intercourse.

Additionally, if older eggs are fertilised, there is an increased risk of congenital abnormality and an increasing risk of miscarriage. About one in three women over 40 are likely to miscarry – this is linked to congenital abnormalities in the baby – and that risk increases. Aged 40, the mother's risk of having a baby with Down's Syndrome is one in 109 babies, which increases to one in 32 at age 45.

The overall message is that though the likelihood of pregnancy is much lower, it's not safe to assume you won't get pregnant. So it's important to use adequate contraception unless, of course, you are happy to have a baby.

Contraceptive options

This guide covers important issues of contraception that are specific for the stage of life around the menopause. But it's not a comprehensive guide to family planning and we recommend you discuss your individual situation with your doctor or gynaecologist.

QUICK GUIDE

For perimenopausal women wishing to avoid pregnancy, there is a simple guideline. If you have your last natural period *after* your 50th birthday, you should take precautions for one year. If you have had your last natural period *before* your 50th birthday, you need contraception for two years. (You can see the value of noting your periods in your diary.)

All artificial forms of contraception are based on disrupting nature. In order to conceive, you need three things: an egg, a sperm and then the two to get together. Whatever contraceptive you choose will aim at preventing one or more of these factors occurring: that is stopping ovulation (the release of an egg), stopping sperm or stopping egg and sperm meeting.

When it comes to deciding on contraception you may wish to talk to your partner first and discuss the question areas below. If you don't have a regular partner, you will probably go straight to your health professional. You need to have a frank discussion about which contraceptive is most suitable for you and your situation. Obviously, if you want to use condoms alone, you may not need to consult your doctor. (Also don't forget that if you have what's called 'casual' sex, you run the risk of infections and pelvic inflammatory disease so it is always sensible to ensure your partner uses a condom.)

The main question areas that you need to talk through with your doctor include the following:

- **Your need for contraception versus any risks**

  - how often do you have sex?
  - what sort of sexual relationship do you have – i.e. is it a stable relationship where your partner will collaborate with contraception, or a casual relationship/s where you may need to consider the risk of sexually transmitted diseases?
  - what would happen if you did get pregnant – would you continue with the pregnancy or consider a termination?

- **Your general health**

  - certain forms of contraception may not be advisable if you have particular health problems or risks such as diabetes, high blood pressure or previous blood clots.

- **Your personal preferences**

  - do you want to be in control rather than leaving it to the man?
  - do you want contraception to be independent of intercourse so you need not worry about it at the time? Or do you not mind?
  - do you want contraception to be non-medical?
  - do you have any cultural or religious factors that need to be considered?

○ do you want contraception to be reversible (i.e. not sterilisation)?

We have listed possible disadvantages and/or risks with each category of contraception below, but remember these are only *possible* and may not affect you at all. Every drug has risks and side effects – usually temporary – but these need to be put into context. There has been a lot of publicity about the risks of the contraceptive Pill and it is certainly not without potential problems. But as you can see from this chart, life is a dangerous business ... and the Pill comes way down.

Risks of dying from various activities

(John Guillebaud, *Contraception: Your Questions Answered* (3rd edition), Churchill Livingstone)

Activity	Deaths per 100,000
Cigarette smoking	167
Hang gliding	150
Scuba diving	22
Road accidents	8
Having a baby (UK/USA)	6
Playing football	4
Accident at home	3
Blood clot on COC (combined oral contraceptive)	0.5
Blood clot not on COC	0.1

METHODS OF CONTRACEPTION

Barrier methods (condoms and caps)

Barrier methods refer to the male condom or sheath and the female cap or diaphragm. The principle behind these methods dates back to Roman times where animal bladders were used not for contraception but to prevent sexually transmitted diseases. Female barrier methods are very ancient with descriptions dating back 1850 BC when crocodile dung was the material of choice ...

How they work

Both condoms and caps work by preventing the sperm entering the uterus and meeting the egg. Today, spermicide (chemical that is toxic to sperm) is also used to help kill sperm. A lot of condoms and caps come with spermicide already placed on the outside or inside.

Barrier methods for both men and women (male sheaths and vaginal sponges containing spermicide) can be bought over the counter or, in the UK, obtained free from Family Planning Clinics. Initially, caps and diaphragms need to be fitted by an expert so you should see a health professional who will be able to give you the correct size and also show you how to fit it for future use.

Female condoms, which are made from polyurethane and line the vagina, need to be inserted prior to intercourse. The downside is that they can be very prominent during foreplay and some women complain of a crackling noise during lovemaking. Not surprisingly, only about half the women who have tried this method find it acceptable.

What do I need to do?

The condom/sheath is put on (by the man or the woman) during intercourse when the penis is erect. The cap/diaphragm needs to be inserted before sex and needs to remain in place for six hours after sex before removal. Initially, the cap/diaphragm needs to be fitted by a trained practitioner (see above).

Effectiveness

In women over 35, the condom and cap have a pregnancy rate of about 2.8/100 women years (that is, 2.8 women in 100 get pregnant over one year using barrier contraception). However, as fertility declines with age, effectiveness improves and by the time you are perimenopausal, the barrier method is as good as most other contraceptives.

Advantages

Condom
* cheap, effective and easily available
* no major medical risks apart from potential latex allergy
* protection against sexually transmitted diseases
* avoids hormones

Cap
* effective (but must be fitted initially by an appropriately trained family planning practitioner or your GP)
* no major medical risks apart from potential latex allergy
* protection against sexually transmitted diseases
* avoids hormones

Disadvantages/Risks

Condom
- may trigger allergy to latex
- may burst
- needs motivation
- decreased spontaneity – putting on interrupts lovemaking

Cap
- may trigger allergy to latex
- needs practice
- decreased spontaneity – needs forward planning before lovemaking
- can be messy

Is It Suitable For Me?

As long as you are aware of the limitations, barrier methods can be useful for older women.

How Long Can I Use It For?

No time limit.

Combined oral contraceptive (COC)

The combined oral contraceptive (COC), launched in the USA in 1960 and in the UK in 1961, is now the most widely used method of reversible contraception. In the past, medical advice was that women should stop taking the COC after the age of 35 years. This is no longer the case unless you smoke, in which case you should stop taking it at 35. Age alone is not a contraindication. If you are healthy, do not smoke nor get migraine then it is reasonable to take the

COC until 50. In 1996, the World Health Organisation stated that the advantages generally outweigh any theoretical or proven risks. However, you should think it through carefully and make sure you have regular consultations with your health professional to review your contraceptive needs and your general health, and survey other options. If you are aged 45 or older and not already on the COC, it might not be the most appropriate choice in the light of diminishing fertility.

How It Works

The COC consists of a mixture of oestrogen (usually ethinyloestradiol) and progestogen (synthetic progesterone). Since it was introduced, the doses of hormones used have been gradually reduced in order to decrease the short- and long-term side effects. (The progestogen-only pill (POP), see below, contains no oestrogen and an even lower dose of progestogen.)

The COC works in several ways. The main action is to stop ovulation (meaning that no egg is released). Additionally, the lack of ovulation means that the ovary does not produce hormones so the lining of the womb (endometrium) does not grow in the usual way, meaning that in the unlikely event that an egg was released and subsequently fertilised, it would not implant. The COC also affects the cervical mucus making it less penetrable to any sperm that reaches it.

What Do I Need To Do?

The COC is usually taken for 21 days followed by a break of seven pill-free days during which a withdrawal bleed (period) is likely. Different products do have different regimes, however, so it's vital to check this with your doctor. It's very important not to forget to take a pill as this will reduce the efficacy.

What To Do If You Miss A Pill

If you are less than 12 hours late taking a pill, don't worry. Just take the delayed pill now, and further pills as usual. That's all.

If you are more than 12 hours late, do the following: take the most recently missed pill now; leave any earlier missed pills in the pack; take your further pills as usual; use extra precautions (e.g. barrier method) for the next seven days. Count up how many pills are left in the pack after the most recently missed pill. If there are seven or more, use extra precautions as above, and when you have finished the pack, leave the usual seven-day break before starting the next pack. If there are fewer than seven pills, use extra precautions for seven days, then when you finish the pack start the next pack immediately without a break. When you get to the end of that, take the seven-day break and if you don't have a withdrawal bleed, see your doctor immediately before starting the next pack to exclude the possibility of pregnancy.

Effectiveness

It's very effective but, like everything, there are always failures. Of 1,000 women across all ages using it for one year, between one and three will get pregnant. Failure is often due to poor compliance – forgetting to take a pill. Research shows that effectiveness does increase as you get older, due mainly to declining fertility and also reduction in the frequency of intercourse.

Advantages

The COC is:

* effective and reliable
* convenient
* non-intercourse related
* reversible

Other positive effects:

* menstrual cycle advantages including:

  - less bleeding
  - less pain with periods
  - reduction of PMS
  - no ovulation pain
  - regular bleeding that can be timed for social convenience by stopping the Pill for a bleed when it suits you.

* the menstrual benefits may help avoid a hysterectomy.
* reduction in ovarian cysts and benign breast disease, plus reduction in risk of endometrial, colorectal and ovarian cancer, also in risk of symptoms of endometriosis.
* reduced risk of pelvic inflammatory disease.
* some protection against osteoporosis: long-term COC users appear to reach the menopause with a bone density two to three per cent higher than non-users but whether this reduces the risk of fracture later on is unknown.
* can improve acne and excessive hair growth if associated with polycystic ovaries.
* reduced risk of benign (i.e. non cancerous) breast disease.

Disadvantages/Risks

Many side effects are temporary (e.g. nausea) and go with time. The risks can be reduced if you and your health professional decide the COC is appropriate for you, having carefully considered your medical and family history.

* may cause weight gain
* possible minor side effects, such as headache, nausea, decreased libido, leg cramps
* increased risk of disorders of blood vessels, especially if you smoke

These include:

○ heart attack
○ stroke
○ high blood pressure
○ clots in veins

BLOOD CLOTS

Venous thromboembolism (VTE) is a condition where a blood clot develops in one of your veins, usually the legs. (You may find it then called a Deep Vein Thrombosis, or DVT. A clot in your lungs is called a pulmonary embolism, or PE.) Women who take the COC are at greater risk of a VTE, especially in the first year of use, which in very rare cases can be fatal.

The risk is smaller than that associated with pregnancy.

General risk in healthy, non-pregnant women of child-bearing age, not taking the oral contraceptive: 5/100,000 women per year:

Risk on COC: 15/100,000 women per year
Risk during pregnancy: 60/100,000 women per year

DVT can also be caused by sitting still for a long time as in air travel. Passengers who don't move around risk so-called Economy Class Syndrome. When you travel, it's essential to move around, do leg exercises and drink lots of water.

- liver disease: the COC increases the risk of:

  - gallstones
  - benign liver tumour hepatic cellular cancer of the liver } both very rare

- small increase in breast cancer risk with prolonged use. The risk goes after you have stopped taking the COC for ten years
- cervical cancer may also be increased with long-term use of the COC but because the causes of this disease are so various (including sexual history) it's not currently possible to be certain. Whatever contraception you are using, please have regular smears (see page 58).

Additionally

- masking the menopause – because you still bleed with the COC, you won't know when you have your last period. Many doctors, including Michael, will advise you to try to avoid taking the COC over 50 years of age as you have a 50 per cent chance of having had your last period. Discuss this with your doctor.
- but if you are 50 or over and still on the Pill, this is what you should do to find out what stage you are at:

○ Take the combined Pill as usual for three weeks.
○ At the end of the following Pill-free week, have a blood test for FSH levels.
○ If these are normal, you will still need to use contraception of some sort (not necessarily the COC because you may not need such a 'strong' contraceptive when the chance of conception is low).
○ If you have a high FSH level, use a barrier method of contraception (see below). Six to eight weeks later, have another FSH test. If this is high, and you have had no natural period, and possibly symptoms such as hot flushes, continue using barrier contraception for 12 months.

Is It Suitable For Me?

Discuss this with your doctor. Your full medical history should be taken into account before starting to take the COC, and should be reassessed on a continuing basis. However there are several absolute contraindications to the COC. These include:

● risk factors for blood clots:

If you have one of the following risk factors for clots it is essential that you discuss it further with your doctor:

○ personal history of blood clot.
○ first-degree family history (parent or sibling) of clots especially if the relative was under 45 and/or if you have any known clotting disorder.
○ overweight/obesity: be cautious if your BMI is greater than 30, and avoid if it's 39 (see page 62 to calculate).
○ long-term immobility.
○ varicose veins.

- transient ischaemic attacks (similar to minor stroke but normal function returns quickly).
- liver disease.
- high blood pressure.
- high blood lipid levels.
- undiagnosed vaginal bleeding.
- smoking (smokers should not take the COC after 35).
- pregnancy.
- migraine, especially with an aura or long-lasting.
- diabetes mellitus.

BE CAREFUL

Reasons to stop taking the Pill (or HRT) immediately
If you experience any of the following symptoms, stop taking the Pill (and HRT) immediately and go to your doctor for investigations. If these prove negative, you can re-start.

- sudden severe chest pain (medical advice is always to dial emergency services and go to hospital immediately)
- sudden breathlessness
- unexplained severe pain in calf
- severe stomach pain
- unusual headache
- loss of vision, hearing or ability to speak
- jaundice
- severe depression
- high blood pressure

How Long Can I Use It For?

See above. If you are healthy, a non-smoker and have no other contraindications, you can take the COC until the menopause. However, we recommend that from the age of 45 you consider if you really want to stay on a strong drug, or would consider an alternative.

Combined contraceptive patch

In 2002, a sticky patch was developed containing the same combined contraceptive as the COC so the advantages and disadvantages are similar – except that a patch is simpler to use. It's often difficult to remember to take a pill. In fact, one study found that almost half of oral contraceptive users missed one or more pills per cycle, leading to the risk of pregnancy. With the patch all you need do is remember to replace it once a week and that has proved much easier and equally as effective as the COC. After three patches (three weeks in all), you have a patch-free week during which you have a bleed. However, as with the COC, the contraceptive effectiveness may be reduced if you weigh more than 90 kg so you need to discuss this with your health professional. Since it is a new product, more research is being carried out to see how well it performs.

Progestogen-only pill (POP/mini pill)

What It Is

The POP contains a very small dose of progestogen. The first POP was introduced in 1969 then withdrawn because it was believed there might be an increase in breast cancer but this is now not believed to be true. The POP is much less popular than the COC, however it has a definite role to play in the years around the menopause and its use should be considered.

Oral (pill or tablet form) progestogen-only preparations may be a suitable alternative contraception when oestrogens are contraindicated. This includes women who have had a venous thrombosis. Overall, the POP does have a higher failure rate than the COC but as you get older – with decreasing natural fertility – the difference may not be that great.

Despite its name, the progestogen content in the POP is actually lower than in the COC. For instance, a typical dose of progestogen in the norethisterone version of the POP is 350 micrograms, compared with 500–1,000 micrograms in the COC; in levonogestrel, it goes down to 30 micrograms in the POP, compared with 150–250 micrograms in the COC.

A different form of synthetic progesterone called desogestrel is now being used in some of the POP products. Desogestrel appears to increase the effectiveness making it comparable to the COC.

How It Works

The POP has an effect on cervical mucus, making it less penetrable to sperm and thus not allowing the sperm to meet the egg. The POP also affects ovulation, decreasing and sometimes stopping it. The main contraceptive effect of desogestrel is to block ovulation.

In most women on the POP, there is a reduction in the number of times you ovulate by about 60 per cent and this percentage increases in older women. Additionally, it reduces the ability of the endometrium to allow any early pregnancy to implant.

What Do I Need To Do?

One tablet is taken daily on a continuous basis, at the same time each day. The timing is very important because a delay of more than three hours may affect the contraceptive effectiveness.

If you miss a pill, the advice is that you take it as soon as you remember and carry on with the next pill at the right time. If the Pill was more than three hours overdue you are not protected. Continue taking subsequent pills as usual but remember that you must also use other contraceptive methods such as a condom for the next seven days.

Effectiveness

The reliability of the POP is dependent on taking it at the same time each day and there is no doubt that the POP has a higher failure rate compared to the COC, although this is less significant in older women, due to decreasing natural fertility.

The quoted failure rate shows that if 100 women use it for a year, between 3 and 4 of all ages will get pregnant. Effectiveness is much better in older women, with some statistics showing the failure rate at 0.3 per 100 women over a year.

There is some evidence of an increased failure rate in women who are overweight. This may be due to the fact that the dose is near the minimum for the drug to be effective and heavier women may need a higher dose. Many doctors advise taking a double dose if you weigh over 70 kg (11 stone) but this may not be necessary for over-45s. Do discuss this with your doctor.

Advantages

- effective, especially in over-35s
- convenient
- non-intercourse related
- can be used in situations where the COC can't be, such as:

  - cancer of the breast or womb
  - history of, or risk of, clots in the veins
  - smokers
  - high blood pressure
  - valvular heart disease
  - diabetes
  - migraine

- fewer minor side effects, such as headache, nausea, decreasing libido, compared with the COC
- reversible on stopping
- may help with difficult menstrual cycle, sometimes stopping periods altogether

Disadvantages/Risks

- less effective than the COC overall but probably as good as women get older and fertility decreases.
- needs to be taken at same time each day: window for forgetting is less than three hours – additional contraception is required if you take it more than three hours late.
- may be less effective in women with higher body weight (over 70 kg/11 stone); this should be discussed with your doctor but since older women are less fertile, it may not be as important.

- may affect menstrual pattern, e.g.:

  - no periods
  - irregular periods
  - bleeding between periods

Interestingly, the more irregular periods become, the less likely is the risk of failure (irregularity indicates a greater effect on menstrual hormones).

- may cause weight gain.
- small increased risk of ovarian cysts.
- small risk (in one to five per cent of women) of headache, acne, breast pain, nausea, dry vagina, painful periods.
- if a pregnancy occurs it is more likely to be ectopic, i.e. when the fertilised egg gets stuck in the Fallopian tube. The risk of fertilisation is greater because ovulation is not always suppressed with POPs, which don't contain desorgestrel and the sperm may get through the cervical mucus; the risk of ectopic pregnancy is increased because progestogens can slow the progress of the egg through the Fallopian tube.

Is It Suitable For Me?

The POP can be used if you have had a previous thrombosis or are at higher risk of one. The higher failure rate may not apply to older women because of their reduced fertility. The POP may offer a very suitable alternative to the COC especially if the COC is contraindicated. If you feel you do not have a good memory for taking pills, the POP is not for you.

How Long Can I Use It For?

If you are well and have no contraindications to the POP, there is no reason why you can't continue to take it until you are menopausal. If you are on the POP and not having periods, you can have your FSH levels tested to see if you are menopausal. But do not forget that you still need contraception for two years after you stop bleeding if you are less than 50, and one year if you are over 50.

Injectable contraception and sub dermal (under the skin) implants

What It Is

These methods use long-acting progestogen hormones that are either injected into your muscle (and so cannot be removed) or contained in a small rod, less than 5 cm long, that is inserted under the skin (and can be removed).

There are now two types:

- **Long-acting intra-muscular injection**: the main one is Depo-Provera (medroxy progesterone acetate), which lasts about 12 weeks and then needs to be repeated.
- **Implants:** this involves a single flexible rod, which lasts for up to three years and can only be removed by a fully trained practitioner. The only brand is Implanon (etonogestrel).

The Depo-Provera intramuscular injection goes back to the 1960s. The implant was introduced in the early 1990s. These types of contraception are used by few women (less than 1 per cent on birth control in the UK) but that may be due to the fact that they are seldom offered rather than not acceptable. Most of the research studies on Implanon were on women under the age of 40, but there appears to be no reason why older women should not use it.

Because these forms of contraception have a prolonged action, it is vital that before insertion you have had full counselling and read the manufacturer's leaflet.

How They Work

Similarly to the COC and POP, they disrupt ovulation, change cervical mucus so that sperm find it more difficult to enter the uterus, and also change the womb lining so that it's less willing to receive the developing embryo.

What Do I Need To Do?

This is the easy part! Your GP or health professional will do it for you. The injection obviously can't be removed but the implant can be removed by an appropriately trained practitioner.

Effectiveness

These forms of contraceptive are effective partly because the problem of forgetting to take the tablet is removed. Research shows that if 1,000 women are on it for a year, one would get pregnant, and similar for Implanon.

Advantages

* effective – even more than the COC since no possibility of missed tablets
* no pills to remember!
* convenient

- reversible
- positive changes in bleeding pattern – although this can be variable:

  - ovulation stopped so no pain from that
  - improvement in any anaemia owing to reduced bleeding
  - reduction in painful periods (if this is a problem)
  - possible reduction in PMS

- decrease in pelvic infection
- may reduce the growth of fibroids (benign growth on the muscle of the uterus)
- may reduce endometriosis
- may reduce risk of endometrial cancer
- no effect on breast-feeding.

Disadvantages/Risks

- insertion and removal of the implant must be performed by a trained individual.
- injected hormones cannot be removed (although implants can be).
- may cause heavy irregular bleeding – 'menstrual chaos'.
- for injectables, there is a delay in return to fertility; periods may not return for up to two years (though this may be less of a problem in menopausal years). There is no delay in return to fertility for the implant once removed.
- possible decreased sex drive.
- slight increase in cases of acne.
- weight gain – all hormones can have an influence on weight; the gain is often explained as fluid retention but this is not the case and diuretics will not help. In a recent study of Implanon, slimmer women (who weighed less

than 50 kg/110 lb at the start) were slightly more likely to put on weight of at least 3 kg/7 lb.
- bloatedness – often due to the gut becoming sluggish; exercise and dietary changes can help.
- headaches.
- vaginal dryness.
- mood changes with associated depression – some women are very sensitive to hormones and this needs to be discussed before starting.
- theoretical concerns about increasing the risk of heart disease although to date this has not been confirmed.
- possible greater risk of losing bone density: there is concern that having no periods can cause low bone density which can lead to osteoporosis; the results of extensive research are somewhat conflicting but it appears that bone density may be reduced in women using Depo-Provera. Those most at risk are young women who use this method for a long time and who smoke. It may be wise to assess bone density in individual women users of Depo-Provera who are at high risk of developing osteoporosis.

Is It Suitable For Me?

This is an effective form of contraception but is not widely popular, mainly because a lot of women don't like the idea of an injection that can't be reversed, or an implant that is difficult to remove – although the most recent form of Implanon is much easier to take out. Don't rule out this form of contraception but do discuss it thoroughly with your doctor and weigh up the pros and cons. For instance, some women really don't like the unpredictable bleeding patterns, which can also mask the menopause. You need to be especially cautious about the injectable form if you are at greater risk of osteoporosis (see page 241 for questionnaire). The bottom line is that there may be a more suitable form of contraception for women over 45.

How Long Can I Use It For?

Once you have been counselled, thought through the pros and cons, try it and if it suits you consider staying on it for five years. Consider how old you will be in five years and remember that there are more suitable options for women over 45. (If, however, your BMI is greater than 35, the implant may not be as effective in the third year, so you should consider replacing it then. Discuss this with your doctor.)

After five years' use, the following questions should be discussed:

Are you getting close to the menopause?
If so, you may want to switch to another contraceptive that isn't so long-acting. Also consider that FSH levels can't be checked while Depo-Provera or Implanon are still active.

Are you getting hot flushes, night sweats, dry vagina, decreased sex drive?
These are all symptoms of decreased oestrogen and it may mean you have a low level of oestrogen in your blood so it may be best to assess your oestrogen level and consider a different contraceptive (Oestrogen levels should be above 100 pmol/l)

Do you smoke?
Smoking reduces the amount of oestrogen and increases your risk of osteoporosis and this needs to be discussed with your health professional

Do you have any other risk factors for osteoporosis? (See page 241.)

Sterilisation

Sterilisation is a permanent method of family planning and is now the most commonly used method of contraception for women in the 40 to 49-year-old age group. About 45 per cent of perimenopausal women in the UK are now sterilised, in contrast to France where the figure is around 11 per cent. Vasectomy (male sterilisation) is more popular for younger couples. Pre-operation counselling is very important for both women and men due to the permanent nature of sterilisation.

How It Works

Sterilisation involves blocking the Fallopian tubes, usually under general anaesthetic as a day case patient, via laparoscopic, or 'keyhole' surgery. Two small 1 cm cuts are made in the abdomen, one in the navel and the other in the pubic hair, so that an endoscope (narrow fibre optic tube) can be fed in to clip off the Fallopian tubes and stop sperm reaching the egg. It may be effective immediately but the cautious approach is to use another form of contraception until the next period.

What Do I Need To Do?

The big plus is that there's nothing more for you to do.

Effectiveness

It is one of the most effective methods of contraception. The failure rate is published as about one pregnancy per year in

200 women but it is much lower when you're older, about one pregnancy per year in 10,000 women. Bear in mind however that other hormonal and non-hormonal methods also get near this effectiveness in women over 45.

Advantages

* once done there's nothing else to do
* permanent
* effective
* no hormones required

Disadvantages/Risks

* initial risks of surgery: anaesthetic (applies in all operations).

  ○ possible damage to bowel, bladder and blood vessels
  ○ if a problem occurs, a larger cut may be needed to sort things out.

* bleeding problems: although heavier periods have been reported they are probably coincidental; they may be more likely to occur if the older method of burning the Fallopian tubes is used, rather than the modern method of clipping with plastic or metal clips. Also many women have often been on the COC before being sterilised and this may have masked an inherent problem with periods.
* regret at irreversibility if you then find a new relationship: you may have heard of women having it reversed but this is a major operation and the success rate is low. For this reason, men should be offered the chance of sperm storage before vasectomy. Michael sees more men who regret having had a vasectomy than women who

regret a sterilisation. IVF (in vitro fertilisation) is possible with female sterilisation but if a man has had a vasectomy, some form of sperm aspiration (extraction) is required before IVF or ICSI (intracytoplasmic sperm injection where the sperm is actually injected into the cell) – hence the advantage of having stored sperm *before the man has a vasectomy*.

- very slight increased risk of ectopic pregnancy if sterilisation fails.

Is It Suitable For Me?

If you want a permanent method which can't be reversed this may be right for you. However, you may not be a suitable candidate for the actual operation if, for instance, you are overweight, unsuitable for an anaesthetic, or have had previous abdominal surgery. All the issues need to be discussed carefully with your doctor.

Intrauterine contraception

What Is It?

There is a range of intrauterine devices (IUD), also known as intrauterine contraceptive devices (IUCD) or the coil. Basically, these are objects that are placed in the uterine cavity (not the vagina) to prevent conception.

The history of IUDs goes back for millennia. Two and a half thousand years ago, Hippocrates put objects in the uterus, in the eighteenth century, Casanova used a golden ball and – wait for it! – stones were placed in the vaginas of female camels to prevent them conceiving. Poor males!

There are many different types of intrauterine device but the two main groups are the copper-containing IUD and the hormonal Intra Uterine System (IUS), marketed as the Mirena coil, which releases a synthetic progestogen.

How It Works

Copper-containing IUD
These coils usually consist of a plastic carrier wound around with copper wire or fitted with copper bands. A newer type of copper coil, Gynaefix, has six copper beads on a thread.

The copper stops the sperm fertilising the egg. It disturbs the action of sperm, affecting its ability both to travel and to fertilise an egg. The copper may also be toxic to an egg. If fertilisation does take place (against the odds), the copper also prevents the implantation of an embryo.

Progestogen-releasing IUS (Mirena coil)
The progestogen-releasing IUS has a little reservoir of a synthetic progestogen, called levonorgestrel, on the coil, which is slowly released into the womb cavity. Although these are in some ways similar to the POP, there are very few side effects because the activity all takes place in that one area, rather than taking a tablet or pill, which affects your whole system. These products work by preventing the growth of the endometrium (womb lining), preventing the thickening of the cervical mucus and in some women stopping ovulation. Also, the actual physical presence of the IUS in the womb cavity contributes to the contraceptive action.

This is the ideal contraceptive if you have heavy and/or painful periods. However, these must be fully investigated first. If no abnormality is found, which should be treated in another way, then this coil is very suitable.

Effectiveness

The failure rate across all ages for the copper-containing IUD ranges from two pregnancies in every 1,000 women and the Mirena coil is one to two per 1,000 women. About one-third of the pregnancies that do occur are due to unrecognised expulsions, especially in the first year. After the age of 35, the failure rate is much lower and, in some expert views, this makes IUDs the method of choice for older women.

Advantages

- effective
- convenient
- not intercourse-related
- reversible
- additionally, the Mirena coil reduces menstrual blood loss by up to 90 per cent. It may also be helpful for women taking oestrogen-only HRT because the progestogen it contains may help protect against endometrial hyperplasia which can become cancer of the lining of the womb or endometrium. So this method has many advantages.
- if a woman does become pregnant, copper IUDs do not increase the risk of an ectopic pregnancy.

Disadvantages/Risks

The risks include:

- heavy and/or irregular bleeding (can occur with all types of intra-uterine conception).
- falling out (you should check regularly which you can do easily).
- displacement in womb – occasionally the coil can turn around in the uterus and may need a scan to confirm

position; if you can't feel the threads which hang from the coil coming from the cervix, it's wise to check with your doctor.

- perforation of the uterus at the time of insertion.
- pain.
- infection.

What Do I Need To Do?

You should discuss the issues fully with your health professional. If you decide to go ahead, the IUD will be inserted by your doctor or gynaecologist. It is important that the person who puts it in is appropriately trained and qualified.

Is It Suitable For Me?

This depends largely on your feelings about having something in your uterus. You should read the Advantages and Disadvantages/risks sections above carefully and discuss it thoroughly with your health professional before making a decision. Remember that if you have heavy vaginal bleeding, the progestogen-containing IUD is very useful because it can help reduce bleeding and so has made many hysterectomies unnecessary.

How Long Can I Use It For?

Because fertility declines with age, a copper IUD fitted in a woman over the age of 40 can remain in the uterus and be effective until the menopause. The Mirena IUS needs replacing every five years.

Natural Family Planning (NFP)

Enormous hormonal changes occur from one menstrual cycle to another, as we describe on page 33. These hormone changes are then reflected in body changes including those in cervical mucus and temperature. Understanding and monitoring these body changes can be used to detect when you ovulate (release an egg) so that you can calculate when you are fertile and when there is a naturally safe time to have unprotected sex.

As Toni Weschler says in her excellent book *Taking Charge of Your Fertility*, NFP can be a challenge. 'If you decide that you want to chart your cycles for birth control,' she writes 'brace yourself for quite a ride.' The advantage is that it gives you a sense of control over your seemingly unpredictable body.

To understand NFP methods you need to know a little bit about the survival times of eggs and sperm. Sperm can survive up to five days, possibly seven, from ejaculation to final ability to fertilise an egg. The potential for an egg to be fertilised is probably only about 24 hours but sometimes you may ovulate twice – that is two eggs – so 48 hours is seen as a cautious estimate. This means that, theoretically, you could become pregnant if you have had intercourse seven days before the egg is released. So the NFP method aims to monitor your body changes to detect ovulation so that you can avoid intercourse from seven days before.

If you're interested, it's worth finding a course on NFP.

Methods of Natural Family Planning

* **The Billings Method:** named after the Australian neurologist, John Billings, who was the first to describe the cervical mucus changes that occur with ovulation. Just

after your period, there is little or no mucus; the egg-white-like substance begins to be produced as you get closer to ovulation. You can do a DIY check by separating your vaginal lips and seeing whether there is any mucus at the lower opening closest to your perineum (the fork between the genitals and the anus). Use your fingers or some tissue paper (if you use paper remember to wipe from front to back to avoid spreading bacteria).

- **Temperature monitoring:** there is a small (0.5°C) rise in temperature at ovulation and this can be used to calculate safe and unsafe times to have unprotected sex. You can buy a fertility (aka ovulation) thermometer over the counter. It needs to be in degrees Fahrenheit because of the tiny changes. Temperature is taken on waking before eating, drinking or teethbrushing. Before ovulation, your temperature is typically around 97 to 97.5° F. Within a day or so of ovulation, rising progesterone levels stimulate a rise to 97.6 to 98.6° F. This increase continues for 12 to 16 days or, if you get pregnant, throughout the pregnancy.

- **Rhythm method:** this method assesses cycle lengths in order to calculate safe and unsafe times but is now virtually obsolete.

- **Symptom-thermal method:** This method combines monitoring your waking temperature and cervical mucus (the Billings Method, see above), as well as ovulation pain and other factors. Many observers think this is the most comprehensive and reliable approach.

- **Persona:** This device, which can be bought over the counter, detects hormonal changes in urine and tells the user whether it's safe to have unprotected sex. However the manufacturers report a six per cent failure rate, which is high.

Advantages

- natural, involves no drugs or artificial methods of any kind.
- free from side effects.
- may be more acceptable to certain religious and cultural groups.
- Requires motivation, planning and co-operation with partner, which can strengthen a relationship.

Disadvantages/Risks

- higher failure rate.
- may require significant amount of abstinence which can put a stress on relationship.
- more difficult if you have irregular periods, which are more common around the menopause.

Post-Coital Contraception (morning-after contraception)

This is used by the woman after intercourse and prevents or disturbs implantation of the embryo. Different folk remedies have been used over the centuries. Around 1500 BC women used wine, garlic and fennel to wash out the vagina. In the fourth century, ground cabbage blossoms were placed in the vagina. Nowadays, the urban myth is that Diet Coke can be used as a douche ... This doesn't work and might be dangerous so please don't try it! Always consult an appropriately trained and qualified health professional. Although there are various effective products available today, emergency contraception should be just that – not used as routine. The types available are:

- **Hormonal emergency contraception**: one tablet of levonorgestrel, a progestogen (synthetic progesterone) is taken as soon after unprotected intercourse as possible (up to 72 hours) and a further tablet 12 hours after that. This combination is now available over the counter in the UK and can be used by women of any age. If vomiting occurs within three hours of taking a tablet, another needs to be taken. (Vomiting happens in about one in ten women, and nausea in one in five.) Barrier forms of contraception should be used until the next period, which may be early or late. Women should always see their doctor if they have any lower abdominal pain which could suggest an ectopic pregnancy. This method is more effective at preventing pregnancy the sooner the tablets are taken after unprotected sex. If taken within 24 hours, this method is about 85 per cent effective, falling to about 65 per cent after 72 hours.

- **Intrauterine device**: inserting a copper IUD is even more effective than the hormonal tablet and can be used up to 120 hours (five days) after unprotected sex. However, there is a risk of infection and antibiotics will often be used to prevent infection.

Advantages

Post-coital emergency contraception may seem an unsatisfactory method but it does have benefits if you have been caught up in a situation beyond your control for whatever reason (overwhelming fit of lust to the head, condom breaking etc.).

- effective – if used correctly the failure rate is very low
- non-intercourse related
- relatively safe
- under your control

Disadvantages/Risks

- possible side effects include nausea and vomiting
- if the copper IUD is used, it needs to be inserted by a doctor
- doesn't protect again infection

FERTILITY

Having a baby may seem the least likely concern for women approaching the menopause but it is proving to be a big issue for many. The way we live now is leading to many couples leaving it very late to start a family. In fact, the whole trend of parenthood has changed in the last decade. Thirty years ago, the average age of new mothers was 26, now it's 30 and climbing rapidly.

Over the decade of the 1990s, the number of babies born annually to mothers over 35 in England and Wales went up to 14 per cent of all births – an eight per cent rise. And double the number of women over 40 gave birth, the percentage rising from one to two per cent. Both here and in America, the number of women having their first child after the age of 35 has seen an extraordinary 50 per cent increase in the last decade.

BABY NUMBER-CRUNCHING

The total number of live births in England and Wales in 2001 (the most recent recorded figures) was 594,634. The number of mums between 35 and 39 was 86,495 (14.54%), between 40 and 44 it was 15,499 (2.6%) and over 45 it was 761 (0.127%).

The last quarter of the twentieth century also saw huge leaps in the technology of assisted conception that enabled many childless parents to have babies by in vitro fertilisation

(IVF) or other techniques. It may seem like a rosy picture –
with headlines like 'Older parents have longed-for babies'
– but for many women over 35 having a baby can be a difficult, emotional and – if they need IVF – costly process.

In Britain and also America, about one-third of women
over 40 who want to be mothers find they are infertile. Overall,
about one in six couples have a problem conceiving but when
the woman is over 40, that goes up to three in six, which has
led to a significant rise in the number of women in their late
30s and 40s seeking infertility investigations and treatment.

HOW BABIES ARE MADE . . .

Conception is a story of transport. Sperm travels up the
vagina, along the uterine cavity and down the Fallopian
tube. The egg jumps from the ovary into the Fallopian
tube to meet the sperm. If and when they get together,
the sperm fertilises the egg and forms an embryo, which
then travels down into the womb to implant. Fascinat-
ingly, the Fallopian tube is the only tube in the body that
is designed to transport things up and down: everything
else is one way only. (If the embryo is stuck in the Fallopian tube, it's called an ectopic pregnancy.)

Is It Safe to Have a Late Baby?

Many older women ask whether there are any medical risks
to women having children at a later age. The simple answer
to this is yes and we have detailed the risks below. But before
you get too anxious, we need to emphasise that this greater
risk is small. You need to weigh up the benefits against the
risks and discuss any concerns you have with your health
professional. (Michael has no medical concerns about a

healthy 45-year-old woman trying to conceive as long as all the implications have been discussed.)

OLDEST WOMAN TO GIVE BIRTH NATURALLY

On 16th July 1969, the Birmingham Evening News reported that Mrs Johanna Due Plessis gave birth to a five lb baby girl in Johannesburg, South Africa at the age of 58. Other reports cited in Records and Curiousities in Obstetrics and Gynaecology (by ILC Ferguson and others, published by Baillieu Tindall in 1982) suggest that women may have given birth aged 62, 72 and even over 100.

OLDEST WOMAN TO GIVE BIRTH VIA IVF

Satyabhama Mahpatra from the eastern Indian state of Orissa became pregnant by IVF and had a healthy three kilogram baby boy by Caesarean section on 8 April 2003 at the age of 65, beating the previous record holder by two years.

OLDER FATHERS

The Nobel Prize winner Saul Bellow had a baby with his fifth wife Janice Freedman when he was 84. In 1996 Anthony Quinn fathered his 13th child, aged 81. Charlie Chaplin had a son at 71 and Paloma Picasso was born when her father Pablo was 78.

Risks of Late Babies

Although most late pregnancies result in healthy babies who bring great joy, it is true that a late unplanned pregnancy can carry a risk to the baby, as well as some risk for the mother. In fact, research shows that 45 per cent of women over 40 in Britain who find themselves pregnant choose to have terminations. This may not always be due to anxiety about physical risks, of course, but to social, emotional or financial concerns.

Congenital abnormality

The main risk is the increased rate of congenital abnormality, namely Down's Syndrome. For a mother of 35, the risk of a baby with Down's Syndrome is one in 365, at 38 it's one in 40, and at 45 the risk is one in 32.

What is Down's Syndrome?

Your entire physical and mental state depends on your chromosomes, the thread-like structures found in every cell in the body. Chromosomes carry genes (segments of DNA), which control the inherited characteristics of every living being. In a normal healthy individual, there are 23 pairs of chromosomes giving a total of 46. Half your chromosomes come from your mother and half from your father. The pairs are numbered 1 to 23. With Down's Syndrome, the person has three chromosomes at 21 (called trisomy 21) instead of two. This leads to the characteristic broad flat face with obliquely placed eyes, small nose and enlarged lips, accompanied by a range of mental disabilities and cardiac problems.

There are a number of screening and diagnostic tests for Down's Syndrome that can be carried out while the baby is in the womb. If the results are positive, you may wish to see a counsellor. (Before embarking on the tests, consider what you would do if the results suggest Down's.) Remember, however, that there is a big difference between screening tests, which are non-invasive and give the odds of the baby being born with Down's Syndrome, and diagnostic tests, which are invasive and give a definitive result. The diagnostic tests carry some risk of triggering miscarriage.

You can think of the difference between a screening test and a diagnostic test in terms of horse racing. Before a race is run, the bookkeepers try to predict the result; their business is to give the odds for and against any individual horse winning. That's like screening. A diagnostic test, however, is actually finding out the result.

Tests for Down's Syndrome

Screening Tests: Used to Assess Risk of Down's Syndrome

- **Nuchal translucency scan**: research shows that babies with Down's Syndrome have an increase in the thickness of the fluid-containing pad at the back of the neck, which is revealed by a nuchal translucency scan at around 12 weeks into pregnancy. This test is non-invasive, takes five to ten minutes and the results are available straight away.
- **Blood screening test**: looking at a range of compounds in blood can indicate the risk of Down's. This is usually carried out at 14 weeks. The 'double' test looks for alpha-feta protein and betaHCG. The 'triple' test looks for alpha-feta protein, betaHCG and oestriol. This test obviously requires a blood test and takes up to five days for a result.
- **Nuchal translucency scan plus blood screening test**: researchers are now combining these tests to give a clearer picture of the risk factors.

- **PAPPA test (pregnancy-associated plasma protein A) and ultra-sound markers:** researchers are now looking at the use of different blood tests and other structural changes in the baby to help screen for Down's Syndrome.

Diagnostic Tests: Invasive and Definitive
Your doctor will offer you one of these tests:

- **Chorionic Villus Sampling (CVS):** the chorionic villi are tiny fine outgrowths from the developing embryo that travel into the womb to get food. Taking a sample of these at about 12 weeks' gestation enables doctors to see the number of your baby's chromosomes and find out whether there is an abnormality of the twenty-first chromosomal pair or any other chromosome. Samples can be obtained either through the cervix of the womb by aspiration (sucking out the villi) or through the abdomen. CVS takes about ten minutes to perform; you are awake and don't need anaesthetic. The sample is then sent to the laboratory and the cells are grown and examined. The risk of losing the pregnancy because of doing this test is about one in 50. The result is available in two to five days.
- **Amniocentesis:** the developing baby is surrounded by fluid, which is called amniotic fluid. Amniocentesis involves taking a sample of this fluid, at around 16 weeks, to assess the chromosomes. This is done with a very fine needle and doesn't need anaesthetic. The risk of losing the pregnancy in this test is about one in 100–200. The result is available in 10 to 14 days.
- **Other Tests:** an ultrasound scan is offered to help exclude other abnormalities including spina bifida and heart defects. These have traditionally been 2D (two dimensional) but technological advances mean they are now 3D and 4D, which obviously gives a more accurate picture.

Other potential risk factors

Blood pressure problems

Higher than average blood pressure is often stated as a 'concern' during pregnancy (which can trigger a rise) but in fact it's normally due to the increase in blood pressure that occurs as you get older. However, even if it is the age-related effect rather than pregnancy, your blood pressure still needs to be carefully monitored. The best thing is forward planning, if possible: so if you're planning on getting pregnant have a blood pressure check first.

Overweight and obesity

The two per cent rise in overweight and obesity in older women can make a pregnancy more difficult to manage and increase the risks including clots in lung or legs.

Smoking

Women who smoke – whatever their age – risk causing the baby's growth to be retarded. Interestingly, the risk is lower with older mothers because they tend not to smoke as much.

Anaemia

Heavy periods are more common as you get older, in turn resulting in more cases of anaemia, which needs to be monitored and treated. You don't want to go into pregnancy anaemic so it's important to check iron levels before trying to get pregnant, or as soon as you know you are. You may need to take an iron supplement. If so, make certain that it's one that suits you and is well absorbed – you need plenty of vitamin C for the iron to be absorbed.

Diabetes

Like hypertension, diabetes occurs more frequently as you get older (type 2 adult onset diabetes) so you should have a check-up to exclude this.

If you find yourself pregnant unexpectedly

Surprise pregnancies do happen – if it's you we suggest the following:

- keep calm ...
- talk to partner and close friends or family who you trust.
- get to see your doctor or gynaecologist as soon as possible.
- ask yourself the following questions and discuss them with your doctor:

  - do I want to continue with the pregnancy?
  - would I consider a termination?
  - would I want tests to see if all is well?
  - what would I do if the tests revealed an abnormality? (If the answer is nothing, you must question whether you want to have the tests at all).

If you want a baby but can't conceive ...

Age undoubtedly brings a decrease in fertility. This is due to several factors:

In the woman:
- decrease in quality of eggs.
- decrease in ovulation (release of eggs) linked to menstrual irregularity leading up to the menopause.
- possible decrease in receptivity of the womb to an implanting embryo.

393

- increase in miscarriage – due to an increase in congenital abnormalities.
- decrease in sexual interest and activity.

In the man:
- decrease in androgen (male hormone) levels leading to decreased desire for sex.

and to ...

- decrease in ejaculation.
- possible decrease in sperm production and motility (movement which enables them to travel up to meet the egg).

Seeking help

As you know, conception needs three things: an egg, a sperm and the two to get together. Good general health is also crucial. In the old days, doctors used to advise women to seek help after one year of trying. But that one year could be crucial if you are in your 40s.

Ideally, we suggest you go and see a doctor the moment you decide you want a baby to ensure you are in good health, have normal blood pressure and no other problems. If you are on any medication you should discuss this with your doctor. Also get your doctor to check that you are immune to rubella (German measles) and start taking folic acid (0.4 mg of folic acid, aka folate, should be taken by all women trying to conceive but if there is a family history or personal history of a previous baby with spina bifida, take 4 mg of folate).

What you can do yourself

At this point, you want to do everything you can to maximise your chances of getting pregnant naturally. If you are trying to conceive, the general health of both you and your partner is crucial. Remember that about one-third of infertility problems originate with the man. It's nothing to do with impotence, but to do with the quality of his sperm. Recent research suggests that a man's fertility starts to decline as he approaches 40, rather than later as previous evidence suggested. So it's essential that your partner joins you in an optimal health regime. The great thing about this is that most of it is totally under your control.

The following factors are important:

Weight

Being under- or overweight can have a significant negative effect on ovulation. Your Body Mass Index (BMI) should be between 20 and 25. (To calculate your BMI, see page 62.) Under 20 indicates you are too thin, and 26 and over you are overweight. A reasonable amount of exercise is vital but remember that, once again, too much or too little can have a negative effect on fertility. As a rule of thumb think of doing at least 30 minutes of good exercise at least five times a week; yoga is really beneficial. (See chapters on exercise and yoga.) There are also specific dietary issues associated with infertility and we suggest you refer to Dr Marilyn Glenville's book *Natural Solutions to Infertility*.

Smoking

Just don't! Smoking in either partner can significantly reduce the chance of conceiving. (Tell your partner that smoking can lead to impotence – fact.)

Alcohol

Drinking alcohol can reduce your fertility by up to 50 per cent. The more you drink the less likely you are to conceive. Women who drink fewer than five units (a unit equals one glass of wine) a week are twice as likely to conceive in six months compared to those who drink more. (Men who drink are much more likely to be impotent – another fact.)

Medication

If you or your partner are taking any pharmaceutical drugs, discuss this with your doctor because they may not only affect your fertility but also might need to be changed if you do conceive.

Stress

It's essential that you try not to worry about conceiving because the more you worry the more stressed you get. And stress is the foremost in the general indirect causes of infertility. (Think of the number of women who have tried to conceive for years and do so only when they cease to try, or adopt a baby.) Firstly stress causes tightness in the neck muscles, which may affect the blood flow to the pituitary gland. When the pituitary gland is not working properly, the follicle stimulating hormones (FSH) that stimulate ovulation are not produced in sufficient quantity. This can lead to delayed ovulation and a longer or erratic menstrual cycle. Stress can also cause significant relationship problems and so a reduction in the frequency of intercourse. Physical stress is also a factor. Sitting in front of a computer for example can cause neck tension, which by affecting the blood flow to the brain as we explain above, may cause psychological stress and hormonal malfunction.

Gentle yoga or walking or swimming can help reduce stress; also see our suggestions on page 99.

Diet

A good balanced diet with lots of vitamin-rich fresh fruit and vegetables is essential. Also make sure you get plenty of protein such as chicken, eggs and fish (ideally organic or in the case of fish reared in clean waters). You want to avoid foods that tend to produce gas – they'll make you feel uncomfortable and may disturb the circulation in the pelvic area. So avoid citrus fruits, a lot of garlic, spicy food, canned products, yeast-containing foods, coffee, alcohol, sugar, fried food and fizzy drinks. Both would-be parents should take a good vitamin and mineral supplement and consider seeing a nutritionist for expert guidance.

FRUITS OF LOVE

Pomegranates are a traditional remedy for infertility in India. The seed actually looks like the womb of a pregnant woman and perhaps this is nature indicating that this fruit is good for women who either are or who want to get pregnant. Pomegranates have a high level of cobalt which is an essential raw material for synthesising blood and thus important for pregnancy.

Exercise

Being fit is a great thing for getting pregnant, both in terms of fitness and libido. The most important thing for women is to learn to listen to your body (it always applies, of course, not just for this). So do exercise that you enjoy but don't get overtired or too hot and don't do contact sports that might disturb an embryo. The best advice is to check with your doctor first if you want to do a particular sport. And if any complications occur, stick to more gentle forms of exercise like walking, yoga and swimming.

'If in doubt, leave it out' is a good motto: we know one husband who went on being upset for years about his wife's miscarriage because he thought it was his fault for urging her to go the gym more to reduce her fat tummy – in fact, neither of them had known she was pregnant and it almost certainly made no difference anyway.

Sex

Michael is often asked how often would-be mothers should have intercourse and when. His general rule is to have intercourse three times a week across the week, i.e. not all on one day! If you and your partner have busy lifestyles and this is not easy, then concentrate on midcycle. Whatever you do – don't create additional stress because that can be (literally) counterproductive.

Complementary Therapies To Try
* massage (mainly for stress)
* acupuncture
* chinese herbal medicine
* homeopathy

NB There is evidence showing that all these can help but it's important to talk to your fertility specialist about what you are doing. See our Co-operation Card on page 19.

In general, read the literature and get as much information as you can and join local and national support groups. Do not be afraid to ask for help. Some fertility clinics have an open access service to a nurse counsellor who has expert knowledge. (But try not to get obsessed.)

AN ALTERNATIVE APPROACH

Dr Mosaraf Ali of the Integrated Medical Centre recommends:

- for stress: practise yoga and give yourself a massage of the head and neck which is very helpful in destressing.
- remedy to improve sperm count:
  - breakfast egg flip: stir a raw organic egg into a glass of hot creamy milk, add salt and pepper to taste and drink at breakfast.
  - other remedies for improving sperm quality, published in peer-reviewed medical journals, include: individualised homeopathy, organic diet, supplementation with vitamin E (400 mg) and selenium (225 micrograms) and also with pycnogenol aka French maritime pine tree bark extract (200 mg).

- traditional advice for women trying to get pregnant is not to do strenuous work like lifting and carrying and avoid high-impact exercises such as weight lifting and jogging.

If you don't conceive

We advise you to seek help early on. (We hope you have already seen a doctor for a general health check and guidance when you first decided you wanted to try for a baby, but if not see one now.) If your doctor refuses to refer you to a fertility expert, either go to another doctor or approach a fertility expert directly. (If you do choose this self-referral route, you must obviously make certain that the doctor you go to is fully qualified and reputable.)

Facing the facts

If you go to see a fertility specialist, it's obvious you are hoping for a baby. The bottom line for any older woman is that she has to face the fact that she may not become a mother easily. There can be huge emotional and financial issues to confront for both partners as well as the ethical concerns for the welfare of the baby. So however much you want a baby, it is essential to try and keep a little bit of perspective. Not least because the stress may add to the factors that prevent you getting pregnant.

It's vital not to turn the hoping into an obsession. As Winnie the Pooh may (according to Michael) have said, 'A problem is a problem because it has a solution' and that's the way you need to approach this. The downside is that the solution may not be the one you thought you wanted. It may be that you will get pregnant and have a lovely baby. If you don't get pregnant, at least you will know that you did everything you possibly could.

What happens at the specialist

The specialist's role is to assess whether you are producing an egg, your partner is producing sperm and whether the two can get together. So the doctor will assess the quality of your eggs and the state of your Fallopian tubes (doctors sometimes talk about whether the Fallopian tubes are 'patent' meaning clear so that the egg can travel down), and also your partner's sperm. The doctor will take a detailed medical history of both of you and your families – including looking at your general health and lifestyle, and also carry out examinations and investigations.

Medical and family history

If you have a family history of Down's syndrome, spina bifida or cardiac defects, this will need to be discussed before embarking on a fertility programme. The doctor will need to know how often you and your partner have sex; if there are problems these need to be addressed. Your general health will be discussed including weight, diet, exercise, stress, smoking, alcohol consumption, prescription drugs and recreational drug intake. Your iron levels should be checked in case you are suffering from anaemia.

Issues to discuss with your fertility specialist

There are several issues that need discussing if you are contemplating fertility treatment. You also need to bear in mind that the treatment options may have no – or very limited – advantage over no treatment at all. You should always question the nature of the treatment and its risks and benefits.

The broad issues fall into four groups: medical, ethical, emotional and financial. You need to discuss all these with your specialist. It's a good litmus test, incidentally, for choosing a specialist; if you don't feel they are really caring for you through this stage, you may want to try someone else.

Here are the question areas we suggest you cover and information about the nature of the answers you may get:

Medical issues
Q How likely am I to get pregnant?
A It's vital to talk to the specialist about how likely you are to get pregnant, the tests you might undergo, the various routes you might take to conception and the exact procedures involved so you have a clear picture. Some women may consult a specialist, discuss the whole situation and then

decide that, actually, they don't want to go ahead with treatment.

One woman we know had a ruptured ectopic pregnancy at the age of 40 and nearly died. Her Fallopian tubes were removed so she became unable to conceive naturally. After talking to two fertility specialists, she realised that, firstly, she needed to get over the emotional scars of losing her baby. Secondly, she came to realise that she could not face taking the fertility drugs with the possible side effects and risk. Then – if the treatment was successful – possibly ending up with twins or triplets.

Q What tests might I or my partner have?
A The key areas for the specialist to investigate are eggs and tubes in women, sperm in men. So the specialist will take your history first of all, then decide on further tests.

History:
Women

* **egg:** if you have regular cycles, the likelihood is that you are ovulating. If you suffer from PMS (premenstrual syndrome) that also strongly suggests you are releasing an egg since the symptoms are linked to ovulation.
* **tubes:** if you have had chlamydia infection in the past this may have resulted in damage to your Fallopian tubes. Tubal damage is permanent but you and your partner need to be screened for infection and any active disease treated. Abdominal surgery, a previous ectopic pregnancy or severe pelvic inflammatory disease may indicate that your tubes are damaged.

Men

If your partner has had operations on his testicles, including an undescended testicle or trauma, there could be a reduction in the sperm count, which would be tested for (see below).

Examinations

- **egg:** examination to see if there are changes in cervical mucus, and a general examination of your pelvis.
- **tubes:** abdominal scans may indicate possible tubal damage.
- **sperm:** examination of the testicles should demonstrate normal-sized testicles. If these are small and feel wasted and/or shrivelled, or if there is a significant difference in size, this may indicate the cause of any infertility.

Investigations

A single investigation only provides a snapshot of a complex and changing situation so doctors often advise doing several different tests, over a period of time.

- **egg:** blood tests for progesterone are done in the second half of your cycle. Counting Day 1 as the first day of your period, progesterone levels should rise in the second half of your cycle. Blood tests are usually done around Day 21. It may be better to have two or three blood tests, usually on Days 19, 21 and 23.

Ultrasound scanning can also be used to assess fertility (as well as pregnancy). Scanning your ovaries throughout the cycle can show the egg growing and then being released.

Urine testing is now available to monitor changes in leutinising hormone (LH) in urine. The LH level surges mid cycle, stimulating the release of the egg (ovulation).

NB Changes in your body temperature can indicate ovulation (as we describe in the section about Natural Family Planning on page 382) but the drawback is that having to take your temperature every single day may lead to your becoming obsessed by the situation and so is not necessarily a wise course of action.

- **Tubes**: tests to see whether the tubes are clear include:

  - hysterosalpingogram X-ray (HSG).
  - hy-cosy: ultrasound scan where fluid is injected into the uterine cavity.
  - laparascopy: keyhole surgery where dye is inserted into the Fallopian tubes to see whether they are open – this is the gold standard test; it also enables the specialist to check for endometriosis and adhesions ('cobwebs' in your abdomen which may reduce fertility and are often due to past infection).

- **Sperm**: investigations of the sperm should be done in a properly approved laboratory. Tests include:

  - motility (movement): this should be 50 per cent or over.
  - morphology (what sperm look like): sperm are like tadpoles – abnormal ones can have an odd-looking head or tail, or even two heads or tails ...
  - number: this should be 20 million or more per ml.
  - antibodies (these make the sperm stick together): should be under 50 per cent.
  - blood tests: these include the hormones LH, FSH, testosterone and prolactin.

Questions to discuss with your doctor
Q *What treatment options are available?*
A Here are the main routes to pregnancy:

Natural Intercourse

What happens?	You know this one ... but never forget, you may conceive naturally
Suitable for	Everyone
Risks	None
Advantages	Lots! Including being good for your relationship
Success rate in 40+	Up to 5 per cent per year

Ovulation induction

What happens?	Tablets or injections to stimulate release of eggs are administered; results monitored by scanning. Tubes and sperm must be normal
Suitable for	Women with normal FSH levels who don't ovulate
Risks	Drugs may induce side effects, e.g. nausea, vomiting, cysts on ovaries; multiple pregnancy; Ovarian Hyperstimulation Syndrome
Advantages	Relatively straightforward
Success rate in 40+	Depends on age but not greater than 5 per cent per year if woman not ovulating before

IVF (In Vitro Fertilisation) using own eggs & ICSI (Intra Cyroplasmic Sperm Injection

What happens?	Eggs are removed from your ovaries and, in IVF, mixed with your partner's sperm, in ICSI the sperm is injected;

	the embryo(s) is then replaced in your womb
Suitable for	IVF is suitable for most women with tubal disease or unexplained infertility; may be trump card if you want to use your own eggs. ICSI is more suitable for severe male infertility
Risks	The risks of both procedures are the same: drug may induce side effects, e.g. nausea, vomiting, cysts on ovaries; multiple pregnancy; Ovarian Hyper-stimulation Syndrome; complications from operation
Advantages	IVF is ideally suited for people with tubal damage and may be more successful for couples who've been trying for a reasonable length of time. If age is a factor, it is important to discuss IVF early on. ICSI has the advantage of being particularly useful in the treatment of male infertility
Success rate in 40+	The same in both procedures: around two to five per cent per go

GIFT *(Gamete Intra Fallopian Transfer)*

What happens?	Eggs removed then placed with sperm (unmixed) in one of your Fallopian tubes, under anaesthetic
Suitable for	Women with unexplained infertility
Risks	As for IVF, plus risk of laparascopy
Advantages	Success may be very slightly greater in 40+ compared to IVF
Success rate in 40+	Around two to five per cent per go

Donor eggs/sperm/embryo

What happens?	A combination of eggs donated by a woman who has gone through the IVF procedure are fertilised with your partner's sperm and placed in your uterus. In sperm donation, the sperm is placed in your womb around the time of ovulation. Or a donated embryo, with donated egg and sperm, may be placed in your uterus
Suitable for	Women over 40 with egg problems
Risks	Emotional and ethical concerns
Advantages	Few drugs; good success
Success rate in 40+	About 25 per cent per go for donated eggs; donor sperm depends on the age of the woman; donated embryo depends on age of donors

Q What drugs do you propose and what are the possible side effects?
A Whatever treatment package you go for, there are associated risks. If you are not ovulating (releasing an egg), it may be due to the fact that there are no eggs left, which is indicated by a high FSH level. If your doctor thinks there are eggs left in your ovaries, drugs called ovulation induction agents such as clomiphine citrate tablets or gonadotrophin injections may be used to try to stimulate their release. These can have significant side effects including ovarian hyper-stimulation syndrome when big cysts grow on your ovaries; this can be a life-threatening event if not picked up early.

Q What surgery do you propose and what are the possible risks?
A Before IVF became more readily available, surgery for

damage to the Fallopian tubes used to be a common option. However, it is still performed and if you are offered tubal surgery you should remember that it is major surgery (although it might be keyhole), and question the value, success and risks.

Q Is there any possibility of multiple pregnancy and what are the risks?
A Multiple pregnancy does increase the risk to both mother and babies. Risks for the mother include:

- greater risk of miscarriage.
- high blood pressure and pre-eclampsia (eclampsia is a potentially crisis state in late pregnancy involving fits or coma; treatment for pre-eclampsia is usually delivery of the baby).
- gestational diabetes (this usually ends with labour but may lead to complications for mother and baby later on)
- low-lying placenta (may lead to Caesarean section).
- surgical delivery (Caesarean section), including anaesthetic.

Risks for the baby include:

- prematurity
- cerebral palsy
- difficult delivery (which may bring problems later)
- gestational diabetes

Ethical issues
Before you commit to any procedure it is important that the welfare of the unborn child is considered by everyone involved. That's why comprehensive counselling is vital; this should be offered by the clinic. One issue that may need to be discussed is your age. The oldest woman who received

successful fertility treatment (egg donation) in this country was 56. However, the majority of specialists will only treat women up to and including 50. So the cut-off date is usually your 51st birthday.

Emotional issues

Don't underestimate this part of your decision-making. Whatever you and your partner decide can drain your emotions and cause significant stress. Consider doing relaxation techniques such as yoga (see Chapter Nine) and having therapies such as massage to help manage the pressure. And don't forget to keep talking to your partner.

Financial issues

It is essential that you get full verbal and written information about the costs involved, which can vary widely.

13

PLANNING AHEAD

Take action in your 40s (or as early as possible) if you want to go smoothly and naturally through the menopause. The two main aims are to balance your body and mind so you are in the best possible state to go through this transition, and to prevent osteoporosis. Remember it's never too early to start looking after your body: these simple lifestyle tips will help you whatever age you are.

- view the menopause positively; see the potential of freedom from periods and pregnancy. Think of it as a new and wonderful opening-up of your life – not a shutting down of your femininity. Remember: thinking positively leads to a positive outcome (it really does!).
- severe pre-menstrual syndrome can become increasingly distressing as you approach the menopause. (Some traditional practitioners say that bad PMS predicts a difficult menopause if not attended to.) If you have PMS, rest as much as you can in the first two days of your period or at least go to bed early. Drink plenty of water and herbal teas, as well as following the other advice on this page and on page 412. Try supplements of vitamin B6, evening primrose oil and trace minerals, particularly magnesium and zinc. Nutritionist Gillian Hamer recommends Femforte by Biocare as an all-in-one product (Take two

410

to four capsules daily depending on the severity of your symptoms).

- remember to check your contraceptive options regularly during your 40s (see Chapter Twelve).

- if osteoporosis runs in your family, or if you have been anorexic, suffered digestive problems such as Crohn's disease or you have not had periods for more than six months at a time, you should always consult a qualified health practitioner. They will test your bone mineral density and prescribe individual therapy.

- don't smoke: smoking lowers blood oestrogen levels and also has a dampening effect on the cells that make new bone so increasing the risk of osteoporosis. It can trigger premature menopause by up to 18 months. Incidentally, nearly half of women smokers die from a smoking-related disease, such as lung cancer, chronic lung disease or heart disease (And just think of the wrinkles you won't have if you don't smoke ...)

- exercise at least 30 to 40 minutes at least five times a week, preferably daily, for general health, weight management and healthy bones: see the chapters on exercise and yoga.

- eat nourishing food regularly – three to five small meals daily rather than one big one – to regulate blood sugar levels and keep your digestion working smoothly.

- lose excess weight but don't get too thin. Your body needs some fat to produce oestrogen, which is produced in fat cells: thin women are more likely to suffer osteoporosis and/or menopausal symptoms. Aim to be within your recommended Body Mass Index; see page 62.

- make sure you are getting enough calcium to help prevent bone loss: the National Osteoporosis Society recommends that women over 40 get 1,500 mg of calcium daily. Always include plenty of fish, dairy products including cheese and yoghurt, seeds, nuts (especially almonds), green leafy vegetables. Tofu (soya) is one of the richest sources of calcium. You also need other minerals, principally magnesium and boron.

- eat slowly and chew your food very thoroughly: nutritionist Kathryn Marsden notes that many women suffering from PMS and also menopausal symptoms like hot flushes have gut problems such as candida. Bolting your food or swallowing over-large morsels can wreak havoc on your sensitive digestive system. Don't eat on the run and always try to sit for at least five minutes at the table after you've finished, then go for five or ten minutes' gentle walk.

- aim to eat fresh, wholesome food; avoid ready prepared food of all sorts.

- avoid white sugar and white flour, which may affect your health and certainly contain no goodness, also salt and salty foods, which may increase the risk of both heart disease and bone loss. Don't add salt to food: use a low salt substitute and/or other flavourings such as herbs, lemon and pepper. Also be aware that many prepared foods contain lots of salt, even sweet products like chocolate pudding.

- if you do have gut problems or constipation, go on an anti-candida diet (see page 263), eat lots of organic natural live yoghurt and take a bio-acidophilus supplement long term.

- eat two to three portions of oily fish weekly for its Essential Fatty Acids, which improve skin and hair and may also improve calcium absorption. Avocadoes are brilliant, too.

- aim for at least five portions of fresh fruit and vegetables daily, preferably organic.

- have fresh vegetable and/ or fruit juices at least twice a week: try organic apple, carrot, celery and ginger. See Chapter Eight.

- cut down on red meat (aim for two to three small portions weekly, preferably organic) and avoid sugar and foods that are spicy, heavy or oily because anything that puts a strain on your digestion will send the blood rushing to the pelvic area and may deprive your brain and your hormonal responses.
- vegans, who eat no animal products, should take specific advice, because they seem to be particularly at risk of bone density loss as well as anaemia.
- avoid constipation because it may be associated with osteoporosis, as well as other problems. When oestrogen levels start to drop, there is a lot of dryness, including in the colon, and the body finds it more difficult to absorb calcium. If you are constipated, drink plenty of still pure water between meals (at least 1.5 litres daily), and eat fruits such as papaya and figs for breakfast. Also take one tablespoonful of linseeds with water or in yoghurt at night before bed.
- if you like a little tipple, drink one to two glasses of good wine daily, preferably red because of the benefits to your heart. Don't go over 14 units a week because it will put on weight and harm your bones as well as making you look older. (One unit equals a glass of wine).
- get out in the sunlight – vitamin D is vital for healthy bones and light is essential particularly in the winter to avoid winter blues (Seasonal Affective Disorder).
- if you're stressed, take up meditation and practise yoga. Develop your own 'bad hair day' strategies for dealing with stressy and/or bluesy days (see page 99).
- consider regular complementary therapy consultations, such as acupuncture and/or homeopathy, which help get your mind and body on an even keel.
- once a week, massage your whole body with organic sesame and mustard oils (two parts sesame to one part

413

mustard) to get the blood into the muscles, and/or have regular deep tissue massages.

- also massage your neck and the back of your skull, as often as you like, to improve the blood flow to the brain. This eases out creaky necks, and may help hormonal function, and to banish water retention.
- look ahead for the next five or ten years: list all the good things and the difficult (or potentially difficult) areas of your life and plan to maximise the good and minimise the difficult ones.
- take a risk or three: as philosopher priest John O'Donohue, author of *Anam Cara: Spiritual Wisdom from the Celtic World*, says, 'The human spirit thrives on risk.' What have you got to lose? Start thinking in terms of living your dream.
  - learn something new: a language, musical instrument, salsa, sport.
  - join a club or choir or book group; or start one!
  - invite new people round for tea – everyone wants to be friends but is often too nervous to make the first move.
  - take off on an adventure.
- take pleasure in small things: tea with a friend, a bunch of flowers, a sunny day, someone saying something nice to you.
- **and finally ... relax ...** Whenever possible give yourself permission to stop working and have fun, or simply rest. You deserve it.

GLOSSARY

Amenorrhoea	not having periods
Androgens	male hormones also produced in much smaller amounts in women
CAM	Complementary and Alternative Medicine
Cervical smear	testing the cells of the cervix (neck of womb) for pre-cancerous changes
Cervix	lower part of the uterus at top of vagina
Climacteric	whole transitional time (or 'change of life'): this may last 15 to 20 years, from the first change in period patterns to the end of symptoms
Deep Vein thrombosis (DVT)	Potentially life-threatening blood clot in leg which travels to lung
Dysmenorrhoea	painful periods
Dyspareunia	pain during intercourse
Ectopic pregnancy	the fertilised egg implants outside the womb, often in the Fallopian tubes where the pregnancy may rupture
Endocrinologist	specialist in hormones
Endocrinology	study of hormones
Endometriosis	bits of lining of the womb (endometrium) growing outside the womb, often leading to pain with intercourse and possible infertility
Fallopian tube (oviduct)	tube between ovary and womb where egg and sperm meet

Fibroids	non-cancerous growth of the muscle of the womb
FSH	follicle stimulating hormone: see gonadotrophin
Gonadotrophins	hormones (FSH and LH) released from the pituitary gland that stimulate the ovaries
Hormones	chemical messengers produced by different glands that run our minds, brains and bodies
HRT (hormone replacement therapy)	replacing hormones – oestrogen, progesterone and sometimes testosterone – that decline around menopause
Hypothalamus	part of the human brain closely linked to pituitary gland; controls body temperature, appetite, blood pressure and sleep; said to be the physical basis of the emotions
Hysterectomy	surgical removal of womb
Subtotal hysterectomy	hysterectomy leaving the cervix
Hysteroscopy	investigating the womb by looking in with a telescope; may be done with or without general anaesthetic
Laparoscopy	looking inside your abdomen with a telescope; usually done with general anaesthetic
LH	luteinising hormone: see gonadotrophins
Libido	sexual drive or desire
Lipids	fats in your body, which may be tested in blood samples
Menarche	your first natural period
Menopause	your last natural period
Menorrhagia	heavy periods
Menstruation	monthly periods
Oestrogen (estrogen)	group of female hormones (oestradiol, oestriol and oestrone) produced principally by the ovaries

Oocyte/ovum/ female gamete	an egg released by the ovary
Oophorectomy	surgical removal of ovaries
Orgasm	climax of making love
Osteoporosis	loss of bone density, mainly after age 50 in women; affects one in three women, one in 12 men
Ova	eggs from ovaries, same as oocytes
Ovarian cyst	benign or malignant growth from ovary, may contain fluid or sometimes solids
Ovarian failure	the ovary stops producing eggs, so ovulation stops, leading to a decline in reproductive hormones (oestrogen and progesterone) and to menopause
Ovaries	female glands which contain and release eggs; testicles are the male equivalent
Ovulation	release of eggs from ovaries
Pelvic inflammatory disease (PID)	infection of the organs within the pelvis
Pituitary	gland at base of brain, which controls hormones
PMS (premenstrual syndrome)	varying symptoms that may affect women in the days leading up to period; used to be called PMT (premenstrual tension)
Polycystic ovaries (PCO)	common condition where ovaries increase in size slightly with multiple small cysts; PCOs may lead to PCO Syndrome (PCOS), which may result in irregular periods, infertility, excessive hair growth (hirsutism) on face and/ or body, acne and obesity
Premature menopause	ovarian failure before the age of 40 to 45

Progesterone	naturally occurring progestogen in female body
Progestogens	group of female hormones, including progesterone, involved with preparing womb lining to receive embryo; also helps control periods
Puberty	beginning of time when you can have babies
Pulmonary embolism (PE)	potentially life-threatening blood clot in lung
Resistant ovary syndrome	disorder of the ovary, closely linked to premature menopause
Surgical menopause	last period caused by removal of ovaries, usually with hysterectomy (sometimes hysterectomy alone can lead to ovaries failing)
Testosterone	male hormone (women have a little)
Thrombosis	a blood clot in a blood vessel
Uterus	womb
Vasomotor symptoms	hot flushes and night sweats
Venous thrombo-embolism (VTE)	blood clot in vein that embolises, i.e. breaks off and travels through the body, usually to the lung

USEFUL BOOKS

Baillie-Hamilton, Dr Paula, *The Detox Diet*, Michael Joseph, 2002

Bourne, Alison, *Colour Breathing*, Energy Press, 2002

Brar, Dr Ali and Jiwan, *Therapeutic Yoga*, Vermilion, 2002

Brown, Bobbi with Wadyka, Sally, *Bobbi Brown Beauty Evolution*, Aurum Press, 2002

Brown, Lynda, *The Insomniac's Best Friend*, Thorsons, 2004

Brown, Marie-Annette and Robinson, Jo, *When Your Body Gets the Blues*, Rodale, 2003

Chevallier, Andrew, *Herbal Medicine for the Menopause*, Amberwood Publishing, 2001

Fairley, Josephine and Stacey, Sarah, *Feel Fabulous Forever: The Antiageing Health & Beauty Bible*, Kyle Cathie, 2002

Glenville, Marilyn, *The New Natural Alternatives to HRT*, Kyle Cathie, 2003

Harper, Dr Jennifer, *Detox Handbook*, Dorling Kindersley, 2002

Harris, Colette and Carey, Adam, *PCOS. A Woman's Guide to Dealing with Polycystic Ovary Syndrome*, Thorsons, 2000

Lane, Roderick and Stacey, Sarah, *The Adam & Eve Diet*, Hodder Mobius, 2002

Lee, Dr Victoria, *Soulful Sex*, Conari Press (USA), 1996

Marber, Ian, *The Food Doctor Diet*, Dorling Kindersley, 2003

Marsden, Kathryn, *The Complete Book of Food Combining*, Piatkus, 2000

Marsden, Kathryn, *Superskin*, Thorsons, 2002

Marsden, Kathryn, *Good Gut Healing*, Piatkus, 2003

O'Donohue, John, *Anam Cara: Spiritual Wisdom from the Celtic World*, HarperCollins, 1998

Puri, Dr Basant K. and Boyd, Hilary, *The Natural Way to Beat Depression*, Hodder Mobius, 2004

Royal College of Obstetrics and Gynaecologists, *Complete Women's Health*, Thorsons, 2000

Sampson, Val, *Tantra, the Art of Mind Blowing Sex*, Vermilion, 2002

Stacey, Sarah and Fairley, Josephine, *The 21st Century Beauty Bible*, Kyle Cathie, 2002

Williamson, Vivien with Tresidder, Dr Andrew, *Bach Remedies and Other Flower Essences*, Select Editions/ Anness Publishing, 2000

DIRECTORY

To call any of the telephone numbers below from any country outside the UK, please dial '00' (used to dial another country), followed by '44' (to dial into the UK), followed by the telephone number you wish to call, remembering to remove the preceding '0' of the area code. E.g. to call 'Hands on Health Acupressure' from abroad you should dial: 00 44 1534 745535.

GENERAL ADVICE IN BRITAIN

British Complementary
  Medical Association
PO Box 5122
Bournemouth
BH8 0WG
Tel: 0845 345 5977
E-mail: web@bcma.co.uk
Website: www.bcma.co.uk

Institute of Complementary
  Medicine
PO Box 194
London
SE16 7QZ
Tel: 020 7237 5165
E-mail:
  info@icmedicine.co.uk
Website:
  www.icmedicine.co.uk

USEFUL ADDRESSES IN BRITAIN

Acupressure

Hands on Health
  Acupressure
Caroline Le Maistre
Industria House
La Route Des Genets
St Brelade
Jersey
JE3 8LD
Tel: 01534 745535
Website: www.polisa.co.uk

Acupuncture

The British Acupuncture
  Council
63 Jeddo Road
London
W12 9HQ
Tel: 020 8735 0400
E-mail:
  info@acupuncture.org.uk
Website: www.acupunc-
  ture.org.uk

British Medical
  Acupuncture Society
12 Marbury House
Higher Whitley
Warrington
Cheshire
WA4 4QW

Tel: 01925 730727
E-mail: Admin@medical-
  acupuncture.org.uk
Website: www.medical-
  acupuncture.co.uk

Alexander Technique

The Society of Teachers of
  the Alexander Technique
  (STAT)
1st Floor
Linton House
39–51 Highgate Road
London
NW5 1RS
Tel: 0845 230 7828
E-mail: enquiries@
  stat.org.uk
Website: www.stat.org.uk

Animal Therapy

Pets As Therapy
3 Grange Farm Cottages
Wycombe Road
Saunderton
Princes Risborough
Bucks
HP27 9NS
Tel: 0870 240 1239
E-mail: reception@petsas
  therapy.org

Website: www.petsas
    therapy.org

Aromatherapy Massage

Aromatherapy and Allied
    Practitioners' Association
    (AAPA)
8 George Street
Croydon
Surrey
CR0 1PA
Tel: 020 8680 7761
Website: www.aroma
    therapyuk.net

Aromatherapy
    Organisations Council
PO Box 6522
Desborough
Kettering
NN14 2YX
Tel: 0870 7743477
Website: www.aocuk.net

Association of Medical
    Aromatherapists (AMA)
Abegare
Rhu Point
Helensburgh
G84 8NF
Tel: 0141 332 4924

The International
    Federation of

Professional
    Aromatherapists
82 Ashby Road
Hinckley
Leicestershire
LE10 1SN
Tel: 01455 637987
E-mail:
    admin@IFPAroma.org
Website: www.ifparoma.org

Register of Qualified
    Aromatherapists
The IFPA
82 Ashby Road
Hinckley
Leicestershire
LE10 1SN
Tel: 01455 637987
E-mail:
    admin@IFPAroma.org
Website: www.ifparoma.org

Ayurvedic

Ayurvedic Medical
    Association UK
59 Dulverton Road
Selsdon
South Croydon
Surrey
CR2 8PJ
Tel: 0208 657 6147

E-mail: Dr N.S.
   Moorthy@ayurvedic.dem
   on.co.uk
Website: www.natural-
   healing.co.uk/ayurvedic-
   medical-association-uk

Beauty

www.beautybible.com
(Sarah Stacey and Josephine
   Fairley's own site)

Bereavement counselling

Cruse Bereavement Care
Cruse House
126 Sheen Road
Richmond
Surrey
TW9 1UR
Tel: 020 8939 9530
Helpline: 0870 167 1677
E-mail: helpline@cruse
   bereavementcare.org.uk
Website: www.cruse
   bereavementcare.org.uk

London Bereavement
   Network
356 Holloway Road
London
N7 6PA
Tel: 020 7700 8134

E-mail:
   info@bereavement.org.uk
Website: www.bereavement.
   org.uk

Biofeedback

Complementary Healthcare
   Information Service – UK
   (To find a practitioner in
   the UK)
Website: www.chisuk.org.uk

Chinese herbal remedies

Register of Chinese Herbal
   Medicine
Office 5
Ferndale Business Centre
1 Exeter Street
Norwich
NR2 4QB
Tel: 01603 623994
E-mail:
   herbmed@rchm.co.uk
Website: www.rchm.co.uk

Chiropractic

British Association for
   Applied Chiropractic
167a London Road
Teynham
Kent

ME9 9QJ
Tel: 01795 520707

British Chiropractic
Association (BCA)
Blagrave House
17 Blagrave Street
Reading
Berkshire
RG1 1QB
Tel: 0118 950 5950
E-mail: enquiries@chiro-
practic-uk.co.uk
Website: www.chiropractic-
uk.co.uk

General Chiropractic
Council
344–354 Gray's Inn Road
London
WC1X 8BP
Tel: 020 7713 5155
E-mail: enquiries@gcc-
uk.org
Website: www.gcc-uk.org

McTimoney Chiropractic
Association
3 Oxford Court
St James Road
Brackley
Northants
NN13 7XY
Tel: 01280 705050

E-mail: admin@mctimoney-
chiropractic.org
Website: www.mctimoney-
chiropractic.org

United Chiropractic
Association
Chichester House
145a London Road
Kingston upon Thames
Surrey
KT2 6SR
Tel: 020 8939 4599
E-mail: uca@bthcc.co.uk
Website: www.united-
chiropractic.org

Counselling and psychotherapy

British Association for
Counselling and
Psychotherapy
BACP House
35–37 Albert Street
Rugby
CV21 2SG
Tel: 01788 568739
E-mail: bacp@bacp.co.uk
Website: www.bacp.co.uk

British Association of
  Psychotherapists
37 Mapesbury Road
London
NW2 4HJ
Tel: 020 8452 9823
E-mail: mail@bap-
  psychotherapy.org
Website: www.bap-
  psychotherapy.org

Counselling and
  Psychotherapy Association
39 Warwick Road
Atherton
Manchester
M46 9TA
Tel: 01942 894885
E-mail: info@counselling.
  ltd.uk
Website: www.counselling.
  ltd.uk

UK Council for
  Psychotherapy
167–169 Great Portland
  Street
London
W1W 5PF
Tel: 020 7436 3002
E-mail: ukcp@psycho
  therapy.org.uk
Website: www.psycho
  therapy.org.uk

Creative visualisation (mental imagery)

www.colourbreathing.com

Dance therapy

Biodanza
48 Clifford Avenue
London
SW14 7BP
Tel: 020 8392 1433
E-mail: martello@biodanza.
  demon.co.uk
Website: www.biodanza.
  co.uk

Flirt therapy

Flirt coach at the flirting
  academy
Tel: 0700 4354 784
E-mail: info@flirtcoach.com
Website: www.flirtzone.com

Flower remedies

The Dr Edward Bach
  Centre
Mount Vernon
Bakers Lane
Sotwell
Oxon
OX10 0PZ

Tel: 01491 834678
Website:
www.bachcentre.com

Healing and spiritual healing

Confederation of Healing
Organisations (govern-
ment-recognised body)
Suite J, Second Floor
The Red and White House
113 High Street
Berkhamsted
Hertfordshire
HP4 2DJ
Tel: 01442 870660

National Federation of
Spiritual Healers
Old Manor Farm Studio
Church Street
Sunbury-on-Thames
Middlesex
TW16 6RG
Tel: 0845 1232777
E-mail: office@nfsh.org.uk
Website: www.nfsh.org.uk

Herbalism

The Herb Society
Sulgrave Manor
Sulgrave

Banbury
OX17 2SD
Tel: 01295 768899
E-mail: info@herb
society.co.uk
Website: www.herb
society.co.uk

International Register of
Consultant Herbalists
32 King Edward Road
Swansea
South Wales
SA1 4LL
Tel: 01792 655 886
E-mail: office@irch.org
Website: www.irch.org

National Institute of
Medical Herbalists
56 Longbrook Street
Exeter
EX4 6AH
Tel: 01392 426022
E-mail:
nimh@ukexeter.freeserve.
co.uk
Website: www.nimh.org.uk

Homeopathy

The Alliance of Registered
Homeopaths
26 Sunningdale Avenue

Leigh-on-Sea
Essex
SS9 1JZ
Tel: 08700 736339
E-mail: info@a-r-h.org
Website: www.a-r-h.org

Faculty of Homeopathy
Hahnemann House
29 Park Street West
Luton
LU1 3BE
Tel: 0870 444 3950
Website: www.trusthomeo
    pathy.org

The Society of Homeopaths
4a Artizan Road
Northampton
NN1 4HU
Tel: 01604 621400
E-mail: info@homeopathy-
    soh.org
Website: www.homeopathy-
    soh.org

The UK Homeopathy
    Medical Association
Administration Office
6 Livingstone Road
Gravesend
Kent
DA12 5DZ
Tel: 01474 560336

E-mail: info@the-hma.org
Website: www.homeopathy.
    org

Hydrotherapy

The Hydrotherapy
    Association
PO Box 30
Godalming
GU8 6WB
Tel: 01483-813 181

The Hydrotherapy
    Association of Chartered
    Physiotherapists
40 Cumbeth Close
Crickhowell
Powys
NP8 1DX
E-mail:
    physio@cheerful.com

Hypnotherapy

Central Register of
    Advanced
    Hypnotherapists (CRAH)
Enquirers seeking CRAH's
    full Register of Practising
    Members, together with
    an explanatory booklet
    on the therapeutic use of
    hypnosis, may write to:
CRAH

PO Box 14526
London
N4 2WG
Your enquiry can be
processed only if you
enclose a stamped and
self-addressed envelope.
Tel: 020 7354 9938

The General Hypnotherapy
Register (GHR)
PO Box 204
Lymington
SO41 6WP
Tel: 01590 683 770
E-mail: info@general-
hypnotherapy-
register.com
Website: www.general-
hypnotherapy-
register.com

The Hypnotherapy Society
PO Box 3511
Wells
BA5 2ZR
Tel: 0845 6024585
E-mail: info@hypnothera-
pysociety.com
Website: www.hypnothera-
pysociety.com

National Council for
Hypnotherapy

PO Box 5779
Burton on the Wolds
Loughborough
LE12 5ZF
Tel: 0800 9520545
Website: www.hypno
therapists.org.uk

Laughter Therapy

The Happiness Project
Elms Court
Chapel Way
Oxford
OX2 9LP
Tel: 01865 244414
E-mail: hello@happiness.
co.uk
Website:
www.happiness.co.uk

Life coaching

Breakthrough Network for
Work Life Coaching
29 Adine Road
London
E13 8LL
Tel: 020 7473 5544
E-mail: andrew.ferguson@
lifeshift.co.uk
Website: www.lifeshift.co.uk

Fiona Harrold Life
  Coaching
The Fiona Harrold
  Consultancy
E-mail: info@fionaharrold.
  com
Website: www.fionaharrold.
  com

Life Coach UK
E-mail:
  info@lifecoachuk.com
Website:
  www.lifecoachuk.com

Light therapy

Outside In Ltd.
31 Scotland Road Estate
Dry Drayton
Cambridge
CB3 8AT
Tel: 01954 211 955
E-mail:
  info@outsidein.co.uk
Website:
  www.outsidein.co.uk

For light therapy products:

Oxyvita Limited
117 Finchley Road
Swiss Cottage
London

NW3 6HY
Tel: 020 8368 7261
E-mail:
  opuroxygen@aol.com
Website: www.lighttherapy
  products.co.uk

A good source of light boxes
  is Boots the Chemist
Website: www.boots.com or
  The Healthy House
Website: www.healthyhouse.
  co.uk

Massage

Massage Therapy UK
E-mail: info@massage
  therapy.co.uk
Website: www.massage
  therapy.co.uk

Meditation and prayer

Brahma Kumaris – world
  spiritual organisation
Global Co-operation House
65 Pound Lane
London
NW10 2HH
Tel: 020 8727 3350
E-mail: london@bkwsu.com
Website: www.bkwsu.com

Transcendental Meditation
Beacon House
Willow Walk
Woodley Park
Skelmersdale
Lancashire
WN8 6UR
Tel: 0870 5143733
Website: www.transcen
dental-meditation.org.uk

Neuro-linguistic programming

The Association for Neuro-
Linguistic Programming
E-mail: info@alnp.org
Website: www.anlp.org

Nutritional therapy

British Association for
Nutritional Therapy
(BANT)
Tel: 08706 061284
E-mail: theadministrator@
bant.org.uk
Website: www.bant.org.uk

The Institute for Optimum
Nutrition
13 Blades Court
Deodar Road
London

SW15 2NU
Tel: 020 8877 9993
Website: www.ion.ac.uk

Society for the Promotion
of Nutritional Therapy
PO Box 47
Heathfield
East Sussex
TN21 8ZX

Women's Nutritional
Advisory Service
PO Box 268
Lewes
East Sussex
BN7 2QN
Tel: 01273 487366
E-mail: NHAS@NHAS.
org.uk
Website: www.wnas.org.uk

Osteopathy

British Osteopathic
Association
Langham House West
Luton
Bedfordshire
LU1 2NA
Tel: 01582 488455
E-mail: enquiries@osteo
pathy.org
Website: www.osteopathy.org

General Osteopathic
  Council
Osteopathy House
176 Tower Bridge Road
London
SE1 3LU
Tel: 020 7357 6655
E-mail: info@osteopathy.
  org.uk
Website: www.osteopathy.
  org.uk

Qigong

The TaiChi-Qigong Health
  Centre
TCQHC
13 Oriel Avenue
Gorleston
Great Yarmouth
Norfolk
NR31 7JH
Tel: 01493 663945
E-mail: contact@taichi-
  qigong.net
Website: www.taichi-
  qigong.net

Tse Qigong Centre
PO Box 59
Altrincham
WA15 8FS
Tel: 0161 929 4485
E-mail:

tse@qimagazine.com
Website:
  www.qimagazine.co.uk

Radionics

The Radionic Association
Tel:01869 338852
E-mail: secretary@radionic.
  co.uk
Website: www.radionic.co.uk

Reflexology

The Association of
  Reflexologists
27 Old Gloucester Street
London
WC1N 3XX
Tel: 0870 5673320
E-mail: info@aor.org.uk
Website: www.aor.org.uk

The British Reflexology
  Association
Monks Orchard
Whitbourne
Worcester
WR6 5RB
Tel: 01886 821207
E-mail: bra@britreflex.co.uk
Website:
  www.britreflex.co.uk

Holistic Association of
   Reflexologists
The Holistic Healing
   Centre
92 Sheering Road
Old Harlow
Essex
CM17 0JW
Tel: 01279 429060

International Federation of
   Reflexologists
78 Edridge Road
Croydon
Surrey
CR0 1EF
Tel: 0208 667 9458
E-mail: ifr44@aol.com

Reiki

The Reiki Alliance
PO Box 114
Stowmarket
Suffolk
IP14 4WA
Tel: 01449 673449
E-mail:
   info@reikialliance.co.uk
Website: www.reikialliance.
   co.uk

The Reiki Association
Cornbrook Bridge House

Clee Hill
Ludlow
Shropshire
SY8 3QQ
E-mail: KateJones@reiki
   association.org.uk
Website: www.reiki
   association.org.uk

UK Reiki Federation
PO Box 1785
Andover
SP11 0WB
Tel: 01264 773774
E-mail:
   enquiry@reikifed.co.uk
Website:
   www.reikifed.co.uk

Sacro-cranial osteo-pathy/cranial osteopathy

The Sutherland Society –
   The UK Organisation for
   Cranial Osteopaths
c/o 15a Church Street
Bradford upon Avon
Wiltshire
BA15 1LN
Tel: 01225 868282
E-mail:
   suthsoc@tiscali.co.uk
Website:
   www.cranial.org.uk

Stress management

The International Stress
  Management Association
PO Box 348
Waltham Cross
EN8 8ZL
Tel: 07000 780430
E-mail: stress@isma.org.uk
Website: www.isma.org.uk

Thought field therapy

Thought Field Therapy
  (TFT) UK
E-mail: listing@thoughtfield
  therapy.co.uk
Website: www.thoughtfield
  therapy.co.uk

Yoga

The British Wheel of Yoga
25 Jermyn Street
Sleaford
Lincolnshire
NG34 7RU
Tel: 01529 306 851
E-mail: office@bwy.org.uk
Website: www.bwy.org.uk

Friends of Yoga
Tel: 01903 741613
E-mail: info@friendsof
  yoga.org
Website: www.friendsof
  yoga.org

Orange Tree Yoga (Hannah
  Lovegrove)
The Ranch House
North Chideock
Bridport
Dorset
DT6 6LG
Tel: 08454 569 826
E-mail: info@orangetree
  yoga.com
Website: www.orangetree
  yoga.com

Yoga Therapy Centre
90–92 Pentonville Street
Islington
London
N1 9HS
Tel: 020 7689 3040
E-mail:
  enquiries.yogatherapy@
  virgin.net
Website:
  www.yogatherapy.org

GENERAL ADVICE IN IRELAND

BCMA Associations:

Association of Registered
  Complementary Health
  Therapists of Ireland
  (ARCHTI)
Main Street
Camolin
Enniscorthy
Co. Wexford
Tel: 00353 54 83425
E-mail: info@complemen-
  tarytherapists.org
Website: www.complemen-
  tarytherapists.org

Natural Healing Centre
Thompson House
McCurtain Street
Cork
Tel: 00353 21450 1600
E-mail: nhc@o2.ie
Website: www.nhc.ie

GENERAL ADVICE IN USA

National Center for
  Complementary and
  Alternative Medicine (NCCAM)
NCCAM Clearinghouse
PO Box 7923
Gaithersburg
MD 20898
Toll Free: 1-888-644-6226
E-mail: info@nccam.nih.gov
Website: www.nccam.nih.gov

GENERAL ADVICE IN AUSTRALIA

BCMA Associations:

Australasian College of
  Natural Therapies
57 Foueaux Street
Surrey Hills
New South Wales 2010
Tel: (0061) 2 9218 8888
UK Toll Free Number:
  0800 028 9931
E-mail: info@acnt.edu.au
Website: www.acnt.edu.au

ICA Associations:

Australian Traditional-
  Medicine Society
PO Box 1027
Meadowbank
New South Wales 2114
Tel: (02) 9809 6800
Website: www.atms.com.au

GENERAL ADVICE IN NEW ZEALAND

Ministerial Advisory
  Committee on
  Complementary and
  Alternative Health

(MACCAH)
E-mail: www.newhealth.
  govt.nz/maccah.htm

PRODUCTS, PRACTITIONERS, HELP GROUPS

If you are having difficulty
finding any of the prod-
ucts mentioned at local
chemists or health food
stores, the Nutri-Centre
below will mail products
all over the world.

The Nutri-Centre
Tel: 020 7436 5122
Website: www.nutricentre.
  com

Ainsworth's Homeopathic
  Pharmacy
Tel: 020 7935 5330

Website: www.ainsworths.
com

Aromatherapy Associates
Tel: 020 8569 7030
Website: www.aromatherapy
associates.com
For heavenly aromatherapy
products, including bath
oils and skin care

Beauty
For beauty product stockist
details, go to www.beauty
bible.com and look in
the Where2find directory

Biocare Ltd UK
Tel: 0121 433 3727
Website: www.biocare.co.uk
Excellent nutritional supple-
ments

Bioforce
Tel: 01294 277344
Website: www.bioforce.
co.uk
Herbal medicines, Alfred
Vogel's Swiss Muesli, Jan
de Vries flower essences

Blackmores (also Apotheke
2020 Jurlique Day Spa)
Tel: 0 8707 700976

Supplements of all kinds
and wonderful beauty
products by Jurlique

Cancer Information Service
CancerBACUP 0808 800
1234
Website: www.cancerbacup.
org.uk

Cancer Screening NHS
Website: www.cancer
screening.nhs.uk

Continence Foundation
Tel: 020 7404 6875
Website: www.continence-
foundation.org.uk

Marilyn Glenville (nutri-
tionist and psychologist
specialising in treating
women's health naturally)
Tel: 0870 5329244
Website: www.marilyn
glenville.com

GNC (General Nutrition
Centre)
Website: www.gnc.co.uk
Supplements, herbs etc

Gillian Hamer (nutritionist/
reflexologist/aura work)

The Wren Clinic
Tel: 020 7283 8908
Website: www.wrenclinic.
   co.uk

The Healthy House
Tel: 01453 752216
Fax: 01453 753533
Website: www.healthy-
   house.co.uk
Mail order company for
   light boxes, water puri-
   fiers, eco-paints and a
   wide variety of low-
   allergen, environmentally
   friendly and organic
   products

The Integrated Medical
   Centre Shop
Tel: 020 7224 5111
Website: www.dr-ali.co.uk
For Ayurvedic medicines
   and other supplies, try
   the shop adjoining Dr
   Ali's Integrated Medical
   Centre

International Flower
   Essence Repertoire
Tel: 01428 741 572
Fax: 01428 741 679
E-mail: flower@atlas.co.uk
For flower essences of all

kinds, and they too will
mail order worldwide

Jenny Jordan (make-up
   artist)
Tel: 020 7483 2222
Website: www.jennyjordan.
   com

Roderick Lane (naturopath/
   nutritionist)
The Eden Clinic, London
Tel: 020 7881 5800
Website: www.roderick
   lane.com

Hannah Lovegrove (yoga
   lessons, weekends, holidays)
Tel: 01297 489 485
Website: www.orange
   treeyoga.com

MedicHerb (Natural
   products)
Tel: 01628 488487
Website: www.medicherb.
   co.uk

Menopause and HRT
   helpline
Tel: 01293 413000

National Endometriosis
Society
Tel: 020 7222 2776
Website: www.endo.org.uk

National Osteoporosis
Society
Tel: 01761 472721
Website: www.nos.org.uk

Neal's Yard Remedies
Tel: 0161 831 7875
Website: www.nealsyard
remedies.com
For aromatherapy essential
oils, herbs and herbal
products, homeopathic
remedies, flower essences
and much more.

OVACOME for informa-
tion about ovarian
cancer
Tel: 020 7380 9589
Website: www.ovacome.
org.uk

The Poundbury Clinic for
Women, Dorchester
Tel: 01305 262626

E-mail: gynaecology2@
hotmail.com

Prince of Wales'
Foundation for
Integrated Health
Tel: 020 7619 6140
Website: www.fihealth.
org.uk

Relate National Marriage
Guidance Council
Helpline: 0845 130 4010
Website: www.relate.org.uk

Savant Health
Tel: 0113 230 1993
Website: www.savant-
health.com
Useful website selling all
manner of health-related
products.

Viridian Nutrition
Tel: 01327 878050
Website: www.viridian-
nutrition.com
Supplements and herbs,
principally.

SCIENTIFIC
REFERENCES

'Use of Botanicals for Management of Menopausal Symptoms', *ACOG Practice Bulletin*, no.28, June 2001

'Postmenopausal hormone therapy increases the risk of venous thromboembolic disease. The heart and estrogen/progestin replacement study', *An Intern Med*, 132, 689–96

'Vitex agnus castus essential oil and menopausal balance: a research update', *Complement Ther Nurs Midwifery*, 2003, Aug; 9(3): 157–60

'Oestrogen, Brain Function and Neuropsychiatric Disorders', a background paper prepared for the Consensus Conference on Hormone Replacement Therapy in Edinburgh, October 2003

'HRT: Update on the risk of breast cancer and long-term safety', *Current Problems in Pharmacovigilance*, 2003; 29: 1–4

'Meta-Analysis of the Efficacy of Hormone Replacement Therapy in Treating Preventing Osteoporosis in Postmenopausal Women', *Endocrine Reviews*, 2002; 23 (4): 529–39

'The effectiveness of low-calorie diet or diet with acupuncture treatment in obese peri- and postmenopausal woman', *Ginekol Pol*, 2003, Feb; 74(2): 102–7

'Effect of Estrogen Plus Progestin on Stroke in Postmenopausal Women: The Women's Health Initiative: A Randomized Trial', *JAMA*, 2003; 289: 2673–84

'Isoflavones in the Management of the Menopause', *Journal of the British Menopause Society*, vol. 7, supplement 1, 2001

'Soy protein has a greater effect on bone in postmenopausal women not on hormone replacement therapy, as evidenced by reducing bone resorption and urinary calcium excretion', *Journal of Clincial Endocrinology Metab*, 2003, Mar; 88(3): 1048–54

'What nonhormonal therapies are effective for postmenopausal vasomotor symptoms?', *Journal of Family Practice*, vol. 52, no. 4, April 2003

'Menopausal hormone therapy after breast cancer', commentary, *Lancet*, 3 February 2004

'International position paper on women's health and menopause: A comprehensive approach', National Heart, Lung, and Blood Institute Office of Research on Women's Health; National Institutes of Health; and the Giovanni Lorenzini Medical Science Foundation, 2002

'Randomised controlled trial of 309 post menopausal women with at least one narrowed coronary artery; Effects of Estrogen Replacement on the progression of coronary-artery atherosclerosis', *New England Journal of Medicine*, 2000, 24 Aug; 343(8): 522–9

'Soy protein consumption and bone mass in early postmenopausal Chinese women', *Osteoporosis Int*, 2003, 14 Aug

'Hormone Replacement Therapy and Venous Thromboembolism', *RCOG*, 1999

Advisory Group on Osteoporosis, Department of Health, 1994

Aksac, B., Aki, S., Karan, A., Yalcın, O., Isıkoglu, M. and Eskiyurt, N., 'Biofeedback and pelvic floor exercises for the rehabilitation of urinary stress incontinence', *Gynecol Obstet Invest*, 2003; 56(1): 23–7. Epub 2003, 14 July

Al-Azzawi, F. and Wahab, M., 'Bleeding patterns and hormone replacement therapy', in Studd, J. (ed.), *The Management of the Menopause*, 3rd edn, pp.159–74

Al-Azzawi, F., 'Pulsed estrogen therapy: from cellular mode of action to tissue effects', in Schneider, H.P.G. (ed.), *Menopause: The State of the Art – in research and management*, 2002, pp.445–8

Albertazzi, P., 'Complementary therapy: Alternative medicines and the menopause – do they work?', *Br J Sexual Med*, 2003; 27:12–17

Albertazzi, P., 'Management of hot flushes without oestrogen', *J of the Br Men Soc*, vol. 8, 2002

Albertazzi, P., 'Soy in the prevention of bone loss', *Osteoporosis Review*, 2002; 10

American Society for Reproductive Medicine, *Guideline for Practice: Age related infertility*, 1995

Ashworth, J.B., Reuben, D.V. and Benton, L.A., 'Functional Profiles of Healthy Older Persons', *Aging*, 1994; 23: 34

Attilakos, G. and Wardle, P., 'Individualising hormone replacement therapy', *Practitioner*, 2002; 246: 295–311

Bair, Yali A., Gold, Ellen B., Greendale, Gail A., Sternfeld, Barbara, Adler, Shelly R., Azari, Rahman and Harkey, Martha, 'Ethnic Differences in Use of Complementary and Alternative Medicine at Midlife: Longitudinal Results from SWAN Participants', *American Journal of Public Health*, vol. 92, no. 11, Nov 2002

Barber, H.R.K., 'Use of herbs in women in the menopause', in Schneider, H.P.G. (ed.), *Menopause: The State of the Art – in research and management*, 2002, pp.374–7

Barlow, D., 'National Osteoporosis Society statement, February 2003: hormone replacement therapy and the Women's Health Initiative study', in Studd, J. (ed.), *The Management of the Menopause*, 3rd edn, pp.13–16

Barlow, D., Samsioe, G. and van Geelan, H., 'Prevalence of Urinary Problems in European Countries', *Maturitas*, 1997; 27: 239–48

Barlow, D.H., 'The menopause: what do women want from their physician? Managing the menopause', *Trends in Urology Gynaecology and Sexual Health*, 1999; 25–8

Barnes, S., 'Phyto-oestrogens and osteoporosis: what is a safe dose?' *Br J Nutri*, 2003, June; 89 supplement 1: S101–8

Barrett, E., Grady, D., Sashegiyi, A. et al., 'Raloxifene and Cardiovascular Events in Osteoporotic Postmenopausal Women', *JAMA*, 2002; 287, 847–57. *Int J Oncol.*, 2003, Nov; 23(5):1407–12

Beardsworth, S.A. and Purdie, D.W., 'Selective oestrogen receptor modulators', *J of the Br Men Soc*, vol. 4, 1998

Black K. and Kubba A., 'What is new in contraception', *Trends in Urology and Sexual Health*, vol. 9, pp. 22–26, 2004

Blacker, C., 'Osteoporosis', *Postgrad Obst & Gyne*, 2001; 21

Blakely, J.A., 'The heart and estrogen/progestin replacement study revisited: hormone replacement therapy produced net harm, consistent with the observational data', *Arch Intern Med*, 2000, 23 Oct; 160(19): 2897–900

Blood clots, *JAMA*, 2003; 289: 2673–84

Bollapragada, S., Panigrahy, R. and Mander, T., 'Hormone replacement therapy and fibroids', *J of the Br Men Soc*, vol. 8, 2002

Breast cancer, *JAMA*, 2000; 283: 485–91, 534–5

British National Formulary, BMA and Royal Pharmaceutical Soc of GB, 6 September 2003

Brown, M.A., Goldstein-Shirley, J., Robinson, J. and Casey, S., 'The effects of a multi-modal intervention trial of light, exercise, and vitamins on women's mood' (LEVITY study), *Women Health*, 2001; 34(3): 93–112

Bull, S.J., Albinson, J.G. and Shambrook, C.J., *The Mental Game Plan. Getting Psyched for Sport*, Sports Dynamics, 1996

Burger, H.G., Davison, S. and Davis, S.R., 'The future of hormone replacement therapy', in Studd, J. (ed.), *The Management of the Menopause*, 3rd edn, pp.1–12

Calvin, M., 'Estrogens and skin repair', in Schneider, H.P.G. (ed.), *Menopause: The State of the Art – in research and management*, 2002, pp.244–7

Caplin, H.S. (ed.), *The New Injection Treatment for Impotence*, Wagner, New York; Brunner, Mazel. 1993: 142

Cassidy, A., 'Dietary phytoestrogens and bone health', *J of the Br Men Soc*, vol. 9, 2003

Cauley, Jane A. et al., 'Effects of hormone replacement therapy on clinical fractures and height loss: the heart and estrogen/progestin replacement study' (HERS), *American Journal of Medicine*, 2001; 110(6): 442–50

Chang, Chueh and Kaohstung, Catherine Hui-Wen Lin, 'Hormone Replacement Therapy and Menopause: A Review of Randomized, Double-blind, Placebo-controlled Trials', *J Med Sci*, vol. 19, no. 6, June 2003 (This lists 110 studies, which the authors investigated)

Chen, L.C., Tsao, Y.T., Yen, K.Y., Chen, Y.F., Chou, M.H. and Lin, M.F., 'A pilot study comparing the clinical effects of Jia-Wey Shiau-Yau San, a traditional Chinese herbal prescription, and a continuous combined hormone replacement therapy in postmenopausal women with climacteric symptoms', *Maturitas*, 2003, 30 Jan; 44(1): 55–62

China Study: personal communication with T. Colin Campbell, PhD and Jacob Gould Schurman, Professor Emeritus of Nutritional Biochemistry, Cornell University

Clarkson, T.B. and Appt, S.E., 'Soy phytoestrogens (isoflavones) for estrogen replacement therapy: strengths and weaknesses', in Schneider, H.P.G. (ed.), *Menopause: The State of the Art – in research and management*, 2002, pp.287–94

Clemett, D. and Spencer, C.M., 'Raloxifene. A Review of its Use in Postmenopausal Osteoporosis', *Drugs*, 2000; 60 (2): 379–411

Clinical Evidence, BMJ Publishing Group, issue 7, 2002

Clover, A. and Ratsey, D., 'Homeopathic treatment of hot flushes: a pilot study', *Homeopathy*, 2002, Apr; 91(2): 75–9

Cohen, A., *Thrombosis and HRT*, Postgraduate Centre Series

Collaborative Group on Hormonal Factors in Breast Cancer, 'Breast cancer and hormone replacement therapy: collaborative analysis of data from 51 epidemiological studies of 52705 women with breast cancer and 108411 women without breast cancer', *Lancet*, 1997; 1047–59

Cooper, J., *Strategies for Managing the Menopause*, 2nd rev. edn, 2000 coronary-artery atherosclerosis', *New England Journal of Medicine*, 2000; 343(8): 522–9

Cronje, W.H. and Studd, J., 'Vaginal estrogens: is there a role for their use?', in Studd, J. (ed.), *The Management of the Menopause*, 3rd edn, pp.213–20

Crosbie, D.I. and Reid, D.M., 'Prevention and correction of osteoporosis', in Studd, J. (ed.), *The Management of the Menopause*, 3rd edn, pp.151–8

Daniels F. and Tedder, A., *A Proper Spectacle. Women's Olympians, 1900–1936*, ZeNaNa Press

Deborah Grady, and others for the HERS Research Group, 'Cardiovascular Disease Outcomes during 6.8 Years of Hormone Therapy. Heart and Estrogen/Progestin Replacement Study Follow-up' (HERS 11), *JAMA*, vol. 288, no. 1, 3 July 2002, 49–57

Delmas, P.D. et al., 'Effects of raloxifene on bone mineral density, serum cholesterol concentrations and uterine endometrium in post-menopausal women', *NEJM*, 1997; 337: 1641–7

Dennerstein, L., Burger, H.G., Randolph, J., Taffe, J. and Clark, M., 'Sexual functioning, dysfunction and the natural menopausal transition', in Schneider, H.P.G. (ed.), *Menopause: The State of the Art – in research and management*, 2002, pp.402–7

Dept of Health, *National Service Framework for Older People Short Summary*, 2001

Deutsch, Helene, *The Psychology of Women*, 1924

Dooley, Michael M. and Brincat, Mark P. (eds.), *Understanding Common Disorders in Reproductive Endocrinology*, Wiley, 1994

Dormire, Sharon L. and Reame, Nancy King, 'Menopausal Hot Flash Frequency Changes in Response to Experimental Manipulation of Blood Glucose', *Nursing Research*, vol. 52, no. 5, Sept/Oct 2003

Ernst, E., 'Herbalism and the menopause', *J of the Br Men Soc*, vol. 8, 2002

Eskin, B.A., (ed.), *The Menopause Comprehensive Management*, 3rd edn, 1994

Faure, E.D., Chantre, P. and Mares, P., 'Effects of a standardized soy extract on hut flushes: a multicenter, double-blind, randomised placebo-controlled study', *Menopause*, 2002, Sept–Oct; 9(5): 329–34

Finn, C., 'Why do women have a menopause?', *J Br Men Soc*, 2002; 10–14 fractures and height loss: the heart and estrogen/progestin replacement study' (HERS), *American Journal of Medicine*, 2001; 110(6): 442–50

Francis, R., 'HRT – the end of the road?', *Osteoporosis Review*, 2002; 10: 2

Gallstone risk 'increased by HRT'. Report from www.News. bbc.co.uk/1/hi/health/1883104.stm

Gardner, C.J., 'Ease through menopause with homeopathic and herbal medicine', *Perianesth Nurs*, 1999, June; 14 (3): 139–43

Gebbie, A., 'Contraception in the Menopause', *Journal of British Menopause Society*, September 2003, 9; 203: 123

Gerhar, I. and Wallis, E., 'Individualized homeopathic therapy for male infertility', *Homeopathy*, 2002, July; 91(3): 133–44

Grady, Deborah, 'A 60-year-old woman trying to discontinue hormone replacement therapy', *Journal of the American Medical Association*, 2002; 287 (16):

Grostein, France, Clarkson, Thomas B. and Manson, JoAnne E., 'Understanding the Divergent Data on Postmenopausal Hormone Therapy', *N Engl J Med*, vol. 348, no. 7, 13 Feb 2003, 645–50

Grube, B. et al., 'St John's Wort Extract: Efficacy for menopausal symptoms of psychological origin', *Advances in Natural Therapy*, vol. 16, no. 4, July/August 1999

Guillebaud, J., *Contraception: your questions answered*, Churchill Livingstone, 1999

Guinness Book of Records, Bantam Books, 2000

Guthrie, J.R. and Dennerstein, L., 'The effects of estradiol and androgens on cardiovascular disease risk factors and bone density', in Schneider, H.P.G. (ed.), *Menopause: The State of the Art – in research and management*, 2002, pp.163–7

Hargarten K.M., 'Menopause: How Exercise Mitigates Symptoms', *The Physician and Sports Medicine*, 1994; 22: 49–67

Hartmann, B. and Huber, J., 'The mythology of hormone replacement therapy', *BJOG*, 1997; 104: 163–8

Hays, Jennifer and others, 'Effects of Estrogen plus Progestin on Health-Related Quality of Life', *N Engl J Med*, 17 March 2003 (from www.nejm.org)

Herrington, David M. et al., 'Effects of estrogen replacement on the progression of *Homeopathy*, 2002, July; 91(3): 133–44

Hope, S., Wager, E. and Rees, M., 'Survey of British women's view on the menopause and HRT', *J Br Men Soc*, 1998; 33–6

Hunter, M., 'Medical problem or natural transition: women's accounts of menopause', *J Br Men Soc*, 1998; 7

Huntley, A.L. and Ernst, E., 'A systematic review of herbal medicinal products for the treatment of menopausal symptoms', *Menopause*, 2003, Sep–Oct; 10(5): 465–76

Hurley, B.F. and Roth, S.M., 'Strength training in the elderly: effects on the risk factors for age-related diseases', *Sports Med*, 2000; 30: 249–68

Husband, A.J., 'Phytoestrogens and menopause', *BMJ*, 2002, 324: 52

Ingamells, S. and Cameron, I.T., 'Menorrhagia in the menopause', *J of the Br Men Soc*, vol. 9, 2003

Jacobs, D., DeMot, W. and Oxley, D., *Laboratory Test Handbook*, Concise 2nd edn, Lexicon, 2002

Jacquote, Y., Rojas, C., Refouvelet, B., Robert, J.F., Leclercq, G. and Xicluna, A., 'Recent advances in the development of phytoestrogens and derivatives: an update of the promising perspectives in the prevention of postmenopausal diseases', *Mini Rev Med Chem*, 2003, Aug; 3(5): 387–400

Jasienska, G., Thune, I. and Ellison, P.T., 'Energetic factors, ovarian steroids and the risk of breast cancer', *European Journal of Cancer Prevention*, 2000; 9: 231–9

Jing, S.Y., Wei, M.L. and Zhongguo Zhong Xi Yi Jie He Za Zhi, 'Clinical study on relationship between memory quotient, estrogen and Chinese nourishing kidney herbs in perimenopausal women', 2002, Jul; 22(7): 494–5

Johnson, A. and Wadsworth, J., 'Heterosexual Practices', in Wellings, K., Field, J. and Johnson, A. (eds.), *Sexual Behaviour in Britain. The National Survey of Sexual Attitudes and Lifestyles*, Penguin Books, 1995, pp.133–77

Jordan, V.C. et al., 'Abstract presented at the American Society of Clinical Oncology Conference, Tuesday 19 May 1998', *Proceedings of ASCO*; vol. 17, 1998

Josefson, Deborah, 'Women taking combination HRT are at greater risk of breast cancer', *BMJ*, 2000; 320: 333 (5 Feb 2000)

Journal of the British Menopause Society, 2003; 9 (supplement I)

Kanis, J.A., 'Clinical use of bone density measurements', in Studd, J. (ed.), *The Management of the Menopause*, 3rd edn, pp.139–50

Keskes-Ammar, L., Feki-Chakroun, N., Rebai, T., Sahnoun, Z., Ghozzi,

H., Hammami, S., Zghal, K., Fki, H., Damak, J. and Bahloul, A., 'Sperm, oxidative stress and the effect of an oral vitamin E and selenium supplement on semen quality in infertile men', *Arch Androl*, 2003, Mar–Apr; 49(2): 83–94

Koh, K.K., 'Observational and randomized controlled studies of secondary prevention of cardiovascular disease', in Schneider, H.P.G. (ed.), *Menopause: The State of the Art – in research and management*, 2002, pp.158–62

Kolomainen, D. and Herod, J., 'Hormone replacement therapy following breast and gynaecological cancer', *O & G*, 2001; 3: 168–72

Kothari, S. and Thacker, H., 'Risk assessment of the menopausal patient', *Med Cl N Am*, 1999; 8: 1489–502

Krinksy, N.I., Landrum, J.T. and Bone, R.A., 'Biologic Mechanisms of the Protective Role of Lutein and Zeaxanthin in the Eye', *Annu Rev Nutr*, 2003, 27 February

Kritz-Silverstein, D., Von Muhlen, D., Barrett-Connor, E. and Bressel, M.A., 'Isoflavones and cognitive function in older women: the Soy and Postmenopausal Health in Aging SOPHIA study', *Menopause*, 2003, May–Jun; 10(3): 196–202

Kronenberg, F. and Fugh-Berman, A., 'Complementary and alternative medicine for menopausal symptoms: a review of randomised, controlled trials', *Ann Intern Med*, 2002, 19 Nov; 137(10): 805–13

Kuh, D.I., Wadsworth, M. and Hardy, R., 'Women's health in midlife: the influence of the menopause, social factors and health in earlier life', *Br J Obstet Gynaecol*, 1997; 104: 923–33

Kunhong, W., Borgatta, L. and Stubblefield, P., 'Low Dose Oral Contraceptives and Bone Mineral Density: An Evidence Based Analysis', *Contraception*, 200; 61: 77–82

Lagro-Janssen, Toine, Rosser, Walter W. and van Weel, Chirs, 'Breast cancer and hormone-replacement therapy: up to general practice to pick up the pieces', commentary, *Lancet*, vol. 362, 9 Aug 2003

Lauritzen, C., 'The menopause in the belletristic literature', in Schneider, H.P.G. (ed.), *Menopause: The State of the Art – in research and management*, 2002, pp.484–91

Lawlor, D.A., Adamson, J. and Ebrahim, S., 'Lay perceptions of a "natural" menopause. Cross sectional study of the British Women's Heart and Health Study', *BJOG*, 2002; 109: 1398–400

Lawton, B., Rose, S., McLeod, D. and Dowell, A., 'Changes in use of hormone replacement therapy after the report from the Women's Health Initiative: cross sectional survey of users', *BMJ*, 11 October, vol. 327; 854–846

Lee, S.J. (ed.), *The Sheffield Protocol for the Management of the Menopause and the Prevention and Treatment of Osteoporosis*, 6th rev. edn, 2000

Leidy, L.E., 'Menopause in evolutionary perspective', in Trevathan, W.R., Smith, E.O. and McKenna, J.J. (eds.), *Evolutionary Medicine*, Oxford University Press, 1999

Leventhal, Alexander J., 'Sexual function and the older woman', in Schneider, H.P.G. (ed.), *Menopause: The State of the Art – in research and management*, 2002, pp.416–19

Lock, M., 'Symptom reporting at menopause: a review of cross-cultural findings', *J of the Br Men Soc*, vol. 8, 2002

Lock, M.M. and Kaufert, P., 'Menopause, local biologies, and cultures of aging', *American Journal of Human Biology*, 2001; 13: 494–504

Lock, M.M., 'Menopause: lessons from anthropology', *Psychosomatic Medicine*, 1998; 60: 410–19

Longmoor, M., Wilkinson, I. and Torok, E., *Oxford Handbook of Clinical Medicine*, 5th edn, Oxford University Press, 2002

Lumsdon, M. and Smith, S., 'Menstruation and Menstrual Abnormalities', in Shaw, R., Suter, P. and Stanton, S. (eds.), *Gynaecology*, Churchill Livingstone, 1993

Lupu, R., Mehmi, I., Atlas, E., Tsai, M.S., Pisha, E., Oketch-Rabah, H.A., Nuntanakorn, P., Kennelly, E.J. and Kronenberg, F., 'Black cohosh, a menopausal remedy, does not have estrogenic activity and does not promote breast cancer cell growth',

Mackey, R. and Eden, J., 'Phytoestrogens', *J of the Br Men Soc*, vol. 4, 1998

Mahady, G.B., Fabricant, D., Chadwick, L.R. and Dietz, B., 'Black cohosh: an alternative therapy for menopause?', *Nutr Clin Care*, 2002, Nov–Dec; 5(6): 293–9

Mander, A., 'Sex and hysterectomy', *BJSM*, 26: 4

Manson, JoAnn E. and Martin, Kathryn A., 'Post-menopausal Hormone-Replacement Therapy: Clinical Practice', *New England Journal of Medicine*, vol. 345, no. 1, 5 July 2001, 34–40

Marsden, J., *HRT and Cancer. Essentials of HRT and the menopause*, Science Press, 2001

McCully, K., Jackson, S., 'HRT and the Bladder', *Journal of the British Menopause Soc.*, 2004, pp32

McNagny, Sally E. and Wenger, Nanette K., *New England Journal of Medicine*, vol. 346, no. 1, 3 Jan 2002

Messina, M. and Hughes, C., 'Efficacy of soyfoods and soybean isoflavone supplements for alleviating menopausal symptoms is positively related to initial hot flush frequency', *J Med Food*, 2003, Spring; 6(2): 1–11

Messinger-Rapport, B.J. and Thacker, H.L., 'Prevention for the older woman. A practical guide to hormone replacement therapy and urogynecologic health', *Geriatrics*, 2001; 56: 32–42

Million Women Study Collaborative Group, 'The Million Women Study: design and characteristics of the study population', *Breast Cancer Res*, 1999; 1: 73–80

Million Women Study Collaborators, 'Breast cancer and hormone-replacement therapy in the Million Women Study', *Lancet*, vol. 362, 9 Aug 2003, 419–27

Million Women Study Collaborators, 'Patterns of use in hormone replacement therapy in one million women in Britain, 1996–2000', *BJOG*, 2002; 109: 1319–30

Morley, J.E., 'Decreased food intake with aging', *J Gerontol A Biol Sci Med Sci*, 2001; 56 (Spec no. 2): 81–8

Mosca, Lori and others, 'Hormone Replacement Therapy and Cardiovascular Disease. A Statement for Healthcare Professionals from the American Heart Association', *Circulation*, 2001; 104: 499

Nadel, E.R. and DiPietro, L., 'Effects of Physical Activity on Function Ability in Older People: Translating Basic Science Findings into Practical Knowledge', *Med Sci Sports Exerc* 1995; 25: S36

National Cancer Institute, *SEER Cancer Statistics Review*, 2001

National Diet and Nutrition Survey, NDNS, vol. 3, 10 July 2003

National Institutes of Health, 'The HERS study results and ongoing studies of women and heart disease', press release, 18 August 1998

National Women's Health Network, *The truth about hormone replacement therapy: How to break free from the medical myths of menopause*, Prima Press, 2002

New York Times, editorial, 'Delusions of Feeling Better'

Newton, Katherine M., Buist, Diana S.M., Keenan, Nora L., Anderson, Lynda A. and LaCroix, Andrea Z., 'Use of alternative therapies for menopause symptoms: results of a population-based survey', *Obstetrics & Gynaecology*, July 2002, 18–25

Ng, C., Hockey, J. and Panay, N., 'The use of hormonal intrauterine systems in menopausal women', in Studd, J. (ed.), *The Management of the Menopause*, 3rd edn, pp.131–8

Notelovitz, M., 'Can exercising prevent or delay aging? The biologic principles', in Schneider, H.P.G. (ed.), *Menopause: The State of the Art – in research and management*, 2002, pp.358–63

Notelovitz, M., 'The Adult Women's Health Plan', in Schneider, H.P.G. (ed.), *Menopause, the State of Art in Research and Management*, Parthenon Publishing Group, 2003, pp.8502–7

O'Brien, S., Ismail, K.M.K. and Jain, K., 'Premenstrual syndrome and the menopause', in Studd, J. (ed.), *The Management of the Menopause*, 3rd edn, pp.111–18

Office of National Statistics, *Population Trends*, Stationery Office, Spring 1997; 87: 17

Panay, N. and Studd, J., 'Pulsed estrogen therapy: a new concept in hormone replacement therapy', in Studd, J. (ed.), *The Management of the Menopause*, 3rd edn, pp.221–8

Panidis, D., Rousso, D., Kourtis, A., Giannoulis, C., Mavromatidis, G. and Stergiopoulos, K., 'Hormone replacement therapy at the threshold of 21st century', *EJOG and Rep Bio*, 99, 2001; 154–64

Parkman, Cynthia, 'The Furor Over Alternative Therapy for Menopause' (review), *TCM*, May/June 2003

Pasqualine, J.R. and Chetrite, G.S., 'Progesterone and progestins: risk or protection?', in Schneider, H.P.G. (ed.), *Menopause: The State of the Art – in research and management*, 2002, pp.65–71

Pitkin, J., 'Compliance with estrogen replacement therapy: current issues', in Schneider, H.P.G. (ed.), *Menopause: The State of the Art – in research and management*, 2002, pp.430–7

Pollard, T.M., 'Sex, gender and cardiovascular disease', in Pollard, T.M. and Hyatt, S.B. (eds.), *Sex, Gender and Health*, Cambridge University Press, 1999

Porzio, G., Trapasso, T., Martyell, S., Sallusti, E., Piccone, C., Mattei, A., Di Stanislao, C., Ficorella, C. and Marchetti, P., 'Acupuncture in the treatment of menopause-related symptoms in women taking tamoxifen', *Tumori*, 2002, Mar-Apr; 88(2): 128–30

Purdie, D., *HRT and Osteoporosis. Essentials of HRT and the menopause*, Science Press, 2001

Purdie, D.W. and Rees, M., 'Parathyroid hormone in osteoporosis', *J of the Br Men Soc*, 2003; 9:175

Rapp, Stephen R. and others, 'Effect of Estrogen Plus Progestin on Global Cognitive Function in Postmenopausal Women. The Women's Health Initiative Memory Study: A Randomized Controlled Trial', *JAMA*, 2003; 289: 2663–72

Read, J., 'Sexual Problems Associated with Infertility, Pregnancy and Aging', in Tomlinson, J. (ed.), *ABC of Sexual Health*, BMJ Books, 1999

Reddish, S., 'Loss of libido in menopausal women', *Aust Family*

Physician, 2002; 31: 427–31

Rees, M. and Purdie, D.W. (eds.), *Management of the Menopause*, BMS Publications, 2002

Rexrode, Kathryn M. and Manson, JoAnn E., 'Postmenopausal hormone therapy and quality of life: no cause for celebration', *Journal of the American Medical Association*, 2002; 287, 5

Robinson, D. and Cardozo, L., 'Urogenital atrophy', in Studd, J. (ed.), *The Management of the Menopause*, 3rd edn, pp.27–40

Roseff, S. J., 'Improvement in sperm quality and function with French maritime pine tree bark extract', *J Reprod Med*, 2002, Oct; 47(10): 821–4

Rosendaal, F.R., Helmerhorst, F.M. and Vandenbroucke, J.P., 'Female Hormones and Thrombosis', *Arteriosclerosis, Thrombosis and Vascular Biology*, 2002; 22: 201

Ross, R., Pagannini-Hill, A., Wan, P.C. and Pike, M.C., 'Effect of hormone replacement therapy on breast cancer risk; estrogen versus estrogen plus progestin', *J Natl Cancer Inst*, 2000; 92: 328–32

Rymer, J. and Richards, J., 'Tibolone (Livial) in the management of menopause', *Prescriber*, 2003

Rymer, J., Wilson, R. and Ballard, K., 'Making decisions about hormone replacement therapy', *BMJ*, 2003; 326: 322–6

Samsioe, G., 'Estrogen therapy for cardiovascular disease', in Studd, J. (ed.), *The Management of the Menopause*, 3rd edn, pp.17–26

Sandberg, M., Wijma, K., Wyon, Y., Nedstrand, E. and Hammar, M., 'Effects of electro-acupuncture on psychological distress in postmenopausal women', *Complement Ther Med*, 2002, Sept; 10(3): 161–9

Santuz, M., Bernardi, F., Driull, L. et al., 'Obesity and the Menopause', in Studd, J. (ed.), *The Management of the Menopause Millennium Review, 2000*, Parthenon Publishing

Sator, M.O., Ferlitsch, K. and Huber, J.C., 'Sex hormones and eye function', in Schneider, H.P.G. (ed.), *Menopause: The State of the Art – in research and management*, 2002, pp.262–4

Schmid, Randolph E, 'US panel adds estrogen to cancer list', Associated Press, 14 Aug 2001 (National Toxicology Program Advisory Committee)

Schneider, H.P.G. (ed.), *Menopause: The State of the Art – in research and management*, 2002

Seely, T., 'Pearls from the British Menopause Society meeting', *Trends in Urology Gynaecology & Sexual Health*, 2002

Seidl, M.M. and Stewart, D.E., 'Alternative treatments for menopausal symptoms. Systematic review of scientific and lay literature', *Can Fam Physician*, 1993, June; 44: 1299–308

Sengupta, A., 'The emergence of the menopause in India', *Climacteric*, 2003, June; 6(2): 92–5

Shimizu, H., 'Leptin in postmenopausal women', in Schneider, H.P.G. (ed.), *Menopause: The State of the Art – in research and management*, 2002, pp.271–8

Shumaker, Sally A. and others, 'Estrogen Plus Progestin and the Incidence of Dementia and Mild Cognitive Impairment in Postmenopausal Women. The Women's Health Initiative Memory Study: A Randomized Controlled Trial', *JAMA*, 2003; 289: 2651–62

Sorenson, M., 'Changes in body composition at menopause – age, lifestyle or hormone deficiency?', *J Br Men Soc*, 2002; 137–40

Sowers, M.F., 'Bone loss in the pre- and perimenopause', in Schneider, H.P.G. (ed.), *Menopause: The State of the Art – in research and management*, 2002, pp.115–17

Speroff, L., 'Alternative therapies for postmenopausal women', in Studd, J. (ed.), *The Management of the Menopause*, 3rd edn, pp.261–74

Spetz, A.E., Hammar, M.L., 'Hot flushes in men: prevalence and possible mechanisms', *J of the Br Men Soc*, vol. 8, 2002

Stanton, S., 'Vaginal Prolapse', in Shaw, R., Sautte, R.P. and Stanton, S. (eds.), *Gynaecology*, Churchill Livingstone, 1993, p.437

Stevenson, J., *HRT and Cardiovascular Disease. Essentials of HRT and the menopause*, Science Press, 2001

Stovall, D.W., Toma, S.K. and Hammond, M.G., 'The Effect of Age on Female Fecundity', *Obstet & Gynaecol*, 1991; 77: 33–6

Strassman, B.I., 'Menstrual cycling and breast cancer: an evolutionary perspective', *Journal of Women's Health*, 1999; 8: 193–202

Studd, J. (ed.), *The Management of the Menopause*, 3rd edn

Studee, David W. and MacLennan, Alastair H., 'Is combined estrogen/progestogen hormone therapy worth the risk?', *Climacteric*, 2003; 6; 177–9

Sturdee, D., 'HRT scare: putting the US study results into a UK perspective', *Trends in Urology Gynaecology & Sexual Health*, 2002

Taunton, J.E., Martin, A.D. and Rhodes, E.C., 'Exercise for Older Women', in Macauley, D. (ed.), *Benefits and Hazards of Exercise*, BMJ Books, 1999

Thompson, E.A. and Reilly, D., 'The homeopathic approach to the treatment of symptoms of oestrogen withdrawal in breast cancer patients. A prospective observational study', *Homeopathy*, 2003, 92: 131–4

Thompson, E.A., 'Homeopathy and the menopause', *J of the Br Men Soc*, vol. 8, 2002

Torgerson, D.J., Bell-Syer, S.E.M. and Porthouse, J., 'Hormone replacement therapy and prevention of fractures: is age of starting therapy important?' in Schneider, H.P.G. (ed.), *Menopause: The State of the Art – in research and management*, 2002, pp.108–14

Vandervoort, A.A. and McComas, A.J., 'Contractual Changes in Opposing Muscles of the Human Ankle Joint with Aging', *Journal of Applied Physiology*, 1986; 61: 361–7

Vastag, Brian, 'Hormone replacement therapy falls out of favor with expert committee', *Journal of the American Medical Association*, 2002; 287, 15

Walsh, B.W. et al., 'Effects of raloxifene on serum lipids and coagulation factors in healthy postmenopausal women', *JAMA*, 1998; 279: 1445–51

Wassertheil-Smoller, Sylvia and others, 'Effect of Estrogen Plus Progestin on Stroke in Postmenopausal Women. The Women's Health Initiative: A Randomized Trial', *JAMA*, 2003; 289: 2673–84

Willett, Walter C., Colditz, Graham and Stampfer, Meir, 'Postmenopausal Estrogens – Opposed, Unopposed, or None of the Above', editorial, *JAMA*, vol. 283, no. 4, 26 Jan 2000

Williamson, J., White, A., Hart, A. and Ernst, E., 'Randomised controlled trial of reflexology for menopausal symptoms', *BJOG*, 2002, Sept; 109(9): 1050–5

Wilson, Robert, *Feminine Forever*, M. Evans, 1966

Women's Health Clinic, *Pros and cons of hormone therapy: Making an informed Women's Health Issues*, 2003, Mar–Apr; 13(2): 74–8

World Health Organisation, *Improving Access to Quality Care in Family Planning. Medical Eligibility Criteria for Contraceptive Use*, WHO/FRH/FPP/96, 9, 1996

Wren, B.G., 'Hormones and breast cancer', in Schneider, H.P.G. (ed.), *Menopause: The State of the Art – in research and management*, 2002, pp.72–5

Writing Group for the PEPI Trial, 'Effects of estrogen or estrogen/progestin regimens on heart disease factors in postmenopausal women. The Postmenopausal Estrogen/Progestin Interventions (PEPI) Trial', *JAMA*, 1995; 273: 199–208

Writing Group for the Women's Health In Initiative Investigators, 'Risks and benefits of estrogen plus progestin in healthy postmenopausal women', *JAMA*, 2002; 288: 321–3

Wu, Chih-Hsing and others, 'Epidemiological Evidence of Increased Bone Mineral Density in Habitual Tea Drinkers', *Arch Internal Med*, 2002; 162: 1001–6

Wuttke, W., Seidlova-Wuttke, D., Balzer, I., Becker, T., Heiden, I., Jarry, H. and Christoffel, V., 'Phytoestrogens: dangerous drugs or soft hormones?', in Schneider, H.P.G. (ed.), *Menopause: The State of the Art – in research and management*, 2002, pp.295–306

Wuttke, W., Seidlove-Wuttke, D. and Gorkow, C., 'The Cimificuga preparation BNO 1055 vs conjugated estrogens in a double-blind placebo-controlled study: effects on menopause symptoms and bone markers', *Maturitas*, 2003, 14 Mar; 44 supplement 1: S17–77

Yoles, I., Yogev, Y., Frenkel, Y., Nahum, R., Hirsch, M. and Kaplan, B., 'Tofupill/Femarelle (DT56a): a new phyto-selective estrogen receptor modulator-like substance for the treatment of post-menopausal bone loss', *Menopause*, 2003, Nov–Dec; 10(6): 522–5

Younus, J., Simpson, I., Collins, A. and Wang, X., 'Mind control of menopause', *Women's Health Issues*, 2003, Mar–Apr; 13(2): 74–8

INDEX

Index

Index

poor 56, 241
  weight gain 260
dieting 105–6
dizziness 44, 145
doctor(s)
  choice of 15–16
  discussing HRT 153–7
  screening 57–62
  things to discuss 56–7
  Western 43, 44
Doisy, Edward 130
Down's Syndrome 352, 389–91,
  401
dowsing 234
driving 75
drug abuse 215
drug companies 14
drug therapy 103
dydrogesterone 158

EAT (Estrogen and Androgen
  Therapy) 159
eating disorders 215, 218
eating plan 266
eclampsia 408
Economy Class Syndrome 363
ectopic pregnancy 387, 402
eggs
  of girl baby in the womb 32
  in menstrual cycle 32–3
embryos 34, 352, 387, 393, 407
Emeleus, Frances 112
endometrial cancer 131, 144,
  171, 180, 373
endometrial hyperplasia 380
endometrial sampling 90, 93, 181
endometriosis 56, 90, 144, 150,
  166, 209, 373, 404
endometrium
  ablation of the 92
  pre-cancer of 180
energy, lack of 40, 41, 69, 164,
  182
energy channels 200
epilepsy 151

EPT (Estrogen and Progestogen
  Therapy) 158
Essential Fatty Acids (EFAs) 68,
  118, 251, 270, 276, 412
ET (Estrogen Therapy) 158
ethinyloestradiol 158, 159, 161,
  359
European Committee for
  Proprietary Medicinal Products
  135
European Expert Working Group
  134, 245
Evidence Based Medicine (EBM)
  14
exercise 48, 49, 56, 68–9, 93,
  104, 156, 236, 241, 247–8,
  256, 266, 278–95, 411
  the baked bean can workout
    292–3
  building up from no exercise
    287
  the exercise mantra 285–6
  fat burning 294–5
  and infertility 397–8
  SMART (Specific, Measurable,
    Adjustable, Realistic, Time)
    282
  three golden rules 281–3
  types of 283–5
  weekly pick 'n' mix exercise
    menu 288–92
  yoga versus pilates 287–8

facials 5
Fairley, Josephine 336
Fairley, Josephine and Sarah
  Stacey: *Feel Fabulous Forever:
  The Anti-ageing Health &
  Beauty Bible* 292, 330
faith 37, 46, 48
faith healing 226
Fallopian tubes 34
  ectopic pregnancy 387, 402
family
  medical history 56, 57

459

Index

Index

Index

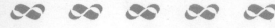

Transform your life
with Hodder Mobius

For the latest information on the best in
Spirituality, Self-Help,
Health & Wellbeing and Parenting,

visit our website
www.hoddermobius.com